Open, Laparoscopic, and Robotic Surgery for Cervical Cancer

Shichao Han • Jun Wang
Editors

Open, Laparoscopic, and Robotic Surgery for Cervical Cancer

Springer

Editors
Shichao Han
Department of Gynecology and Obstetrics
Second Affiliated Hospital of Dalian Medical University
Dalian, China

Jun Wang
Department of Obstetrics and Gynecology
Second Affiliated Hospital of Dalian Medical University
Dalian, China

ISBN 978-981-97-7686-3 ISBN 978-981-97-7687-0 (eBook)
https://doi.org/10.1007/978-981-97-7687-0

Jointly published with People's Medical Publishing House, PR of China

This Springer imprint is published by the registered company Springer Nature Singapore Pte Ltd.
The registered company address is: 152 Beach Road, #21-01/04 Gateway East, Singapore 189721, Singapore

Preface

"A surgeon's surgical skill is a moral commitment to the patient!"—Te Linde's

The enhancement of surgical skills is the lifelong pursuit of every surgeon, as well as the greatest assurance for achieving optimal treatment outcomes for patients. Cervical cancer, a gynecological malignancy that poses a serious threat to women's health, still relies primarily on surgery as the initial treatment approach for early-stage cases. However, due to the complexity of surgical anatomy and the high level of technical difficulty involved, standardized surgical procedures for cervical cancer have not been widely disseminated.

In 2008, Querleu-Morrow proposed a new classification method for cervical cancer surgery, which was subsequently updated in 2017. Following the revision of the International Federation of Gynecology and Obstetrics (FIGO) staging for cervical cancer in 2018 and the publication of the cervical cancer laparoscopic surgery trial, there have been new developments in the indications, surgical approaches, and techniques for cervical cancer surgery. The National Comprehensive Cancer Network (NCCN) guidelines in the United States (2022) and the Chinese Expert Consensus on Quality Control of Surgical Treatment for Cervical Cancer (2022) have both been revised accordingly. The Q-M classification has now become the "gold standard" for quality control in clinical practice internationally.

However, the surgical techniques and practices based on the Q-M classification combined with the Chinese expert consensus have not yet been effectively disseminated. Therefore, our team has preliminarily summarized some surgical techniques and experiences through learning from domestic and international experts and repeated clinical practices. We are willing to share them with fellow colleagues and look forward to receiving feedback and criticism to guide mutual progress.

Key features of this book:

1. Covers open, laparoscopic, and robotic surgical approaches, guided by the concept of fascial dissection.
2. Utilizes the fusion fascial plane between different embryonic compartments as the surgical pathway.
3. Fully demonstrates the relationships between fusion fascial planes and highlights the key points of separation, resection, and preservation of important structures.

4. Provides preliminary explanations of the principles of tumor-free surgery based on embryonic origins.

The description of surgical steps combines continuous images (resembling animations) with explanatory text. Additionally, surgical videos are integrated to elucidate the technical key points of each surgical approach. This includes the coordination between the surgeon and assistants, positioning of instruments, avoidance of injury, and application of tumor-free principles. The complex surgical procedures are broken down into manageable and reproducible actions, each with imitable and repeatable characteristics. This approach ensures surgical safety while preventing beginners from blindly following complex procedures. Furthermore, it enhances accessibility and generalizability for novice learners.

Due to the distinct anatomical theoretical systems of "in situ anatomy" and "surgical anatomy of dissecting planes," combined with the support of the concept of tumor-free boundaries based on embryonic origins and fascial dissection theory, the theoretical framework of this book becomes more comprehensive and has been further validated through the practical experience of our team. However, there are currently no authoritative works available that address the interplay between these theoretical frameworks, both domestically and internationally. As a result, this book may contain certain ambiguities and unclear expressions. We kindly request colleagues and experts to provide valuable feedback while understanding the author's thought process.

On the path of improving surgical skills and pursuing academic excellence, our team has dedicated ourselves to continuous learning and extensively studying numerous works. During this process, we have come to realize that the "confusions" and "unexpected discoveries" encountered during surgery have long been mentioned in the works of our predecessors. This realization has humbled us and filled us with a sense of inadequacy and humility. It has also instilled a deep reverence for our predecessors, further motivating us to continue moving forward and exploring new frontiers.

On the occasion of its completion, we sincerely thank every member of our writing team who has shown great passion for exploring and innovating beyond traditional boundaries in the pursuit of enhancing surgical skills and the application of techniques. Each surgery has strived for the utmost achievement of "bloodless visualization and precise dissection." Apart from innate talent and understanding, it is primarily the result of sweat and dedication that has contributed to the creation of this book, ensuring its comprehensibility, visual appeal, and widespread accessibility through diagrams and videos.

Dalian, China

Shichao Han
Jun Wang

Contents

Part I Anatomy Related to Radical Hysterectomy

1 **Anatomy of Abdominal and Pelvic Vessels** 3
Shichao Han and Xinyou Wang

2 **Nerve Anatomy** 19
Jun Wang and Yuemei Cui

3 **Lymphatic Anatomy** 27
Jun Wang and Junling Lu

4 **Anatomy of Space of Pelvic Sidewall** 35
Jun Wang and Shichao Han

5 **Anatomy of Spaces of Paracervix** 39
Shichao Han, Jun Wang, and Jing Na

6 **Anatomy of Landmark Structures** 45
Jing Na and Ya Li

7 **Re-recognition of Membrane Theory of Ontogenetic Anatomy** 49
Shichao Han and Jun Wang

Part II Illustration of Radical Hysterectomy for Cervical Cancer Under QM Classification

8 **Type QM-A Radical Hysterectomy** 65
Shichao Han and Jing Na

9 **Type QM-B Radical Hysterectomy** 83
Jun Wang and Ya Li

10 **Type QM-C1 Radical Hysterectomy** 103
Shichao Han, Jun Wang, Jing Na, and Ya Li

11 **Type QM-C2 Radical Hysterectomy** 147
Jun Wang, Shichao Han, Jing Na, and Ya Li

12 **Fertility-Sparing Radical Trachelectomy for Cervical Cancer** 183
Shichao Han, Jun Wang, Jing Na, Ya Li, and Xinyou Wang

13 **Robot-Assisted Radical Hysterectomy** 193
Jun Wang, Shichao Han, Jing Na, Ya Li, and Xinyou Wang

Part III Lymphadenectomy for Cervical Cancer

14 **Pelvic Lymphadenectomy** 205
Jun Wang and Jing Na

15 **Parametrial Lymphadenectomy** 245
Shichao Han and Ya Li

16 **Lymphadenectomy of the Abdominal Aortic Region** 253
Shichao Han and Xinyou Wang

17 **Sentinel Lymph Node Mapping and Dissection** 281
Shichao Han, Jun Wang, Jing Na, Ya Li, and Xinyou Wang

Part IV Complications and Postoperative Care

18 **Complications Related to Radical Hysterectomy Surgery and Postoperative Care** 299
Jun Wang, Junling Lu, and Yuemei Cui

Contributors

Yuemei Cui Department of Gynecology and Obstetrics, Dalian Municipal Central Hospital, Affiliated of Dalian University of Technology, Dalian, China

Shichao Han Department of Gynecology and Obstetrics, Second Affiliated Hospital of Dalian Medical University, Dalian, China

Ya Li Department of Gynecology and Obstetrics, Second Affiliated Hospital of Dalian Medical University, Dalian, China

Junling Lu Department of Gynecology and Obstetrics, Second Affiliated Hospital of Dalian Medical University, Dalian, China

Jing Na Department of Gynecology and Obstetrics, Second Affiliated Hospital of Dalian Medical University, Dalian, China

Jun Wang Department of Gynecology and Obstetrics, Second Affiliated Hospital of Dalian Medical University, Dalian, China

Xinyou Wang Department of Gynecology and Obstetrics, Second Affiliated Hospital of Dalian Medical University, Dalian, China

Part I

Anatomy Related to Radical Hysterectomy

Anatomy of Abdominal and Pelvic Vessels

1

Shichao Han and Xinyou Wang

1.1 Abdominal Vasculature

1.1.1 Arterial Anatomy of the Abdominal Cavity

1.1.1.1 Abdominal Aorta

Anatomy The abdominal aorta is located slightly to the left in front of the lower border of the 12th thoracic vertebra. It enters the retroperitoneal space through the aortic hiatus of the diaphragm, descends along the left anterior side of the spine, and bifurcates into the left and right common iliac arteries at the level of the lower border of the fourth lumbar vertebra. The total length of the abdominal aorta is about 14–15 cm, with a diameter of approximately 2.9–3.0 cm [1].

Clinical Significance The abdominal aorta rarely exhibits variations and serves as an anatomical landmark for dissecting lymph nodes in the region. Clinically, the opening of the posterior peritoneum is guided by the abdominal aorta. By doing so, the inferior vena cava, inferior mesenteric artery, and both ureters are exposed on the left and right sides, respectively (Fig. 1.1).

S. Han (✉) · X. Wang
Department of Gynecology and Obstetrics, Second Affiliated Hospital of Dalian Medical University, Dalian, China

1.1.1.2 Ovarian Artery

Anatomy The ovarian artery originates from the abdominal aorta or renal artery at the level of the second lumbar vertebra. It descends diagonally toward the caudal direction and crosses over the ureter at the level of the third lumbar vertebra. At the pelvic inlet, it passes over the iliac vessels, approximately 2 cm anterior to the ureter [2].

Clinical Significance The right ovarian artery is relatively slender and runs on the surface of the inferior vena cava, making it easily recognizable. In contrast, the left ovarian artery is generally larger and commonly originates from the abdominal aorta, although some arise from the left renal artery. When performing lymph node dissection in the region lateral to the abdominal aorta and cephalad to the inferior mesenteric artery, it's crucial to identify the left ovarian artery originating from the abdominal aorta. Due to its origin from the abdominal aorta, the ovarian artery's vascular wall is subjected to higher pressure. Accidental injury to this artery could lead to profuse bleeding. The use of bipolar electrocoagulation for hemostasis is not recommended in such cases. Employing vascular clamps for ligation provides more effective hemostatic results (Fig. 1.2).

1.1.1.3 Inferior Mesenteric Artery

Anatomy The inferior mesenteric artery originates approximately at the level of the third lum-

S. Han, J. Wang (eds.), *Open, Laparoscopic, and Robotic Surgery for Cervical Cancer*,
https://doi.org/10.1007/978-981-97-7687-0_1

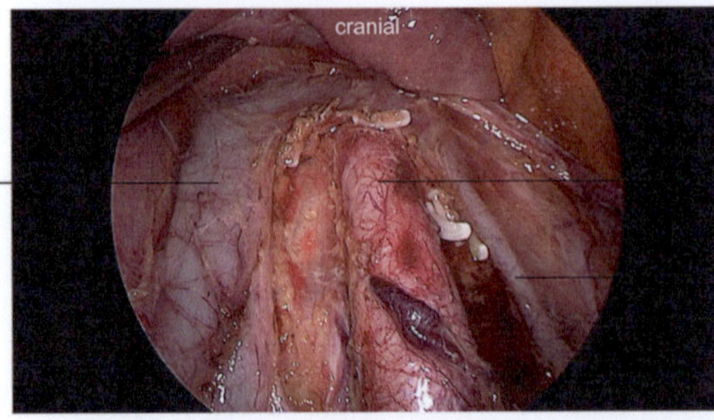

Fig. 1.1 Abdominal aorta

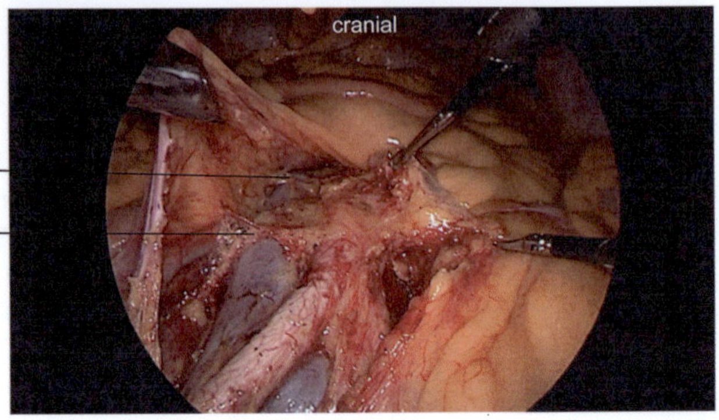

Fig. 1.2 Ovary artery

bar vertebra, about 3–4 cm above the bifurcation of the aorta. Arising from the anterior wall of the abdominal aorta, it traverses the retroperitoneum along the deep surface of the mesentery, coursing downward and to the left. It enters the left iliac fossa and proceeds within the root of the mesentery of the sigmoid colon, descending into the pelvic cavity, where it transitions into the superior rectal artery. The length of the inferior mesenteric artery from its origin to the point of emergence of its first branch is approximately 34.7 mm. There are three major branches: the left colic artery, sigmoid artery, and superior rectal artery, providing blood supply to the descending colon, sigmoid colon, and upper portion of the rectum [2].

Clinical Significance The inferior mesenteric artery serves as a landmark for lymph node dissection in the higher and lower regions of the abdominal aorta. Adequate exposure of the inferior mesenteric artery facilitates the visualization and removal of lymph nodes in the higher and lower regions of the abdominal aorta. It's not recommended to skeletonize the inferior mesenteric artery, especially at its root. The inferior mesenteric artery originates from the surface of the abdominal aorta at an acute angle. Excessive skeletonization, particularly at the root, could lead to inadvertent detachment of the artery during the lymph node removal process. This could result in uncontrollable bleeding (Fig. 1.3).

1.1.1.4 Common Iliac Artery

Anatomy There is one left and one right common iliac artery, which are the two major terminal branches of the abdominal aorta. The left common iliac artery is slightly longer and thinner than the right. The superior hypogastric plexus and the ureter pass in front of the common iliac artery. The common iliac artery travels bilaterally and divides into the external iliac artery and internal iliac artery upon entering the pelvic cavity [3].

Clinical Significance During pelvic lymph node dissection, when opening the peritoneum over the surface of the common iliac artery, caution is necessary due to the common occurrence of the ureter crossing over the common iliac artery and entering the pelvic region. Therefore,

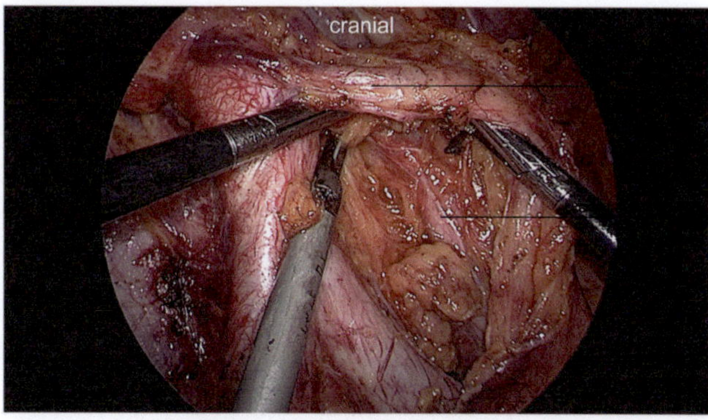

Fig. 1.3 Inferior mesenteric artery

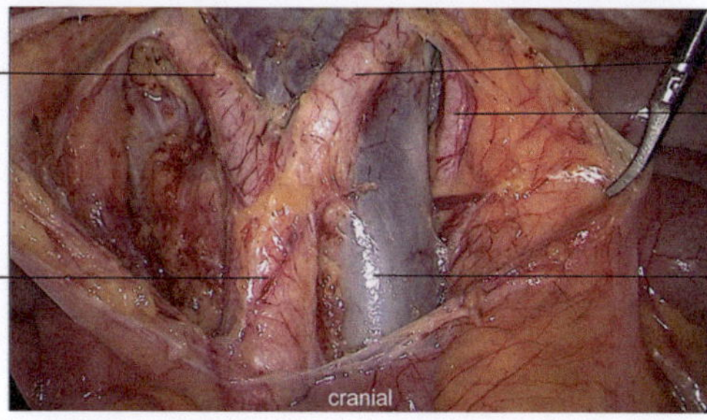

Fig. 1.4 Common iliac artery

it is essential to open the peritoneum while directly visualizing the ureter to expose the common iliac artery, preventing inadvertent damage to the ureter. On the left side, the common iliac artery is often covered by the sigmoid colon and its mesentery. In such cases, it's necessary to open the mesentery on the medial side of the sigmoid colon, push the inferior mesenteric artery, ureter, and sigmoid colon sufficiently laterally, thereby revealing the left common iliac artery (Fig. 1.4).

1.1.1.5 Median Sacral Artery

Anatomy The median sacral artery originates from the posterior aspect of the terminal abdominal aorta and is relatively slender. Upon its emergence, it descends anteriorly in front of the fourth and fifth lumbar vertebrae, the sacrum, and the coccyx, ultimately reaching the coccygeal body. Anteriorly, it is crossed by structures such as the left common iliac vein and the presacral nerves [2, 4].

Clinical Significance Arising from the posterior aspect of the terminal abdominal aorta, the median sacral artery is not easily exposed.

1.1.1.6 Lumbar Artery

Anatomy The lumbar arteries typically occur in four pairs and arise from the posterior-lateral aspect of the abdominal aorta. They individually course along the anterior or lateral aspects of the bodies of the first to fourth lumbar vertebrae, often accompanied by the lumbar veins [2].

Clinical Significance During the removal of lymph nodes in the left region of the abdominal aorta, the lumbar arteries may come into view. Since these arteries often closely follow the anterior aspect of the lumbar vertebrae, caution should be exercised to avoid direct proximity to the anterior surface of the lumbar vertebrae while excising lymph nodes in this area. This precaution is necessary to prevent uncontrollable bleeding (Fig. 1.5).

1.1.2 Venous Anatomy of the Abdominal Cavity

1.1.2.1 Inferior Vena Cava (IVC)

Anatomy The inferior vena cava is the body's largest vein, playing a critical role in gathering

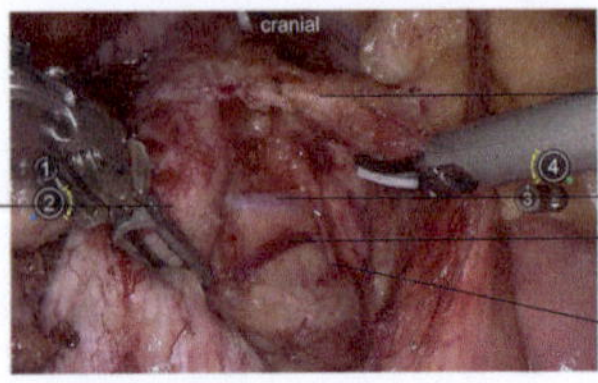

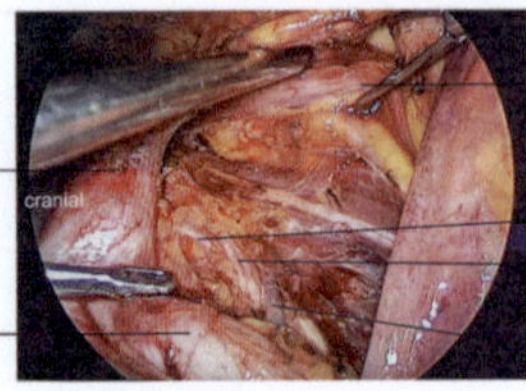

Fig. 1.5 (**a**, **b**) Lumbar artery

deoxygenated blood from the lower body, abdomen, and pelvis, and transporting it to the right atrium of the heart. The inferior vena cava forms as the left and right common iliac veins converge. Typically, this convergence occurs at the level of the fifth lumbar vertebra, occasionally at the fourth lumbar vertebra. Positioned to the right anterior aspect of the spine, the inferior vena cava ascends along the right side of the abdominal aorta. It traverses the hepatic venous groove of the liver and the diaphragmatic caval foramen before ultimately entering the posterior-inferior portion of the right atrium [2].

Clinical Significance The inferior vena cava can exhibit anatomical variations, with occasional instances of it being located to the left of the abdominal aorta. It is particularly crucial for gynecologists to thoroughly review imaging before surgery. On the surface of the inferior vena cava, there are often several small perforating veins connecting with lymphatic adipose tissue. This area is considered a hazardous zone for lymph node dissection on the surface of the vena cava. Precise handling is required in this region. In cases of inadvertent detachment of these perforating vessels at their roots, hemostasis may necessitate the use of 4-0 or 5-0 vascular sutures. During suturing, it's essential to sew in a perpendicular direction to the axis of the vessel to avoid exerting excessive force that could lead to secondary catastrophic damage (Fig. 1.6).

1.1.2.2 Renal Vein

Anatomy The renal veins originate from the renal hilum and traverse horizontally along the ventral aspect of the renal arteries, joining the inferior vena cava on its medial side. The left renal vein is approximately three times longer than the right renal vein (7.5 mm and 2.5 mm respectively). In most cases, the left renal vein courses along the ventral aspect of the abdominal aorta (with a few instances along the dorsal aspect of the abdominal aorta), ultimately merging into the inferior vena cava. The left renal vein receives the left adrenal vein and the left ovarian vein [2].

Clinical Significance The left renal vein serves as a crucial anatomical landmark for lymph node dissection in the higher region of the abdominal aorta. When performing lymph node dissection in this area, the surface of the left renal vein often harbors multiple prominent lymphatic vessels. To mitigate the risk of postoperative chyle leakage, it is recommended to securely ligate or apply vascular clips to these larger lymphatic vessels. Whether dissecting the left renal vein through open surgery or laparoscopy, meticulous attention is imperative due to the intricate surrounding anatomical structures. Blind manipulation should be avoided. Importantly, the left renal vein can occasionally traverse along the dorsal aspect of the abdominal aorta, underscoring the significance of thorough preoperative imaging review by gynecologists (Fig. 1.7).

1.1.2.3 Lumbar Vein

Anatomy The lumbar veins typically exist in four pairs and collect blood from the lumbar vascular supply region, including the posterior, lateral, and anterior abdominal walls. Paired lumbar ascending veins connect with their respective lumbar veins. Lumbar veins of the third and fourth levels usually converge from the posterior aspect into the inferior vena cava at the corresponding vertebral bodies. The left lumbar vein takes a longer course along the dorsal external

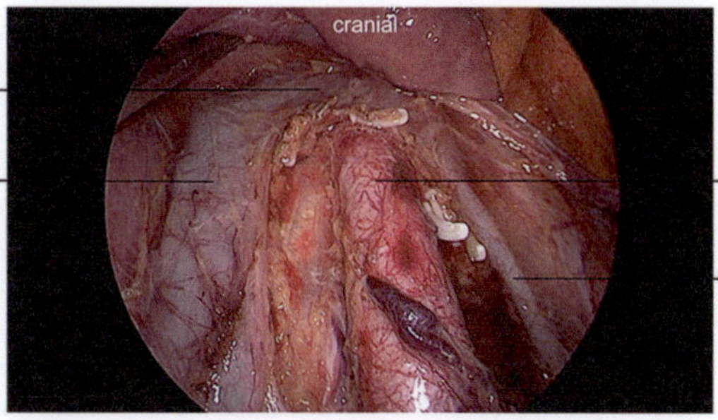

Fig. 1.6 Inferior vena cava

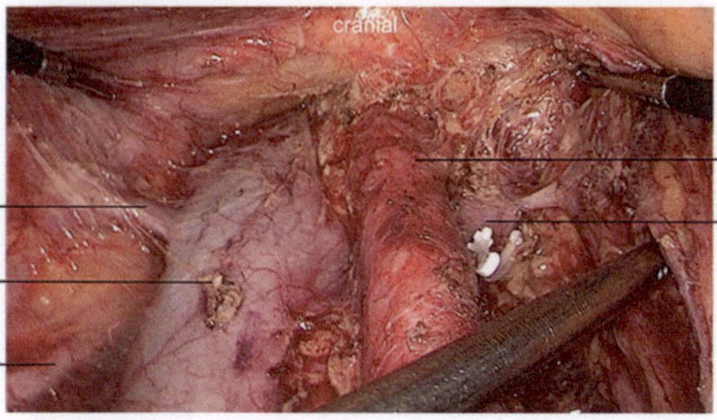

Fig. 1.7 Left renal vein

aspect of the abdominal aorta. Lumbar veins of the first and second levels exhibit more variability, as they can drain into the inferior vena cava, lumbar ascending vein, hemiazygos vein, or azygos vein. Lumbar veins communicate with the extraspinal venous plexus, thereby connecting with the intraspinal venous plexus [2].

Clinical Significance During the excision of lymph nodes in the left side of the abdominal aorta region, lumbar veins might be encountered. As these veins often course closely along the anterior aspect of the lumbar vertebrae, caution should be exercised to avoid close manipulation to the anterior side of the lumbar vertebrae while removing lymph nodes in this area. This precaution is taken to prevent occurrences of uncontrollable bleeding.

1.1.2.4 Ascending Lumbar Vein

Anatomy The longitudinal communicating branches between the lumbar veins are known as the ascending lumbar veins. These veins are paired structures coursing medially within the psoas major muscle. They connect with the ipsilateral common iliac vein, iliolumbar vein, and lumbar vein. Additionally, they communicate upwardly with the renal veins and subcostal veins. The course and connections of the ascending lumbar veins exhibit considerable variability, and they can occasionally be absent on the one side or the other. The ascending lumbar veins on both sides, respectively, pass through the left and right crus of the diaphragm, transforming into the hemiazygos vein on the left side and the azygos vein on the right side before ultimately joining the superior vena cava. Consequently, the ascending lumbar veins constitute one of the collateral circulatory pathways connecting the superior and inferior vena cava systems [5].

Clinical Significance During lymph node dissection in the higher region of the abdominal aorta, particularly when removing lymph nodes below the left renal vein, careful attention should be paid to the exposure of the ascending lumbar veins to prevent inadvertent injury (Fig. 1.8).

1.1.2.5 Ovarian Vein

Anatomy The ovarian veins on both sides ascend from the pelvic sidewalls, accompanying their respective arteries. The right ovarian vein obliquely joins the inferior vena cava, while the left ovarian vein ascends almost vertically to join the left renal vein.

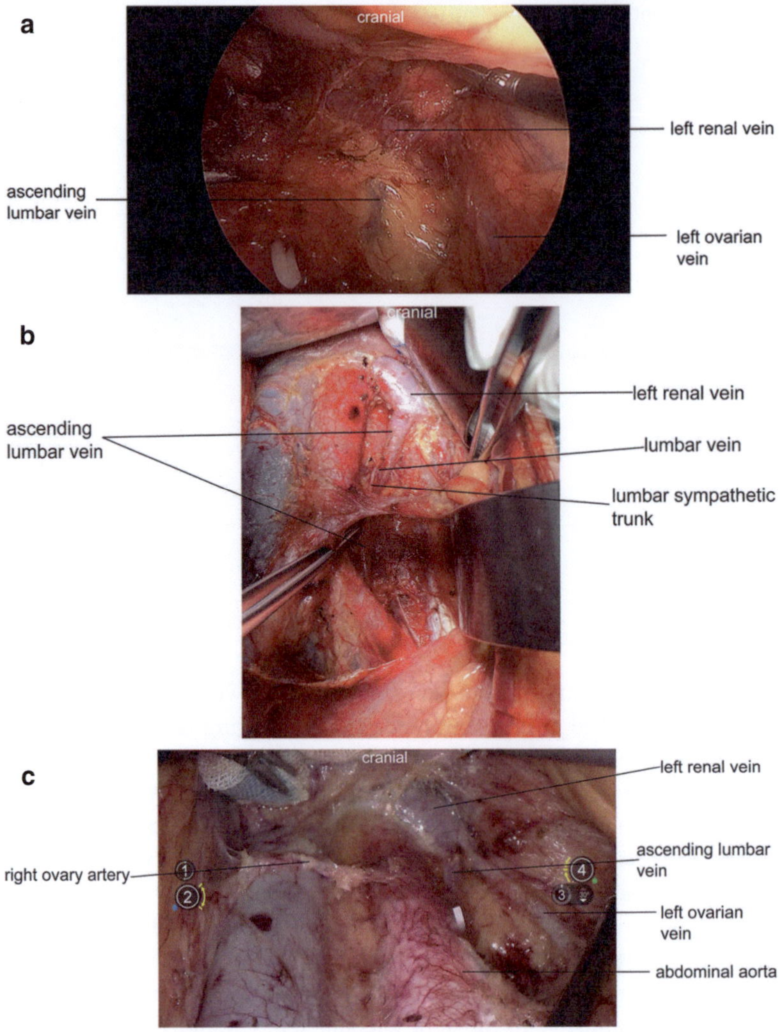

Fig. 1.8 (a–c) Ascending lumbar vein

Clinical Significance The right ovarian vein typically drains into the lateral aspect of the inferior vena cava, slightly below the left renal vein by about 2 cm in adults. Occasionally, it may drain into the right renal vein. When removing lymph nodes in this area, caution is necessary to avoid potential bleeding from this vein. On the other hand, the left ovarian vein mainly drains into the left renal vein (Fig. 1.9).

1.1.2.6 Inferior Mesenteric Vein

Anatomy The inferior mesenteric vein collects blood from the superior rectal vein, several branches of the sigmoid veins, and the left colic vein. It typically joins the splenic vein after passing behind the lower margin of the pancreas and in front of the left renal vein. However, it can also join the splenic vein at the confluence of the splenic vein and the superior mesenteric vein, or it may directly drain into the superior mesenteric vein. The inferior mesenteric vein is located within the posterior mesenteric space to the left of the inferior mesenteric artery. It then ascends, passing posterior to the left psoas major muscle and in front of the left ureter. This vein can either pass over the ovarian vessels or ascend within their medial aspect [6].

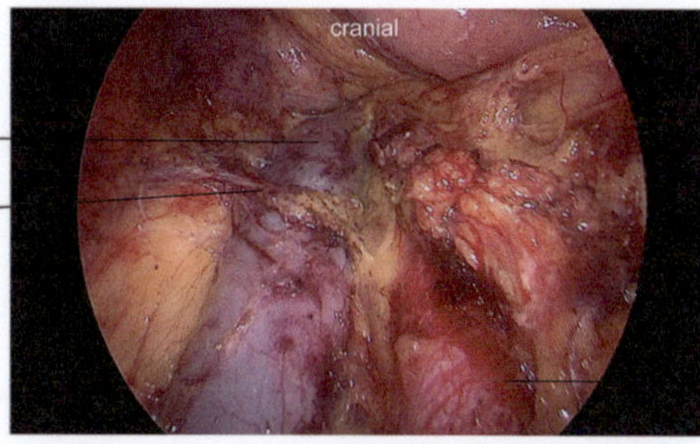

Fig. 1.9 Ovary vein

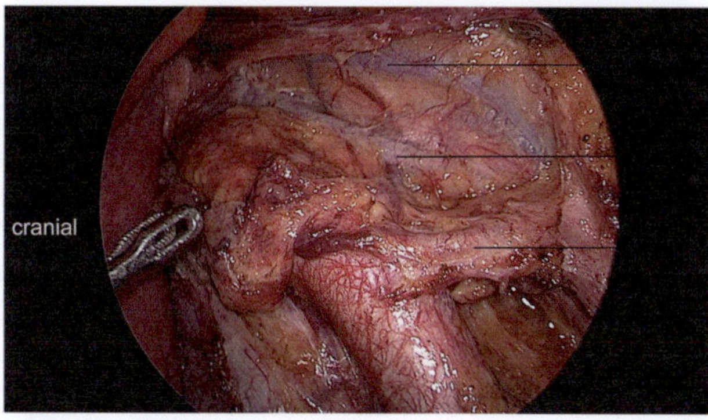

Fig. 1.10 Inferior mesenteric vein

Clinical Significance The inferior mesenteric vein is situated laterally to the duodenojejunal flexure and may occasionally be positioned posterior to it. This anatomical characteristic serves as a reference point during surgical procedures. It does not accompany the inferior mesenteric artery. When opening the posterior peritoneum to expose the abdominal aorta and superiorly mobilizing the duodenum, care should be taken to avoid injury to this vessel (Fig. 1.10).

1.1.2.7 Common Iliac Vein

Anatomy The common iliac vein is formed by the convergence of the external iliac vein and internal iliac vein in front of the sacroiliac joint. It ascends diagonally inward and upward, uniting at the level of the fifth lumbar vertebra to form the inferior vena cava.

Clinical Significance There are small veins within the lymphatic adipose tissue that directly drain into the common iliac vein. When removing lymphatic tissue on the surface of the common iliac vein, it is important to avoid blunt tearing as it can cause damage to the vein wall and result in significant bleeding. The left common iliac vein often courses obliquely over the surface of the lumbar vertebrae, so caution must be exercised when performing lymph node dissection in this area. In the event of vascular injury, suturing becomes extremely challenging.

1.1.2.8 Median Sacral Vein

Anatomy The median sacral veins typically exist as two separate veins that accompany the corresponding arteries in front of the sacrum. These veins subsequently merge to form a single vein, which often joins the left common iliac vein. Occasionally, it terminates at the confluence of the common iliac veins [2].

Clinical Significance This vein is the vessel that needs to be exposed during the removal of presacral lymph nodes. Care should be taken to avoid damaging it (Fig. 1.11).

Fig. 1.11 Median sacral vein

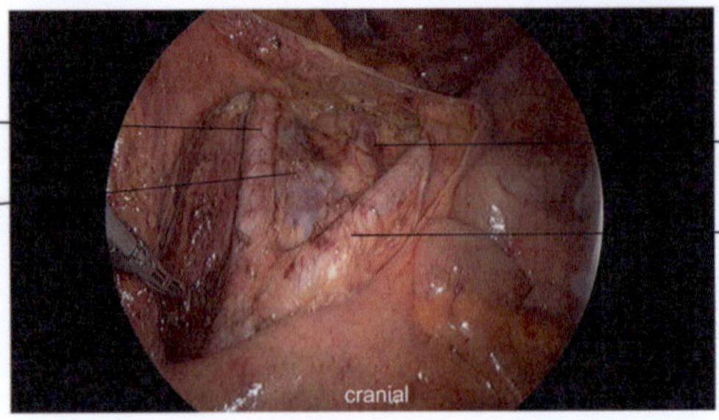

1.2 Pelvic Vasculature

1.2.1 Arterial Anatomy of the Pelvic Cavity

1.2.1.1 External Iliac Artery

Anatomy The external iliac artery arises from the bifurcation of the common iliac artery. It descends along the medial border of the psoas major muscle and passes behind the inguinal ligament at the junction of the inner and middle thirds. It then transitions into the femoral artery in the anterior thigh. The length of the external iliac artery is approximately 100–115 mm. The ventral side of the left external iliac artery is adjacent to the sigmoid colon, while the proximal portion of the right external iliac artery is crossed by the ureter. Above the inguinal ligament, the external iliac artery gives off the inferior epigastric artery, which enters the sheath of the rectus abdominis muscle and anastomoses with the superior epigastric artery, providing nourishment to the rectus abdominis muscle. Posterior to the inguinal ligament, the deep circumflex iliac artery branches off.

Clinical Significance The external iliac artery is the main arterial supply to the lower limb and should be protected from injury. In the event of injury, it is crucial to seek experienced medical professionals for management. Avoidance of postoperative vascular stenosis is important to ensure adequate blood supply to the lower limb. If necessary, the internal iliac artery can be used for anastomosis or artificial graft placement. Maintaining a patent flow in the external iliac artery is essential to prevent lower limb ischemia and necrosis. Examination of dorsalis pedis artery pulsations can be performed to assess the patency of the external iliac artery and the success of surgical anastomosis following injury (Fig. 1.12).

1.2.1.2 Internal Iliac Artery

Anatomy The internal iliac artery originates from the bifurcation of the common iliac artery. It courses downward anterior to the lumbosacral disc and the sacroiliac joint. Its distal segment terminates and continues as the lateral umbilical ligament [7]. The branches of the internal iliac artery are complex and can be generally categorized based on their vascular supply areas into visceral branches (including the umbilical artery, superior vesical artery, uterine artery, inferior rectal artery, internal pudendal artery, and vaginal artery), parietal branches (including the iliolumbar artery and lateral sacral artery), and branches to the lower limb and perineum (including the superior gluteal artery, inferior gluteal artery, and obturator artery) [8, 9].

Clinical Significance During pelvic lymph node dissection, the internal iliac artery and its anterior branches, particularly the umbilical artery, are among the critical anatomical structures that need to be carefully mobilized first (see Fig. 1.12).

Anterior Trunk of the Internal Iliac Artery

Uterine Artery

Anatomy The uterine artery descends anteriorly along the pelvic sidewall behind the peritoneum. It passes through the base of the broad ligament,

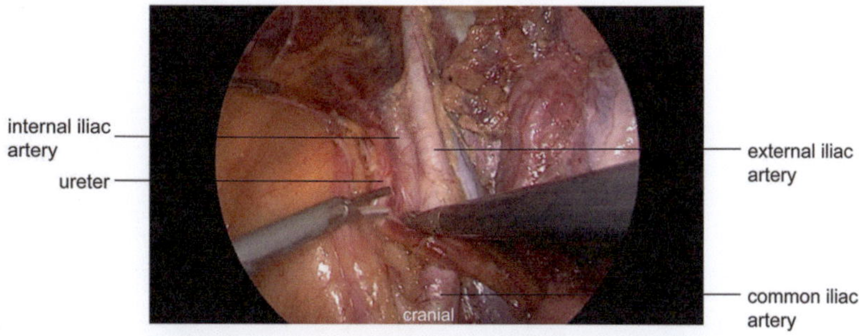

Fig. 1.12 External iliac artery, internal iliac artery

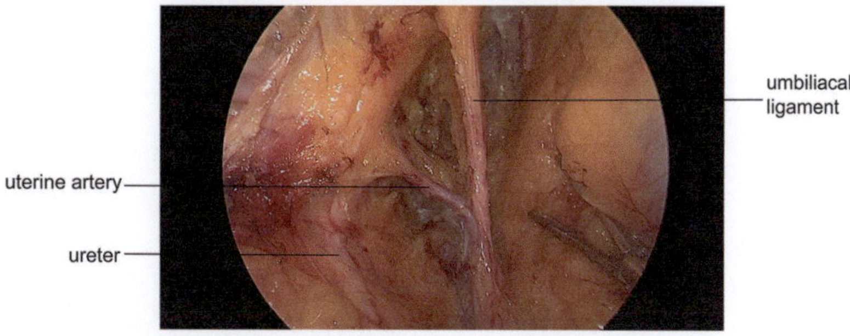

Fig. 1.13 Uterine artery

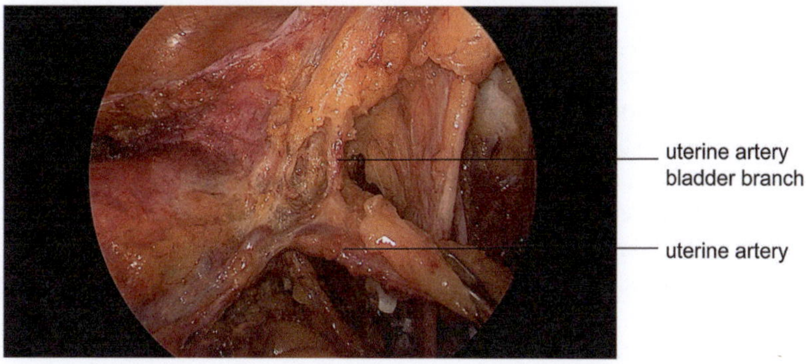

Fig. 1.14 Uterine artery bladder branch

reaches the lateral aspect of the uterus through the parametrial tissue, and crosses the ureter at approximately 2 cm from the level of the internal os to reach the uterine edge (Fig. 1.13) [10]. The main trunk of the uterine artery gives off branches including the uterine fundal branch (supplying the uterine fundus), ovarian branch (anastomosing with the distal branches of the ovarian artery), and tubal branch (supplying the fallopian tube). At the level of the internal os, the uterine artery gives off several collateral branches that supply the bladder, upper vagina, and cervix, including bladder branches (Fig. 1.14), ureteral branches (Fig. 1.15), and cervicovaginal and cervical branches. The bladder branches are slender and arise anterior to the ureteral crossing, extending along the uterine cervix segment within the cardinal ligament, and extending to the base of the bladder and lateral fornix of the vagina. The ureteral branches arise at the ureteral crossing and travel along the ureteral wall.

Clinical Significance The uterine artery is particularly important in radical hysterectomy procedures. It serves as an important anatomical landmark for identifying the lateral parametrial tissue. By identifying the uterine artery, the lateral rectal compartment can be dissected from the bladder compartment, allowing for optimal exposure of the lateral parametrial tissue.

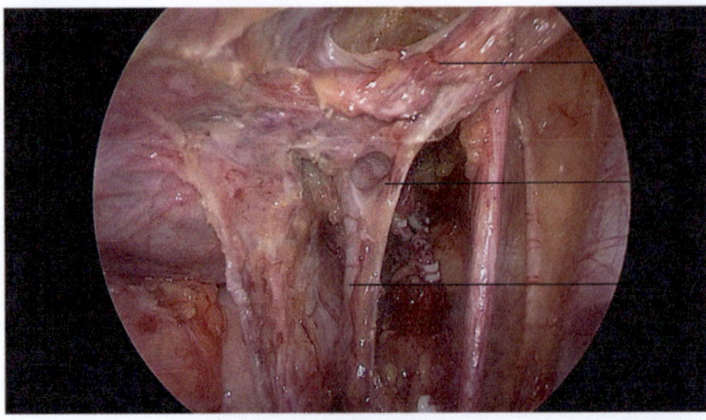

Fig. 1.15 Uterine artery ureteral branch

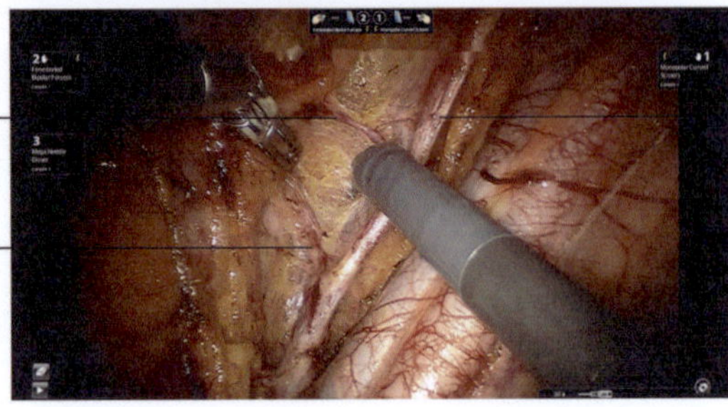

Fig. 1.16 Umbilical ligament

Although less commonly mentioned in clinical practice, the bladder branches of the uterine artery have anatomical significance during surgical dissection. The location of the ureteral tunnel entrance is located on the medial side of the bladder branch of the uterine artery and serves as an anatomical landmark during the exposure of the ureteral tunnel entrance.

Superior Vesical Artery. Superior vesical artery arises from the umbilical artery and descends inwardly, supplying the upper and middle parts of the urinary bladder (Fig. 1.16) [2].

Inferior Vesical Artery. Arises from the anterior division of the internal iliac artery, runs posteriorly and inferiorly to the obturator artery, and then turns medially to supply the base of the urinary bladder and the lower segment of the ureteral pelvic region.

Umbilical Artery. It is the first branch of the anterior division, and its distal portion closes to form the medial umbilical ligament.

Obturator Artery

Anatomy The obturator artery is a branch of the internal iliac artery. It runs closely along the pelvic wall in the direction of the obturator foramen, passes through the obturator canal into the pelvic cavity, and reaches the medial aspect of the thigh. Its branches provide blood supply to the surrounding muscles and the hip joint. The obturator artery can also originate from the internal pudendal artery, inferior epigastric artery, superior gluteal artery, or external iliac artery. Before traversing the obturator canal, the obturator artery gives off the pubic branch, which anastomoses with the branches of the inferior epigastric artery (pubic branch), and sometimes this anastomosis can be relatively large, forming an abnormal obturator artery. The obturator vein is a tributary of the internal iliac vein and accompanies the course of the obturator artery [2, 11, 12].

Clinical Significance The obturator artery is a lateral branch of the internal iliac artery and mostly runs posteriorly along the pelvic wall in close proximity to the obturator nerve. Therefore, during the dissection of the internal iliac artery and the umbilical artery, it is safer to dissect along their lateral sides, as it reduces the risk of obturator artery injury. During surgery, if the obturator vessels interfere with lymph node dis-

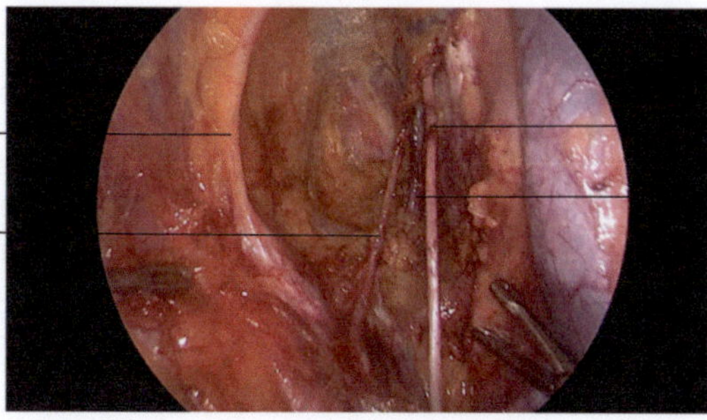

Fig. 1.17 Obturator artery

section or if the lymph nodes are significantly enlarged, the obturator artery and vein can be ligated without intentional preservation (Fig. 1.17).

Accessory Obturator Artery

Anatomy The accessory obturator artery is a variant of the obturator artery. It refers to any artery directly or indirectly arising from the external iliac artery or femoral artery, constituting the accessory obturator artery. Typically, it denotes the anastomotic branch between the obturator artery and either the external iliac artery or the inferior epigastric artery. It is situated posterior to the pubic symphysis, at an average distance of 6 cm (ranging from 4.0 to 9.6 cm) from the symphysis. Numerous studies have emphasized that inadvertent transection of this artery can result in unmanageable profuse bleeding and patient mortality. Hence, it is also referred to as the "artery of death" [13]. Over 50% of accessory obturator arteries exit the pelvic cavity through the femoral ring, lateral to the lacunar ligament, while a minority exits medially or centrally through the femoral ring [14].

Clinical Significance During pelvic lymph node dissection, it is essential to be attentive to vascular variations in the origin, course, and branching of the accessory obturator artery to prevent hemorrhage.

Inferior Rectal Artery Most commonly arises from the internal iliac artery, but can also originate from the internal pudendal artery. It passes through the lateral ligament of the rectum and branches to supply the lower part of the rectum.

Internal Pudendal Artery It is the terminal branch of the internal iliac artery. It traverses the lesser sciatic foramen, located posterior to the ischial spine. Medially, it is accompanied by the pudendal nerve, superior rectal nerve, and inferior rectal vessels. Laterally, it is accompanied by the sciatic nerve, inferior gluteal nerve, coccygeal nerve, and posterior femoral cutaneous nerve. After bypassing the ischial spine, the internal pudendal artery enters the ischiorectal fossa, pierces the perineal membrane, and enters the deep perineal pouch. At the level of the perineal transverse ligament, it gives off two branches: the deep artery of the clitoris and the dorsal artery of the clitoris. The deep artery of the clitoris enters the root of the corpus cavernosum and courses through the center of the corpus cavernosum. The dorsal artery of the clitoris descends below the perineal transverse ligament, passes through the suspensory ligament of the clitoris, and gives off branches to the anterior bladder, posterior union of the pubic bones, anterior union of the pubic bones, and skin.

Inferior Gluteal Artery It is a branch of the anterior trunk of the internal iliac artery and is relatively large. After passing through the lesser sciatic foramen, it supplies the inferior gluteal region and the upper part of the posterior thigh tissues.

Posterior Trunk of the Internal Iliac Artery

With an internal diameter of approximately 8 mm, it increases in thickness with age. It gives rise to the iliolumbar artery, lateral sacral arteries (superior and inferior), and superior gluteal artery. The iliolumbar artery ascends along the iliac fossa and anastomoses with the fifth lumbar artery and the deep branch of the lateral sacral artery. The superior lateral sacral artery enters the pelvic cavity through the first sacral foramen. The inferior lateral sacral artery gives off branches to the sacral foramina of S2, S3, and S4. The superior gluteal artery passes through the greater sciatic foramen and distributes to the gluteal region [15].

1.2.2 Venous Anatomy of the Pelvic Cavity

1.2.2.1 External Iliac Vein

Anatomy The external iliac vein accompanies the external iliac artery and is a direct continuation of the femoral vein. Its main trunk and tributaries run parallel to the corresponding arteries. The left external iliac vein runs entirely medial to the artery, while the right external iliac vein initially runs medial to the artery and gradually shifts posteriorly as it ascends. The external iliac vein crosses over the uterosacral ligament and ovarian vessels. Its tributaries include the abdominal wall veins, deep circumflex iliac vein, and pubic vein [2].

Clinical Significance It is the main vein through which lower limb blood returns to the pelvic cavity. In case of injury, it is crucial to seek experienced medical professionals for precise repair to avoid postoperative complications such as vascular stenosis or tortuosity, which can lead to impaired lower limb venous return, leg swelling, venous thrombosis, and other complications. In most cases, 4-0/5-0 vascular suture thread can be used for repair and closure. Additionally, during the surgical procedure, caution should be taken to avoid clamping the veins and causing damage to the intima of the vein wall, which can lead to postoperative thrombus formation.

1.2.2.2 Internal Iliac Vein

Anatomy The internal iliac vein originates from the upper part of the greater sciatic foramen and runs posterior and medial to its corresponding artery. It ascends to the anterior aspect of the sacroiliac joint where it joins the external iliac vein. Veins are more closely adhered to the pelvic wall compared to arteries and are covered by arteries. Therefore, arteries are usually positioned on the medial and anterior superior aspect of the veins. The internal iliac vein exhibits more variations and complex course compared to the internal iliac artery. While veins generally accompany arteries, there are rich venous plexuses surrounding the pelvic organs. These venous plexuses, including the vaginal venous plexus, bladder venous plexus, rectal venous plexus, and uterovaginal venous plexus, are composed of branches of the internal iliac vein. These venous plexuses are located within loose connective tissue surrounding the organs, forming an interlacing network with extremely thin vessel walls. Arteries often traverse through the venous plexuses, creating a sponge-like space. The internal iliac vein and its plexuses are usually deeply embedded in the pelvic floor and are not encountered during routine gynecological surgeries. However, they become exposed during pelvic lymph node dissection, and due to the extensive distribution and numerous branches of the internal iliac vein, significant uncontrollable bleeding may occur if injured [2, 16].

Clinical Significance During the excision of lymph nodes in the region of the ischial spine, the lateral aspect of the internal iliac vein becomes visible, while the medial aspect of the vein is exposed during the management of lateral parametrial tissues. The bifurcation of the internal and external iliac veins is one of the most vulnerable sites during pelvic lymph node dissection, and it is commonly referred to as the "tiger's mouth" in traditional surgery, indicating the hazardous nature of handling lymph nodes in that region. Dissection of the lymphatic fatty tissue in this area, which lies lateral to the common iliac vein, allows for visualization of the internal iliac vein and the pudendal nerve (Fig. 1.18).

Superior Uterine Vein

Accompanies the uterine artery (Fig. 1.19).

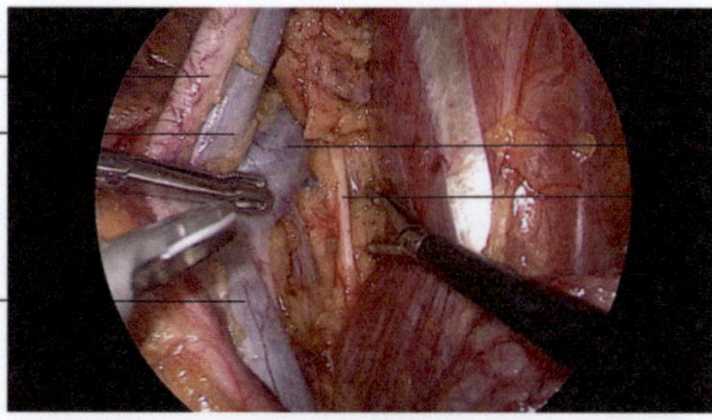

Fig. 1.18 Internal iliac vein

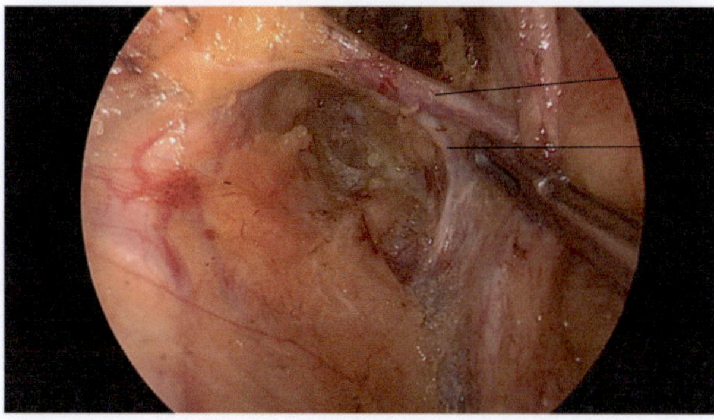

Fig. 1.19 Superficial uterine vein

Deep Uterine Vein

Anatomy It mainly collects venous blood from the body of the uterus and runs along the vascular portion of the broad ligament (surface of the broad ligament), ultimately draining into the uterine vein. The bladder's superior (Fig. 1.20), middle, and inferior veins join along the course. Between the vascular portion of the broad ligament and its inferior ligamentous portion, branches of the pelvic visceral nerves pass through and join the inferior hypogastric plexus [17].

Clinical Significance The deep uterine vein is an important anatomical landmark during radical hysterectomy of the QM-C type [18]. Its caudal aspect is associated with the pelvic splanchnic nerve plexus. The deep uterine vein is typically multiple, occasionally single, and can be dissected along with the vesical venous plexus to expose the neurovascular plane formed by the convergence of the pelvic splanchnic nerve plexus and the inferior hypogastric plexus, known as the "crossing of the nerves." When dealing with the lateral parametrial tissues, it is recommended to directly ligate and dissect the deep uterine vein to avoid the risk of tumor cell dissemination during surgery (Fig. 1.21).

Obturator Vein

Anatomy In normal circumstances, the obturator vein is typically a single vessel that collects blood from the adductor muscle group. It runs upward between the pectineus and adductor brevis muscles, passes through the obturator canal, and reaches above the obturator foramen. It accompanies the obturator artery and ascends along the lateral wall of the pelvis, ultimately draining into the internal iliac vein [2, 19].

Clinical Significance The obturator vein does not have any specific significance. In challenging situations during lymph node dissection, it can be ligated and divided. The veins below the obturator nerve often form a complex network and may have significant size and collateral connections. In traditional open abdominal surgery, the posterior aspect of the obturator nerve has been referred to as the "wolf's den" due to the difficulty in achieving hemostasis if injured, often

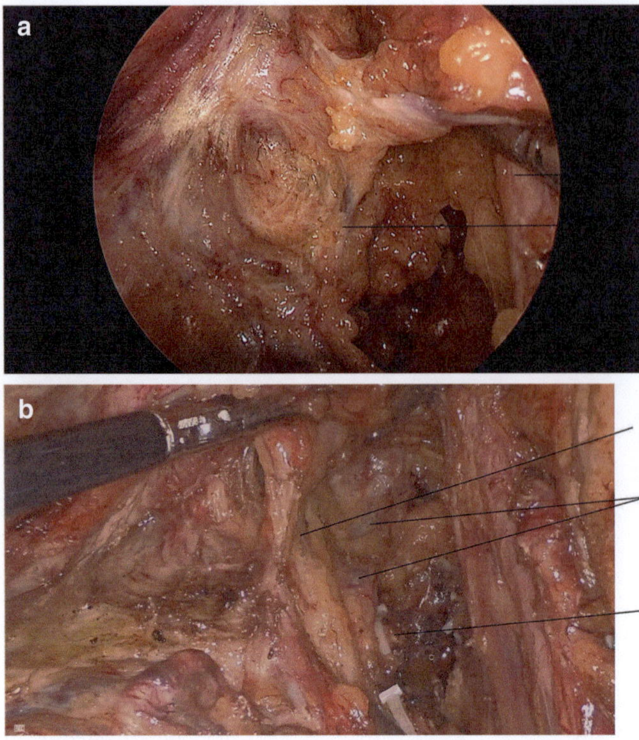

Fig. 1.20 (**a**, **b**) Superior vesical vein

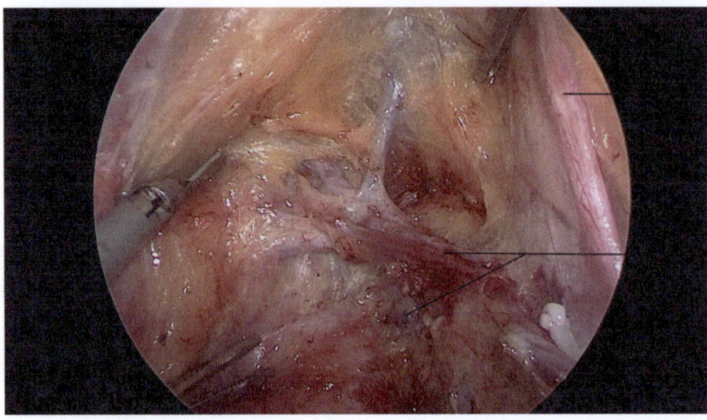

Fig. 1.21 Deep uterine vein

requiring compression for hemostasis. However, in laparoscopic procedures, there are advantages in visualization and bipolar coagulation, making the management of bleeding in this area relatively easier. In cases of profuse bleeding, suturing may be required for hemostasis.

Accessory Obturator Vein

Anatomy The accessory obturator vein is a venous branch that emerges from the obturator region and drains into the external iliac vein. It is distributed along the pelvic wall [19].

Clinical Significance The accessory obturator vein is a relatively fixed branch of the external iliac vein and often does not have a corresponding artery. In most cases, bipolar coagulation is sufficient for hemostasis if this vein is injured (see Fig. 1.22).

Vesical Venous Plexus

Anatomy The vesical venous plexus is the largest venous plexus in the pelvis, located around the base of the bladder within the bladder uterine vaginal ligament. It collects venous blood from

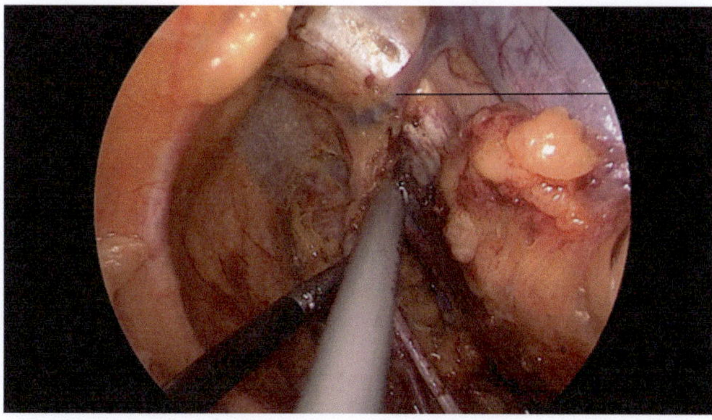

Fig. 1.22 Accessory obturator vein

the bladder, urethra, and vagina. Bladder venous plexus comprises the bladder superior vein, bladder middle vein, and bladder inferior vein. Due to variations within the bladder venous plexus, different scholars have varying interpretations and understandings of their anatomy. Japanese scholar Yoshihiko Yabuki suggests that, in terms of anatomical location, the bladder superior vein often accompanies the bladder superior artery and primarily drains into the deep uterine vein. In most cases, the bladder middle vein directly joins the internal iliac vein, while in a minority of cases, it flows into the deep uterine vein before joining the internal iliac vein. As for the bladder inferior vein, in the majority of cases, it drains into the rectal middle vein before joining the internal iliac vein [20]. Professor FUJI from Japan, however, contends that the bladder superior vein, bladder middle vein, and bladder inferior vein all primarily drain into the deep uterine vein [21].

Clinical Significance The vesical venous plexus plays an important role in the venous drainage of the pelvic organs. It is involved in the circulation of blood from the bladder, urethra, and vagina. Our team, based on extensive surgical exploration, believes that the bladder superior vein runs within the vesicocervical ligament and primarily drains directly into the deep uterine vein. In most cases, the bladder middle vein runs on the surface of the paracolpium and drains into the deep uterine vein, while in some cases, it runs on the outside of the paracolpium and directly joins the internal iliac vein. The bladder inferior vein, due to its initial drainage into the rectal middle vein before joining the internal iliac vein, is rarely involved in cervical cancer surgery.

References

1. Mirjalili SA, McFadden SL, Buckenham T, et al. A reappraisal of adult abdominal surface anatomy. Clin Anat. 2012;25:844–50.
2. Standring S. Gray's anatomy, the anatomical basis of clinical practice. 41st ed. New York: Elsevier; 2016.
3. Roberts WH, Krishingner GL. Comparative study of human internal iliac artery based on Adachi classification. Anat Rec. 1967;158:191–6.
4. Dimov I, Sobczak S, Grabs D, et al. The median sacral artery in rectal blood supply: a cadaveric study. Clin Anat. 2021;34:342–7.
5. Lolis E, Panagouli E, Venieratos D. Study of the ascending lumbar and iliolumbar veins: surgical anatomy, clinical implications and review of the literature. Ann Anat. 2011;193:516–29.
6. Graf O, Boland GW, Kaufman JA, et al. Anatomic variants of mesenteric veins: depiction with helical CT venography. AJR Am J Roentgenol. 1997;168:1209–13.
7. Gupta NP, Kumar M, Karan SC, et al. Lower ureteral obstruction due to a persistent umbilical artery. Urol Int, 1999, 63: 249–251.
8. Selçuk İ, Yassa M, Tatar İ, et al. Anatomic structure of the internal iliac artery and its educative dissection for peripartum and pelvic hemorrhage Turk J Obstet Gynecol, 2018, 15: 126–129.
9. Bleich AT, Rahn DD, Wieslander CK, et al. Posterior division of the internal iliac artery: anatomic variations and clinical applications. Am J Obstet Gynecol, 2007, 197: 658.e1–658.e5.
10. Paulsen F, Waschke J. Sobotta clinical atlas of human anatomy. 15th ed. Germany: Elsevier/Urban & Fischer; 2013.
11. Rajive AV, Pillay M. A study of variations in the origin of obturator artery and its clinical significance. J Clin Diagn Res. 2015;9(8):Ac12–5.

12. Brachini G, Matteucci M, Sapienza P, et al. Systematic review and meta-analysis of the variants of the obturatory artery. J Clin Med. 2023;12(15):4932.
13. Sarikcioglu L, Sindel M, Akyildiz F, et al. Anastomotic vessels in the retropubic region: corona mortis. Folia Morphol (Warsz). 2003;62:179–82.
14. Al Talalwah W. A new concept and classification of corona mortis and its clinical significance. Chin J Traumatol. 2016;19(5):251–4.
15. Selçuk İ, Uzuner B, Boduç E, et al. Step-by-step ligation of the internal iliac artery. J Turk Ger Gynecol Assoc. 2019;20:123–8.
16. Beran BD, Shockley M, Arnolds K, et al. Anatomy of the internal iliac vein: implications for uterine transplant. J Minim Invasive Gynecol. 2018;25:329.
17. Li H, Jia J, Xiao Y, et al. Anatomical basis of female pelvic cavity for nerve sparing radical hysterectomy. Surg Radiol Anat. 2015;37:657–65.
18. Querleu D, Cibula D, Abu-Rustum NR. Update on the Querleu-Morrow classification of radical hysterectomy. Ann Surg Oncol. 2017;2017(24):3406–12.
19. Căpîlna ME, Szabo B, Rusu SC, et al. Anatomical variations of the obturator veins and their surgical implications. Eur J Gynaecol Oncol. 2017;38:263–5.
20. Yabuki Y. New theory and technique for nerve-sparing radical hysterectomy. 1st ed. Tokyo: Medical View; 2009.
21. Fujii S. Precise neurovascular anatomy for radical hysterectomy. 1st ed. Singapore: Springer; 2020.

2 Nerve Anatomy

Jun Wang and Yuemei Cui

The pelvic and abdominal nerves consist of sympathetic and parasympathetic nerves. The distribution of sympathetic nerves follows the path of the abdominal aorta and its major branches from top to bottom, while the parasympathetic nerves travel from the outer to inner regions of the pelvic cavity. During lymphadenectomy for malignant gynecological tumors, the highest level of lymph node dissection along the abdominal aorta is usually at the level of the renal veins, which ensures that the abdominal plexus and mesenteric plexus above this level are not damaged. The main nerves associated with surgical injury are located below the abdominal plexus.

The autonomic nervous system in the pelvic region mainly includes the sympathetic and parasympathetic nerves. The sympathetic nerves originate from the visceral nerves of the abdominal aorta and converge in front of the abdominal aorta to form the abdominal plexus. These nerves descend along the front of the abdominal aorta and form the upper hypogastric plexus after branching from the internal iliac arteries. They then continue to descend along the outer sides of the rectum, forming the lower hypogastric plexus. At the level corresponding to the vagina, they merge with the pelvic visceral nerves primarily composed of the parasympathetic nerves originating from S2-4, forming the inferior hypogastric plexus that innervates the pelvic organs, including the bladder, uterus, vagina, and rectum [1].

2.1 Abdominal Nerves

2.1.1 Abdominal Aortic Plexus

Anatomy The abdominal aortic plexus is a continuation of the abdominal sympathetic plexus and ganglia, receiving fibers from the visceral nerves of L1 and L2. It is situated bilaterally and anteriorly to the abdominal aorta, between the origins of the superior and inferior mesenteric arteries. Some fibers are distributed anteriorly to the inferior vena cava, leading to its alternate name, the intermesenteric plexus. It extends downward to form the superior hypogastric plexus [2].

Clinical Significance When performing lymph node dissection in the lower abdominal aortic region for cervical cancer, the concept of preserving nerves becomes essential. The abdominal aortic plexus, a sympathetic nerve structure, is composed of a network of nerves of varying sizes arranged in front of the abdominal aorta, easily

J. Wang (✉)
Department of Gynecology and Obstetrics, Second Affiliated Hospital of Dalian Medical University, Dalian, China

Y. Cui
Department of Gynecology and Obstetrics, Dalian Municipal Central Hospital, Affiliated of Dalian University of Technology, Dalian, China

S. Han, J. Wang (eds.), *Open, Laparoscopic, and Robotic Surgery for Cervical Cancer*,
https://doi.org/10.1007/978-981-97-7687-0_2

identifiable during laparoscopic procedures. The lymph nodes located on the left, anterior, and right sides of the abdominal aorta need to be removed. However, since the abdominal aortic plexus is interwoven with these lymph nodes, there is a risk of damaging it. Yet, due to its mesh-like structure, careful manipulation can allow for partial preservation of the plexus while preventing bleeding complications (Fig. 2.1).

2.1.2 Lumbar Sympathetic Trunks

Anatomy It consists of 3 to 5 pairs of ganglia along with their interganglionic branches, situated on the anterior and lateral aspects of the lumbar vertebral bodies, medial and anterior to the psoas major muscle. Covered by the deep fascia, it is superiorly connected to the sympathetic trunk in the thorax and inferiorly crosses over the pelvic inlet, continuing as the sacral sympathetic trunk posterior to the iliac vessels. There are transverse communicating branches between the left and right lumbar sympathetic trunks. The right lumbar sympathetic trunk is situated posterior to the inferior vena cava, lumbar lymph nodes, and the right ureter, hidden by the inferior vena cava. The left lumbar sympathetic trunk lies adjacent to the left margin of the abdominal aorta, often concealed by the abdominal aorta and left lumbar lymph nodes. Both lumbar sympathetic trunks course anteriorly to the lumbar arteries and veins, with the genitofemoral nerve traveling along their lateral sides [2].

Clinical Significance During the left-sided abdominal aortic lymph node dissection procedure, there exists a potential risk of injuring the lumbar sympathetic ganglia. In the event of such injury, patients may experience symptoms such as elevated skin temperature, skin redness, and dryness on the same side of the lower limb. Concurrently, they may report a decrease in skin temperature on the contralateral lower limb (Fig. 2.2).

2.1.3 Superior Hypogastric Plexus

Anatomy The direct continuation of the celiac plexus, located anterior to the sacral promontory, is often referred to as the presacral plexus or presacral nerves. The superior hypogastric plexus is predominantly distributed within the triangular region between the bifurcation of the abdominal

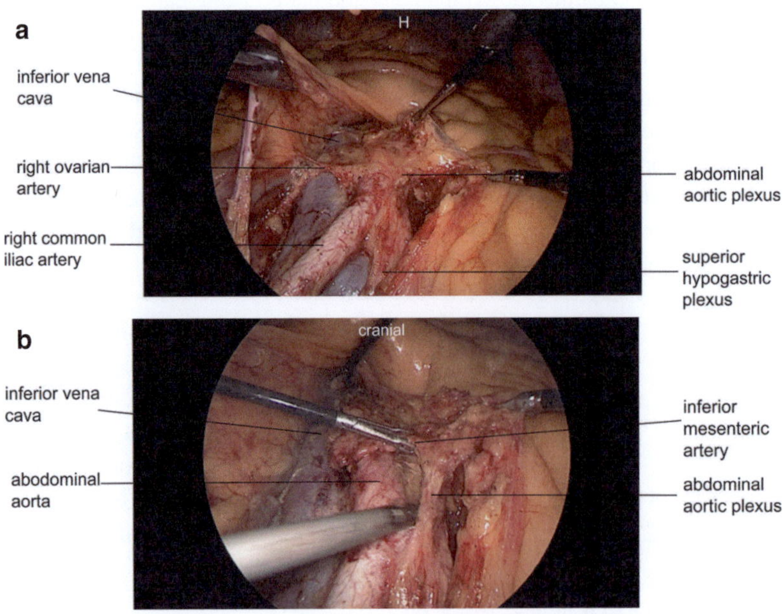

Fig. 2.1 (a, b) Abdominal aortic plexus

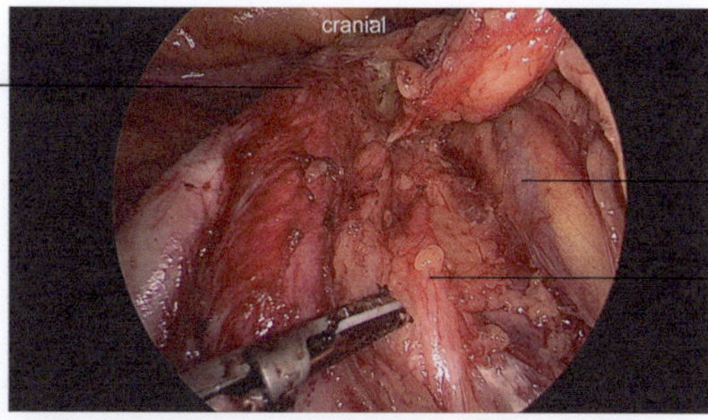

Fig. 2.2 Lumbar sympathetic trunk

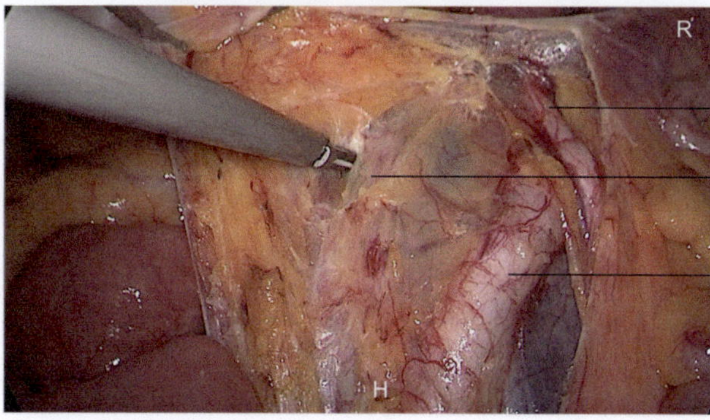

Fig. 2.3 Superior hypogastric plexus

aorta, the bilateral common iliac arteries, and the sacral promontory. It forms an irregular meshwork closely adhering to the peritoneal wall and divides into left and right hypogastric nerves at the level of the sacral promontory or below. The main components of the superior hypogastric plexus are sympathetic nerve fibers originating from the celiac plexus, inferior mesenteric plexus, and visceral nerves of the L3 and L4 sympathetic ganglia. These fibers descend as the left and right hypogastric nerves to join the left and right pelvic plexuses, with additional smaller branches extending to the ureteric plexus, ovarian plexus, and internal iliac vascular plexus (Fig. 2.3) [3, 4].

2.2 Pelvic Nerves

2.2.1 Genitofemoral Nerve

Anatomy The genitofemoral nerve is composed of fibers from the anterior branches of the first lumbar nerve and the majority of fibers from the anterior branch of the second lumbar nerve. It descends anteriorly to the psoas major muscle and divides into the femoral branch and the genital branch. The femoral branch innervates the skin sensation of the inner one-third of the thigh, while the genital branch accompanies the round ligament of the uterus, passes through the inguinal canal, and branches to the labia majora [5].

Clinical Significance During pelvic lymph node dissection, it is important to preserve the genitofemoral nerve to avoid functional impairment of the skin sensation on the inner aspect of the thigh. In some patients, neuralgia of this nerve may manifest as a burning pain in the inguinal region, radiating to the external genitalia and upper inner thigh. Pain exacerbation may occur during walking and excessive extension of the thigh, but most patients gradually recover within several months (Fig. 2.4).

2.2.2 Obturator Nerve

Anatomy The obturator nerve is formed by the branches of the second to fourth lumbar

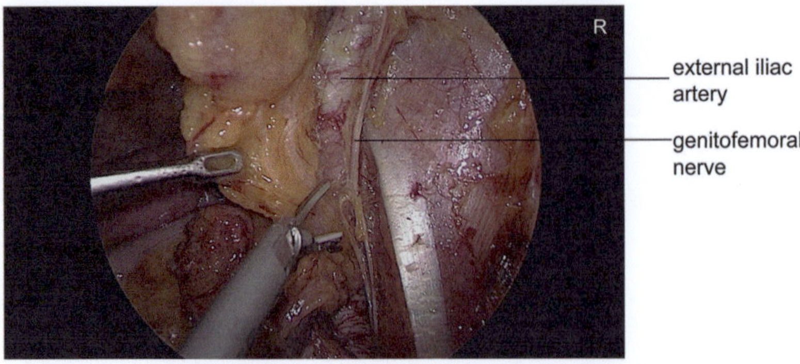

Fig. 2.4 Genitofemoral nerve

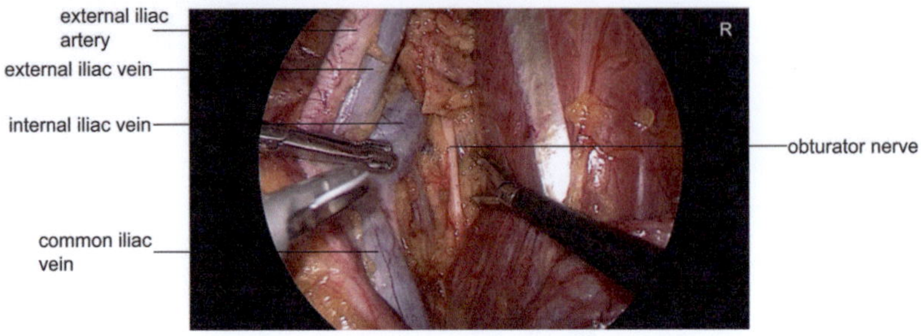

Fig. 2.5 Obturator nerve

anterior rami. It passes through the medial border of the psoas major muscle and posterior to the external iliac vessels, entering the lesser pelvis. It runs above the obturator vessels, through the obturator canal, and reaches the thigh. It innervates the adductor muscles of the thigh and provides sensory supply to the medial two-thirds of the thigh. Damage to this nerve results in paralysis of the adductor muscle group of the thigh, difficulty in crossing the legs, and weakness in thigh external rotation. Prompt repair and reconnection are necessary after nerve injury [6, 7].

Clinical Significance The obturator nerve is located within the obturator canal, and care should be taken to avoid injury during the excision of obturator lymph nodes. Clinical manifestations of obturator nerve injury include: (1) Loss of sensation in the lower one-third of the medial thigh and (2) paralysis and atrophy of the adductor muscles of the affected limb, resulting in weakness of adduction. Studies have shown that 70% of the obturator nerves have no function (Fig. 2.5) [8].

2.2.3 Accessory Obturator Nerve

Anatomy The incidence of the accessory obturator nerve is 3.44%, while some reports from foreign countries suggest a rate of 29%, and it is more commonly observed in high-level lumbar plexus. The accessory obturator nerve is relatively small and is mostly composed of the ventral branches of the third and fourth lumbar anterior divisions. In some cases, it may arise from the obturator nerve or the femoral nerve and occasionally from the fifth lumbar anterior division. It descends along the medial aspect of the psoas major muscle, adjacent to the obturator nerve, crosses over the pubic branch of the ischium, and divides into three branches within the deep surface of the adductor muscles. In extremely rare cases, the accessory obturator nerve may pass through vessels at the base of the obturator canal and then join the obturator nerve [9].

Clinical Significance Occasionally, the lumbosacral trunk is mistakenly identified as the accessory obturator nerve. The distinction between the obturator nerve, accessory obturator nerve, and lumbosacral trunk can be made based on the anatomical position relative to the iliolumbar vein. The obturator nerve and accessory obturator nerve are located on the ventral side of the iliolumbar vein, while the lumbosacral trunk is located on the dorsal side of the iliolumbar vein.

2.2.4 Lumbosacral Trunk

Anatomy The lumbosacral trunk is formed by the small portion of the anterior branch of the fourth lumbar nerve and the entire anterior branch of the fifth lumbar nerve. It is located posterior and medial to the psoas major muscle, close to the sacral wing. It passes behind the common iliac vessels and reaches the medial side of the obturator nerve, with the internal iliac vein separating the lumbosacral trunk from the obturator nerve [2].

Clinical Significance The lumbosacral trunk is an important anatomical structure that needs to be exposed during the removal of deep iliac lymph nodes. During electrocoagulation hemostasis in this area, attention is often given to protect the familiar obturator nerve, while the deeper lumbosacral trunk nerve may be easily overlooked. If the lumbosacral trunk is damaged, the symptoms can be more severe than obturator nerve injury. It mainly manifests as difficulty in walking, progressive limping, atrophy of the calf muscles, and inability to dorsiflex the toes (Fig. 2.6).

2.2.5 Hypogastric Nerves

Anatomy The upper part of the hypogastric plexus descends at the level of the sacral promontory or below the sacral promontory and divides into the left and right hypogastric nerve bundles, which are symmetrically located on both sides. The hypogastric nerves descend into the pelvic cavity through the extraperitoneal connective tissue and run along the medial side of the internal iliac artery and on both sides of the rectal ampulla. The branches of the hypogastric nerve bundles, along with the pelvic visceral nerves, form the pelvic plexus [2].

Clinical Significance The hypogastric nerve bundles are primarily sympathetic nerves that regulate urinary storage function. These nerve bundles travel on the posterior side of the ureteric mesentery and then run closely along the posterior side of the rectal mesentery. By opening the lateral space of the rectum (Goligher's plane), the hypogastric nerve bundles can be observed on the outer side of the uterosacral ligament, running beneath the ureter, and reaching the level of the uterine artery where they join the pelvic visceral nerves to form the pelvic plexus (Fig. 2.7) [10].

2.2.6 Pelvic Splanchnic Nerves

Anatomy The pelvic visceral nerves arise from the anterior branches of the S2–S4 sacral nerves through the anterior sacral foramina. The branches of the pelvic visceral nerves ascend

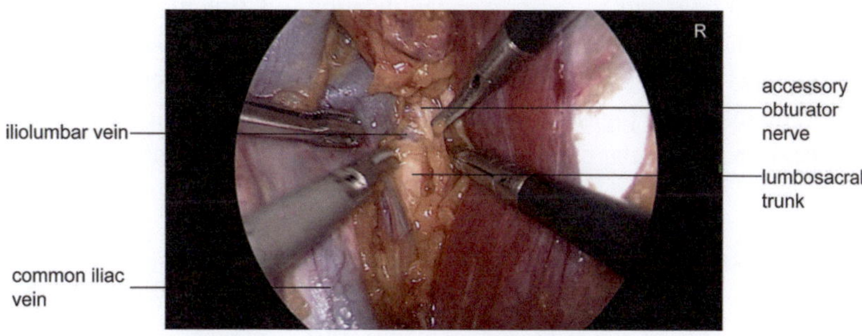

Fig. 2.6 Accessory obturator nerve, lumbosacral trunk

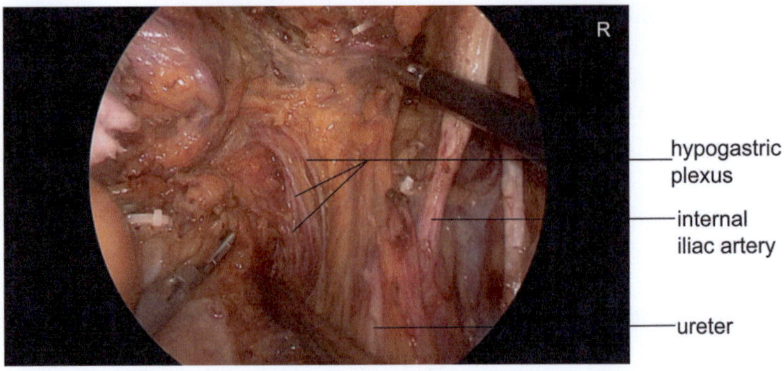

Fig. 2.7 Hypogastric plexus

within the lower hypogastric plexus and give off visceral motor fibers that supply the sigmoid colon, descending colon, splenic flexure, and distal transverse colon. Some studies have indicated that the branches of the pelvic visceral nerves, after emerging from the anterior sacral foramina, fan out through the presacral fascia and travel anteriorly between the pelvic cavity and the pelvic wall fascia. They then pass through the fascial layers of the pelvic cavity wall and proceed in a lateral and anterior direction, where they join the hypogastric nerves to form the pelvic plexus. The length of this course is approximately 25–30 mm, with its initial segment located outside the internal iliac vessels and its middle to distal segment running along the medial side of the internal iliac vessels [11].

Clinical Significance The pelvic splanchnic nerve plexus is located posterior to the deep uterine veins. During QM-C1 type surgeries, it is necessary to preserve this nerve plexus, which requires careful handling of the deep uterine veins to avoid bleeding that may interfere with the surgical field and hinder nerve identification. It is important to exercise caution when operating in this area and when dissecting blood vessels, avoiding the use of high-energy instruments. The application of vascular clamps is recommended.

2.2.7 Inferior Hypogastric Plexus

Anatomy Also known as the pelvic plexus (PP), this plexus is a large and dense autonomic nerve network located in the extraperitoneal connective tissue. In females, the pelvic plexus is situated lateral to the rectum, cervix, and vaginal vault, posterior to the bladder, and extends into the base of the broad ligament of the uterus. Its lateral aspect is bordered by the internal iliac vessels and their branches, the levator ani muscle, coccygeus muscle, and the internal sphincter ani. Posteriorly, it is adjacent to the sacral plexus, and anteriorly and superiorly, it is related to the superior vesical arteries and obliterated umbilical arteries. Due to the passage of pelvic venous branches through the pelvic plexus to reach pelvic organs, the fiber density of the plexus varies, forming an irregular mesh-like structure. Nerve fibers originating from this plexus, accompanying the branches of the internal iliac artery and vein, form secondary nerve plexuses, giving rise to the ureteral plexus, uterovaginal plexus, vesical plexus, and rectal plexus. These plexuses supply the ureters, uterine body, uterine cervix, vagina, clitoris, bladder, and rectum, directly or indirectly regulating the functions of these organs [12].

Clinical Significance The pelvic plexus (Figs. 2.8 and 2.9) is formed by the convergence of the inferior hypogastric plexus and the visceral nerves within the pelvic cavity, creating a "cross-shaped" nerve plexus (Fig. 2.10) located laterally to the extraperitoneal portion of the vaginal cuff complex. The pathways of the vesical and rectal plexuses closely related to QM-C1 type radical hysterectomy are as follows: (1) the vesical plexus is situated on both sides of the bladder, originating from the pelvic plexus and receiving parasympathetic nerve fibers from S3 and S4.

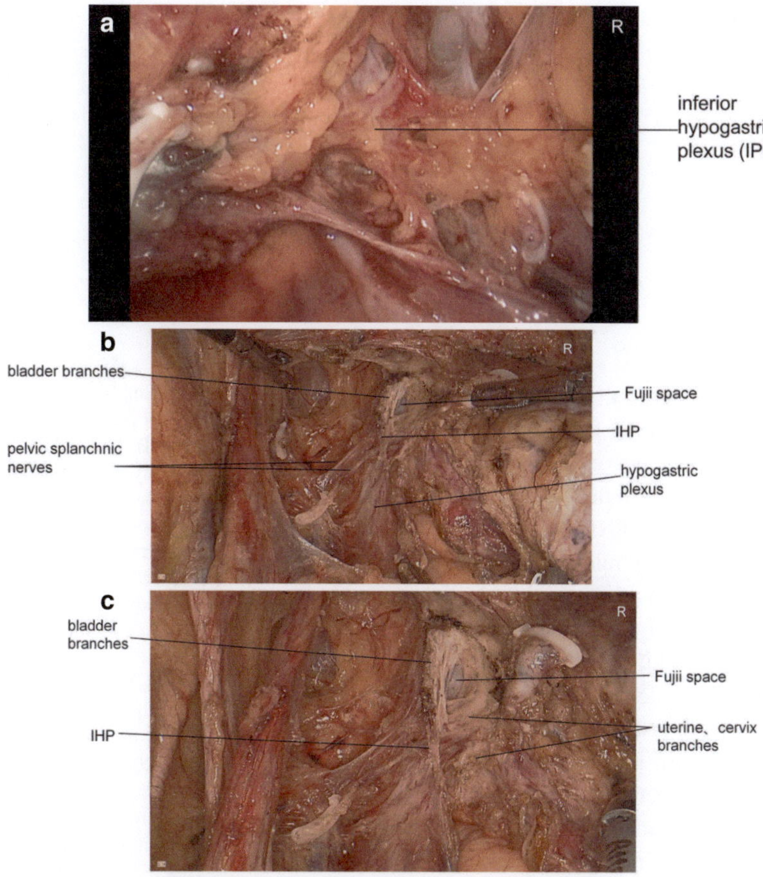

Fig. 2.8 (**a**–**c**) Inferior hypogastric plexus (IPH)

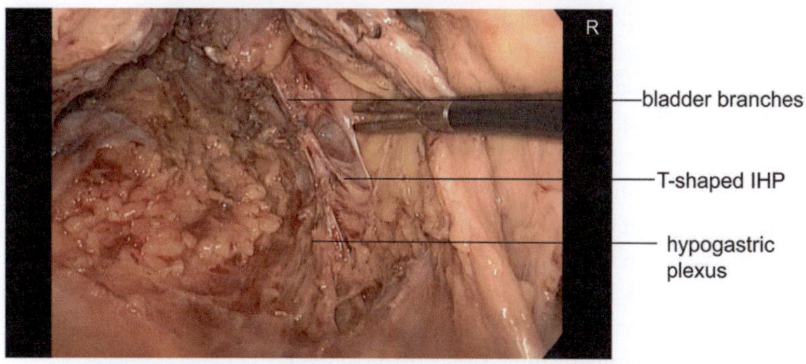

Fig. 2.9 Pelvic splanchnic nerves

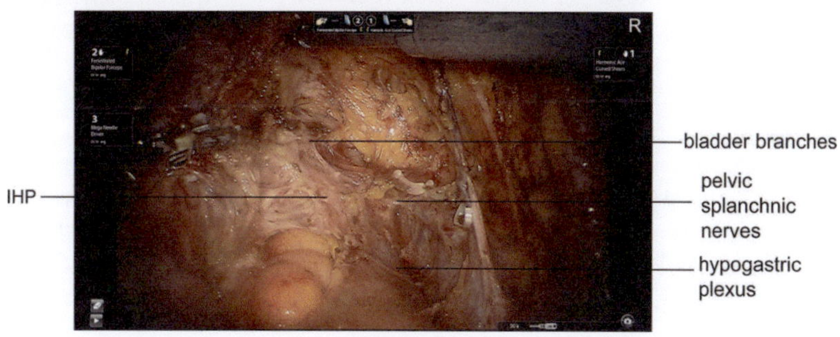

Fig. 2.10 "Cross-shaped" nerve plexus

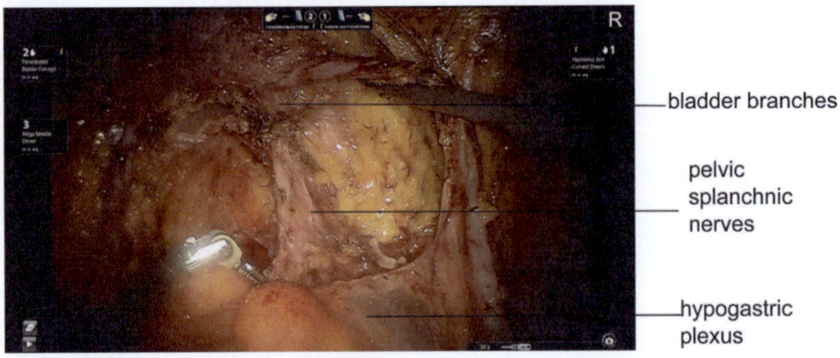

Fig. 2.11 "T-shaped" configuration

The bladder wall and internal sphincter receive dual innervation from the sympathetic and parasympathetic nerves. Parasympathetic fibers cause impulses that induce contraction of the detrusor muscle and relaxation of the urethral sphincter, controlling the micturition function. Sympathetic fibers have a primary role in maintaining bladder fullness and increasing the muscle tone of the internal sphincter, thus inhibiting urination. (2) The rectal plexus arises from the upper part of the pelvic plexus, follows the inferior rectal artery to the rectum, and connects with fibers from the superior rectal plexus. These fibers distribute downward to the internal anal sphincter. The innervation of the rectum and anal canal is derived from the superior rectal plexus, inferior rectal plexus, and pudendal nerve. Sympathetic fibers cause relaxation of the rectum and contraction of the internal anal sphincter, while parasympathetic fibers cause contraction of the rectum and relaxation of the internal anal sphincter. Surgery involving the preservation of the pelvic autonomic nerves requires identification of the visceral nerves within the pelvic cavity, including the uterine and bladder branches. The uterine branches are divided while preserving the bladder branches, transforming the "cross-shaped" configuration into a "T-shaped" configuration (Fig. 2.11) [13].

References

1. Alkatout I, Wedel T, Pape J, et al. Review: pelvic nerves–from anatomy and physiology to clinical applications. Transl Neurosci. 2021;12:362–78.
2. Standring S. Gray's anatomy, the anatomical basis of clinical practice. 41st ed. New York: Elsevier; 2016.
3. Kutlu B, Guner MA, Akyol C, et al. Comprehensive anatomy of the superior hypogastric plexus and its relationship with pelvic surgery landmarks: defining the safe zone around the promontory. Tech Coloproctol. 2022;26:655–64.
4. Baader B, Herrmann M. Topography of the pelvic autonomic nervous system and its potential impact on surgical intervention in the pelvis. Clin Anat. 2003;16:119–30.
5. Rab M, Ebmer And J, Dellon AL. Anatomic variability of the ilioinguinal and genitofemoral nerve: implications for the treatment of groin pain. Plast Reconstr Surg. 2001;108:1618–23.
6. La RA, Sayegh AS, Perez LC, et al. Obturator nerve injury in robotic pelvic surgery: scenarios and management strategies. Eur Urol. 2023;83:361–8.
7. Tipton JS. Obturator neuropathy. Curr Rev Musculoskelet Med. 2008;1:234–7.
8. Andan C, Bakır MS, Şen S, et al. Concurrent primary repair of obturator nerve transection during pelvic lymphadenectomy procedure via laparoscopical approach. Int J Surg Case Rep. 2018;53:394–6.
9. Archana BJ, Nagaraj DN, Pradeep P, et al. Anatomical variations of accessory obturator nerve: a cadaveric study with proposed clinical implications. Int J Anat Res. 2016;4(2):2158–61.
10. Seracchioli R, Mabrouk M, Mastronardi M, et al. Anatomic cartography of the hypogastric nerves and surgical insights for autonomic preservation during radical pelvic procedures. J Minim Invasive Gynecol. 2019;26:1340–5.
11. Shoja MM, Sharma A, Mirzayan N, et al. Neuroanatomy of the female abdominopelvic region: a review with application to pelvic pain syndromes. Clin Anat. 2013;26:66–76.
12. Moawad GN, Wu C, Klebanoff JS, et al. Pelvic neuroanatomy: an overview of commonly encountered pelvic nerves in gynecologic surgery. J Minim Invasive Gynecol. 2021;28:178.
13. Fujii S, Sekiyama K. Precise neurovascular anatomy for radical hysterectomy. 1st ed. Singapore: Springer Nature; 2020.

3 Lymphatic Anatomy

Jun Wang and Junling Lu

3.1 Lymph Nodes in the Abdominal Aortic Region

3.1.1 Lymph Nodes on the Lateral Side of the Abdominal Aorta

Anatomy The lymph nodes along the left side of the abdominal aorta are arranged from the diaphragmatic aortic hiatus superiorly to the continuation with the left common iliac lymph nodes inferiorly at the termination of the abdominal aorta. These lymph nodes primarily collect lymphatic fluid from the para-aortic region, uterus, ovaries, fallopian tubes, and other organs in the abdomen. The efferent lymphatic vessels from the lymph nodes located on the outer side of the aorta form the left lumbar lymph trunk (Figs. 3.1 and 3.2) [1, 2].

3.1.2 Pre-aortic Lymph Nodes

Anatomy Located anterior to the abdominal aorta, these lymph nodes primarily gather lymphatic fluid from the gastrointestinal organs, pancreas, liver, spleen, and mesentery. The efferent lymphatic vessels of the pre-aortic lymph nodes drain into the lateral side of the abdominal aorta lymph nodes and the lymph nodes between the abdominal aorta and the inferior vena cava (Fig. 3.3) [1].

3.1.3 Retro-aortic Lymph Nodes

Anatomy Located behind the abdominal aorta, in front of the first to fourth lumbar vertebrae, it primarily collects lymphatic fluid from the deep abdominal wall and lymphatic fluid output from the lateral side of the aorta.

3.1.4 Lymph Nodes Between the Aorta and the Vena Cava

Anatomy Located between the abdominal aorta and the inferior vena cava, typically below the level of the renal artery origin. It primarily collects lymphatic fluid from organs such as the uterus, ovaries, fallopian tubes, and right kidney (Fig. 3.4).

3.1.5 Para-caval Lymph Nodes

Anatomy Para-caval lymph nodes are arranged in a chain along the right side of the inferior vena cava. They extend superiorly to the diaphragm and inferiorly to the origin of the inferior vena cava. They primarily collect lymphatic fluid from

J. Wang (✉) · J. Lu
Department of Gynecology and Obstetrics, Second Affiliated Hospital of Dalian Medical University, Dalian, China

S. Han, J. Wang (eds.), *Open, Laparoscopic, and Robotic Surgery for Cervical Cancer*,
https://doi.org/10.1007/978-981-97-7687-0_3

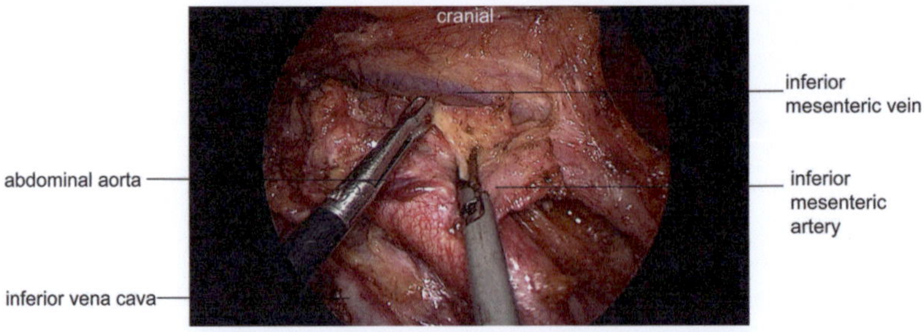

Fig. 3.1 Lymph nodes on the lateral side of the abdominal aorta

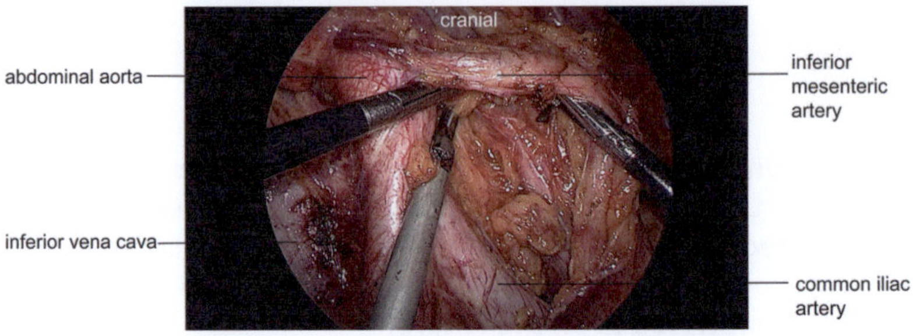

Fig. 3.2 Lymph nodes on the lateral side of the abdominal aorta

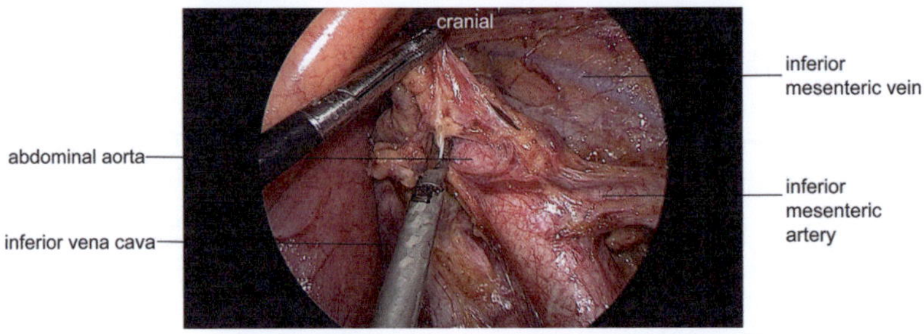

Fig. 3.3 Pre-aortic lymph nodes

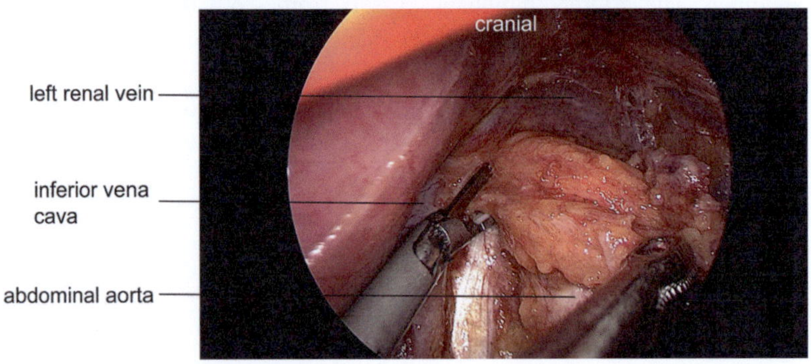

Fig. 3.4 Lymph nodes between the aorta and the vena cava

the right common iliac lymph nodes as well as lymphatic fluid from the uterus, ovaries, and fallopian tubes. The efferent lymphatic vessels of the para-caval lymph nodes drain into the retrocaval lymph nodes or directly into the right lumbar trunk.

3.1.6 Pre-caval Lymph Nodes

Anatomy The pre-caval lymph nodes are located anterior to the inferior vena cava, below the origin of the right renal artery. They primarily collect lymphatic fluid from the right kidney and ovaries, as well as the output lymph from the iliac lymph nodes. The efferent lymphatic vessels of the pre-caval lymph nodes drain into the intercaval lymph nodes and the para-caval lymph nodes (see Figs. 3.5 and 3.6).

3.1.7 Retrocaval Lymph Nodes

Anatomy Located behind the inferior vena cava, extending from the level of the right renal vein to the bifurcation of the abdominal aorta, the retrocaval lymph nodes primarily collect lymphatic fluid from the right kidney and ovaries. Their efferent lymphatic vessels form the right lumbar lymphatic trunk.

Clinical Significance In cervical cancer surgery, when pelvic lymph nodes are positive and lymph node staging surgery is required for patients with stage IIB to IV, lymph nodes in the region of the abdominal aorta need to be removed. However, unlike ovarian and endometrial cancer, usually only the lower abdominal aortic lymph nodes need to be excised [3, 4]. The lymph nodes in the abdominal aortic region can be divided into seven groups [5]. In the absence of specific indications from preoperative imaging examinations, typically only lymph nodes on the surface of the inferior vena cava, between the inferior vena cava and abdominal aorta, in front of the abdominal aorta, and on the left side of the abdominal aorta are removed. Among them, the removal of lymph nodes on the left side of the abdominal aorta and the proximal side of the mesenteric artery is the most challenging. This region has a relatively high rate of lymph node metastasis. In order to better expose and completely remove lymph nodes in this region, the lateral peritoneum is pulled toward the abdomen and outward. The junction between the descending mesocolon and the lymph nodes becomes visible. Sharp dissection is performed at the junction to reveal the gap between them. Continued dissection along the gap toward the dorsal side gradually exposes the gap between the lymph nodes and the renal fat, revealing the inferior mesenteric vein, left ovarian vein, and left ureter in the process.

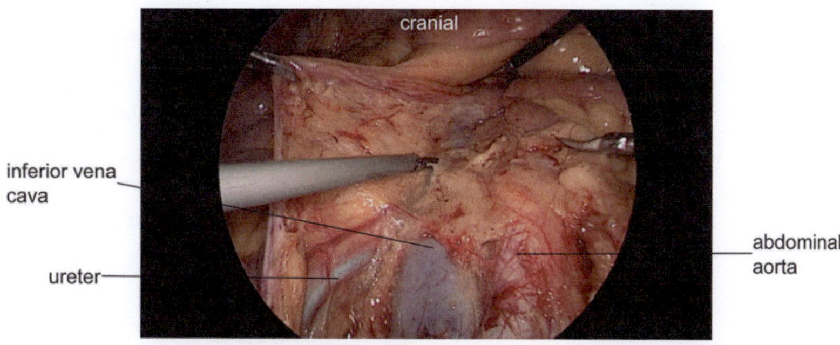

Fig. 3.5 Pre-caval lymph nodes

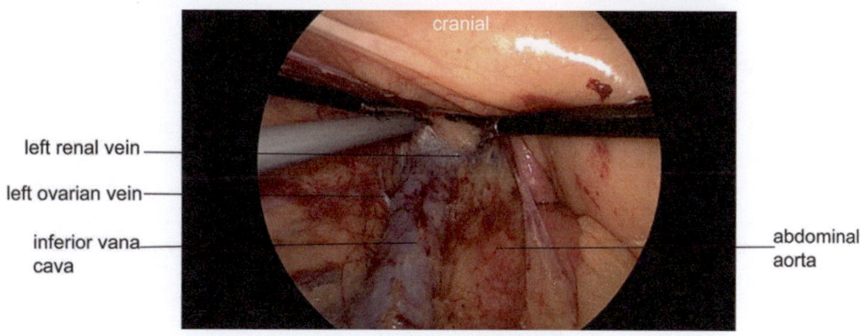

Fig. 3.6 Pre-caval lymph nodes

3.2 Pelvic Lymph Nodes

3.2.1 Common Iliac Lymph Nodes

Anatomy The iliac lymph nodes are located around the common iliac vessels and receive lymphatic drainage from the external iliac, internal iliac, and presacral lymph nodes. They collect lymphatic fluid from the lower limbs, perineum, external genitalia, and pelvic organs [6, 7].

The Medial Lymph Nodes Located on the medial side of the common iliac artery or anterior to the common iliac vein (Fig. 3.7).

The Lateral Lymph Nodes On the left side, they are located between the left common iliac artery and the psoas major muscle, while on the right side, they are situated on the outer side of the right common iliac artery and anterior to the right common iliac vein (Figs. 3.8 and 3.9).

Deep Common Iliac Lymph Node Located on the posterior side of the common iliac artery and vein, and medial to the iliolumbar muscle.

Clinical Significance One of the pathways of pelvic lymph node drainage is the lymphatic vessels crossing over the internal iliac artery, traversing the presacral region, and continuing cranially to reach the posterior side of the bifurcation of the internal and external iliac veins, where the deep common iliac lymph node region is located [8]. Therefore, thorough excision of lymph nodes in this region is particularly important. The anatomy of this region is complex, and lymph node dissection must be performed with caution to avoid damage to important anatomical structures such as the sacral nerve, lumbosacral trunk, common iliac vein, and internal and external iliac veins (Fig. 3.10).

3.2.2 Presacral Lymph Node

Anatomy The presacral lymph nodes are located in front of the sacrum, typically arranged along the midline artery of the sacrum, without extending above the sacral promontory. They receive lymphatic drainage from the lower portion of the cervix, lower uterine body, upper vagina, rectal mucosa, and posterior pelvic wall, and drain into the inferior mesenteric lymph nodes. The efferent lymphatic vessels of the infe-

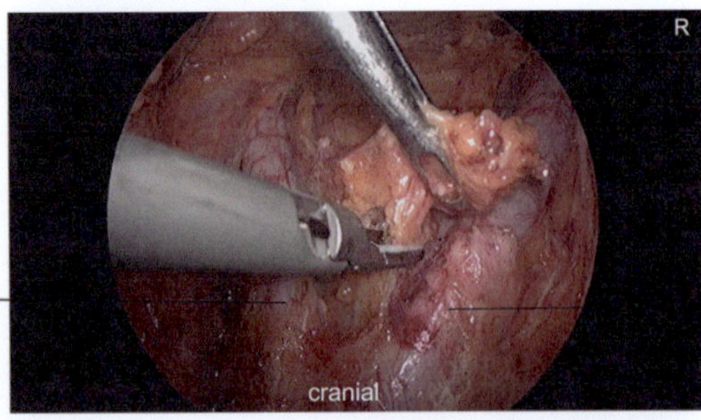

Fig. 3.7 The medial lymph nodes

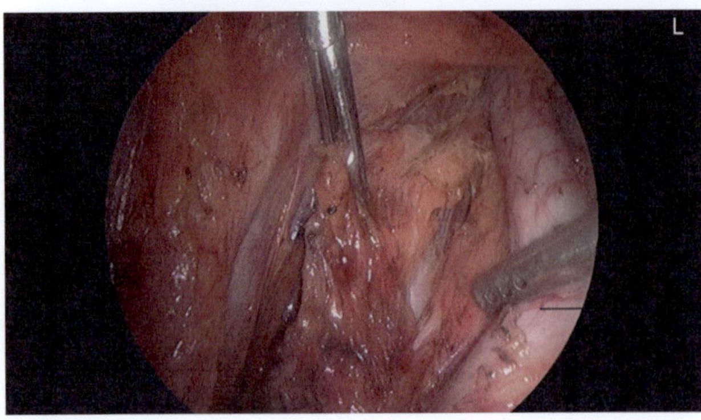

Fig. 3.8 The lateral lymph nodes (L)

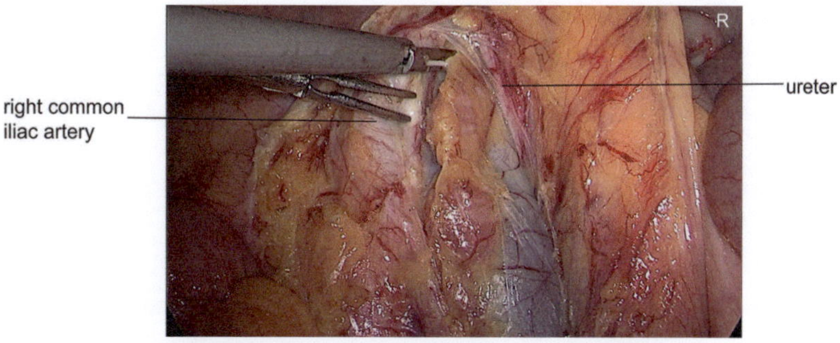

Fig. 3.9 The lateral lymph nodes (R)

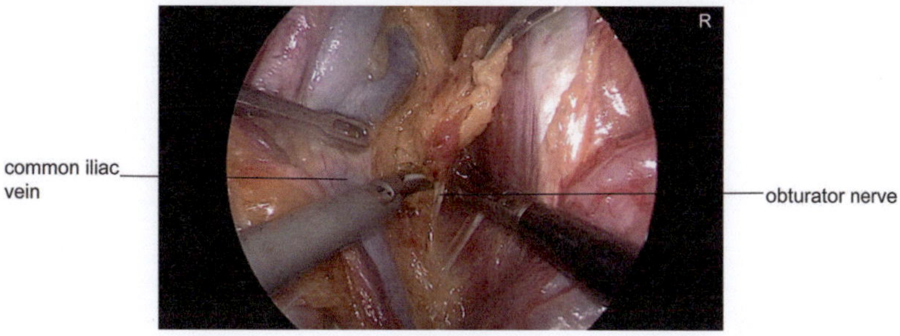

Fig. 3.10 Deep common iliac lymph node

rior mesenteric lymph nodes then either join the pre-aortic lymph nodes or the para-aortic lymph nodes.

Clinical Significance Some researchers consider the lymph nodes in the region between the left and right common iliac arteries as presacral lymph nodes, although strictly speaking, they should be classified as part of the lymph nodes in the region of the abdominal aorta [9]. If we adhere to this anatomical definition of presacral lymph nodes, they would not be involved in surgical procedures for cervical cancer (Fig. 3.11).

3.2.3 External Iliac Lymph Nodes

Anatomy The external iliac lymph nodes often comprise three subgroups, situated in the lateral, medial, and anterior regions of the iliac vessels. They drain lymph from the lower abdominal wall below the umbilicus, bladder, cervix, lower uterine body, and upper vagina, among other areas. Additionally, they receive the efferent lymphatic vessels from the superficial and deep inguinal lymph nodes (lymph from the lower limb, perineum, anus, and external genitalia). Their efferent lymphatic vessels converge into the common iliac lymph nodes [1, 7] (Fig. 3.12).

3.2.4 Internal Iliac Lymph Nodes

Anatomy Arranged along the internal iliac artery and its branches. Mainly collects lymph from pelvic organs, perineum, and buttock region. It consists of two groups: the gluteal group and the sacral group. The gluteal group of lymph nodes collects lymph from the rectum, deep perineal region, and gluteal region [10]. The sacral group of lymph nodes is distributed along the lateral side of the sacrum, close to the anterior aspect of the second and third sacral foramina, adjacent to the sacral plexus. It collects lymph from the rectum and cervix. This group includes the paracervical lymph nodes, located on both sides of the cervix near the crossing of the uterine artery and ureter, receiving lymphatic vessels from the cervix and lower uterine body, and draining into the common iliac lymph nodes [1].

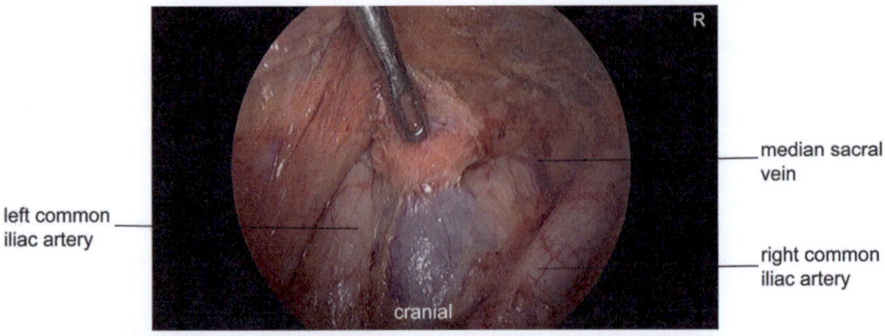

Fig. 3.11 Presacral lymph node

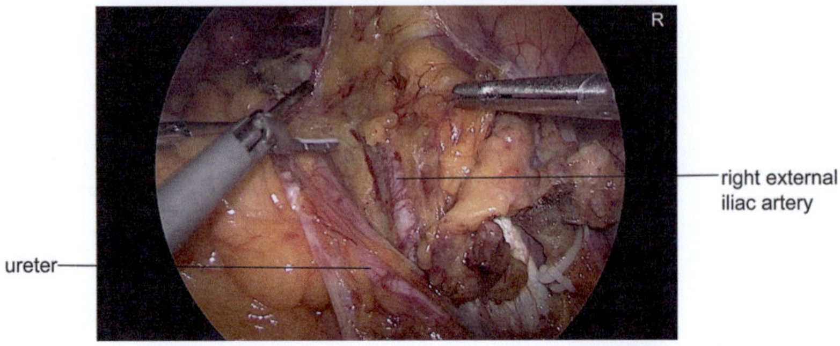

Fig. 3.12 External iliac lymph nodes

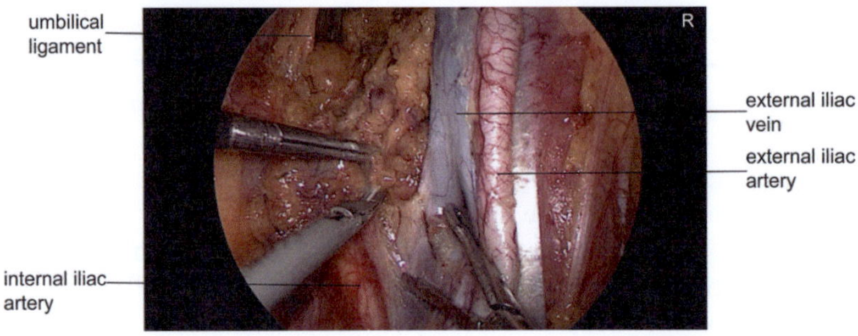

Fig. 3.13 Internal iliac lymph nodes

Clinical Significance Typically, the lymph nodes in the outer region of the internal iliac vessels are removed during pelvic lymphadenectomy. However, the lymph nodes in the inner region of the internal iliac vessels belong to the lower paracervical pathway of lymphatic drainage. In QM-C and QM-B2 surgeries, these lymph nodes may need to be completely or separately removed (Fig. 3.13) [11].

3.2.5 Obturator Lymph Node

Anatomy The obturator lymph nodes are distributed along the obturator artery and are often arranged around the obturator nerve. They primarily receive lymphatic drainage from the bladder, ureters, uterus, and vagina and drain into the internal and external iliac lymph nodes as well as the common iliac lymph nodes. They are the most common lymph nodes for metastasis in cervical cancer.

Clinical Significance The obturator lymph nodes are the most common lymph nodes for metastasis in cervical cancer and are also frequently identified as sentinel lymph nodes (SLNs) [12]. During the removal of these lymph nodes, it is important to preserve the integrity of the obturator nerve (Fig. 3.14).

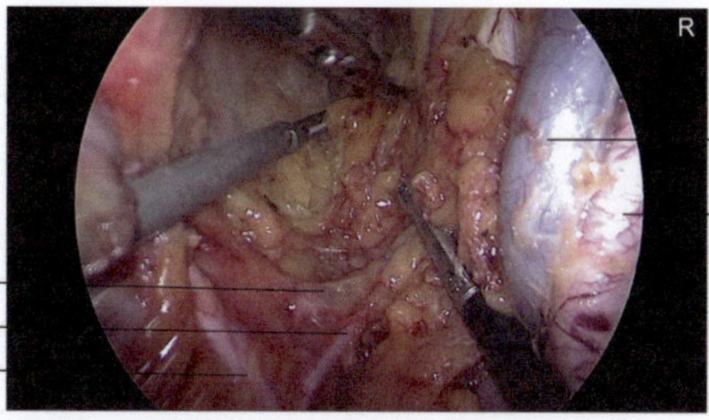

Fig. 3.14 Obturator lymph node

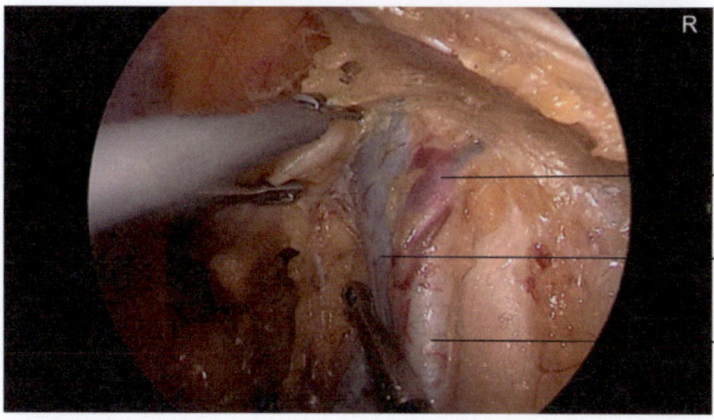

Fig. 3.15 Deep inguinal lymph nodes

3.2.6 Deep Inguinal Lymph Nodes

Anatomy Located within the femoral canal and medial to the femoral vein, the deep inguinal lymph nodes receive lymphatic drainage from the uterine corpus. They are connected to the superficial inguinal lymph nodes via the uterine round ligament and the inguinal lymph nodes. The efferent lymphatic vessels of the deep inguinal lymph nodes drain into the external iliac and obturator lymph nodes [6, 13].

Clinical Significance According to the anatomical definition provided here, the deep inguinal lymph nodes are not involved in cervical cancer surgery (Fig. 3.15).

References

1. Standring S. Gray's anatomy, the anatomical basis of clinical practice. 41st ed. New York: Elsevier; 2016.
2. Panici PB, Scambia G, Baiocchi G, et al. Anatomical study of para-aortic and pelvic lymph nodes in gynecologic malignancies. Obstet Gynecol. 1992;79:498–502.
3. Thelissen AAB, Jürgenliemk-Schulz IM, van der Leij F, et al. Upstaging by para-aortic lymph node dissection in patients with locally advanced cervical cancer: a systematic review and meta-analysis. Gynecol Oncol. 2022;164:667–74.
4. Sakuragi N, Satoh C, Takeda N, et al. Incidence and distribution pattern of pelvic and paraaortic lymph node metastasis in patients with stages IB, IIA, and IIB cervical carcinoma treated with radical hysterectomy. Cancer. 1999;85:1547–54.
5. Hu JL, Deng L, Tang YB, et al. Advances of robotic surgical system in gynecological para-aortic lymph node dissection. Chin J Robot Surg. 2021;2(05):335–41.
6. Mangan CE, Rubin SC, Rabin DS, et al. Lymph node nomenclature in gynecologic oncology. Gynecol Oncol. 1986;23:222–6.
7. Zlotta AR. Limited, extended, superextended, mega-extended pelvic lymph node dissection at the time of radical cystectomy: what should we perform? Eur Urol. 2012;61:243–4.
8. Cibula D, Abu-Rustum NR. Pelvic lymphadenectomy in cervical cancer-surgical anatomy and proposal for a new classification system. Gynecol Oncol. 2010;116:33–7.
9. Querleu D, Ferron G, Rafii A, et al. Pelvic lymph node dissection via a lateral extraperitoneal approach: description of a technique. Gynecol Oncol. 2008;109:81–5.

10. Henriksen E. The lymphatic spread of carcinoma of the cervix and of the body of the uterus; a study of 420 necropsies. Am J Obstet Gynecol. 1949;58:924–42.
11. Querleu D, Morrow CP. Classification of radical hysterectomy. Lancet Oncol. 2008;9:297–303.
12. Daraï E, Lavoué V, Rouzier R, et al. Contribution of the sentinel node procedure to tailoring the radicality of hysterectomy for cervical cancer. Gynecol Oncol. 2007;106:251–6.
13. Herrell SD, Trachtenberg J, Theodorescu D. Staging pelvic lymphadenectomy for localized carcinoma of the prostate: a comparison of 3 surgical techniques. J Urol. 1997;157:1337–9.

4 Anatomy of Space of Pelvic Sidewall

Jun Wang and Shichao Han

4.1 Lateral Retroperitoneal Space [1–3]

Clinical Significance The lateral retroperitoneal space offers an optimal and secure pathway for pelvic lymph node dissection, ureter exposure, handling the suspensory ligament of the ovary, as well as addressing lateral pelvic organ exposure and treatment. By medially pulling the suspensory ligament of the ovary and laterally and cranially manipulating the round ligament, the lateral retroperitoneal space becomes accessible between the external iliac artery and the psoas major muscle. Gradual sharp dissection of this space unveils the suspensory ligament and the ureter, enabling the safe transection of the suspensory ligament along the iliac vessel surface. Further dissection within this space toward the posterior and caudal direction gradually reveals the internal iliac artery and the lateral umbilical ligament, laying the groundwork for subsequent exposure and management of the obturator space and lateral parametrium (Fig. 4.1).

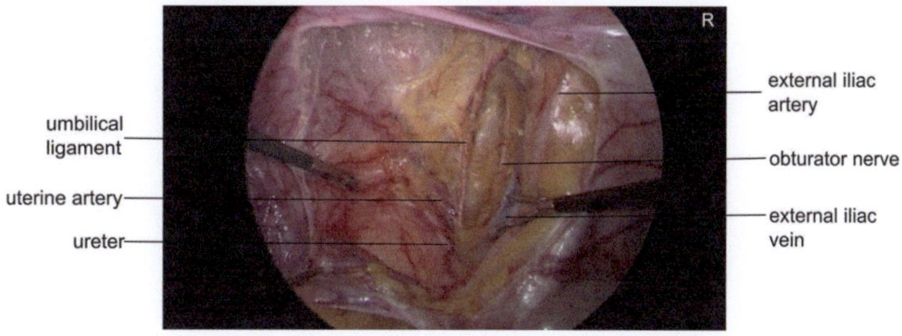

Fig. 4.1 Lateral retroperitoneal space

J. Wang (✉) · S. Han
Department of Gynecology and Obstetrics, Second Affiliated Hospital of Dalian Medical University, Dalian, China

S. Han, J. Wang (eds.), *Open, Laparoscopic, and Robotic Surgery for Cervical Cancer*,
https://doi.org/10.1007/978-981-97-7687-0_4

4.2 Iliopsoas and External Iliac Vessel Space [1–3]

Clinical Significance The establishment of this space is primarily for the exposure of the lymph nodes in the lateral region of the external iliac vessels and the deep lymph nodes of the common iliac vessels. By gradually exposing the common iliac vein, the internal iliac vein, and the iliolumbar vein, as well as important anatomical structures such as the pelvic segment of the obturator nerve, the accessory obturator nerve, and the lumbosacral trunk, after fully exposing these important anatomical structures, the deep lymph nodes of the common iliac vessels can be gradually freed toward the caudal direction. Finally, the lymph nodes in this region can be safely moved to the medial side of the bifurcation of the internal and external iliac veins, greatly reducing the risk of vascular and nerve injury associated with handling lymph nodes directly at the medial side of the bifurcation (Fig. 4.2).

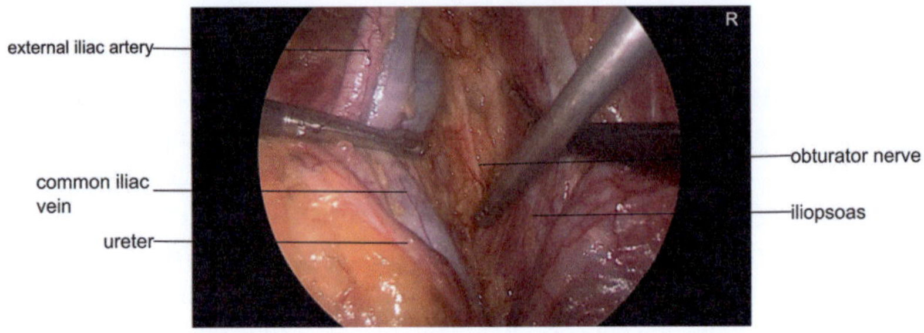

Fig. 4.2 Iliopsoas and external iliac vessel space

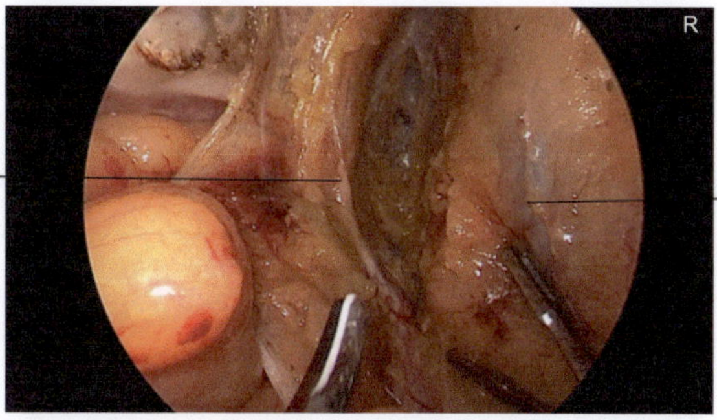

Fig. 4.3 Obturator space

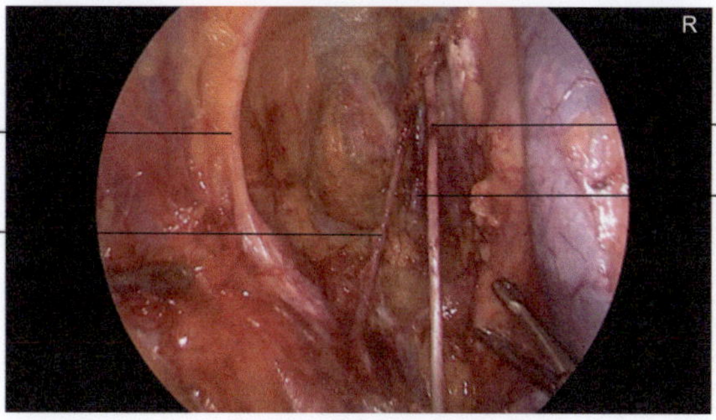

Fig. 4.4 Obturator space

4.3 Obturator Space [1–3]

Clinical Significance The obturator space is primarily used to expose the obturator nerve and obturator vessels and facilitate the removal of lymph nodes in this region. It helps to avoid unnecessary bleeding and nerve damage during lymph node dissection in the area. In clinical surgery, some surgeons prefer to perform a radical hysterectomy first, followed by pelvic lymph node dissection. The medial border of this space can be used to mobilize the internal iliac artery and the uterine artery. Subsequently, pulling the internal iliac artery and uterine artery laterally helps provide sufficient tension during the exposure of the lateral pelvic sidewall structures (Figs. 4.3 and 4.4).

References

1. NCCN. NCCN clinical practice guidelines in oncology—cervical cancer. (2022-12-23) [2023-03-15]. https://www.nccn.org/professionals/physician_gls/pdf/cervical.pdf
2. Querleu D, Cibula D, Abu-Rustum NR. Update on the Querleu-Morrow classification of radical hysterectomy. Ann Surg Oncol. 2017;2017(24):3406–12.
3. Querleu D, Morrow CP. Classification of radical hysterectomy. Lancet Oncol. 2008;9:297–303.

Anatomy of Spaces of Paracervix

5

Shichao Han, Jun Wang, and Jing Na

5.1 Ventral Parametrium [1–3]

5.1.1 Vesicocervical Space

Clinical Significance The exposure of this space is primarily important for the subsequent visualization of the vesicovaginal space. The vesicocervical space is typically easily identifiable. After opening the reflected peritoneum, the bladder is adequately pulled toward the ventral side, and the space is sharply dissected within the white, loose connective tissue. Occasionally, when there is severe adhesion of the bladder reflection, and the anatomical layers of this space are unclear, it is recommended to identify the lateral wall of the bladder and open this space from the lateral side toward the midline (Fig. 5.1).

5.1.2 Vesicovaginal Space

Clinical Significance The vesicovaginal space is an extension of the vesicocervical space. During extensive type C hysterectomy, it is important to dissect this space thoroughly. Deepening the space allows for the removal of an adequate length of vaginal wall, while widening the space on both sides facilitates better visualization of the paravaginal space. Adequate exposure of the paravaginal space is essential for safe management of the vesicocervical ligaments (Fig. 5.2).

5.1.3 Paravaginal Space

Clinical Significance The adequate and bloodless exposure of the paravaginal space is a key factor in performing bloodless dissection of the ureteral "tunnel." Our team has summarized the key points for managing this space, which include deep and wide dissection of the vesicovaginal space. Under direct visualization of the knee of the ureter, the bladder is pulled toward the abdominal and lateral sides. Using a sharp and precise technique with the ultrasonic scalpel, the surface tissues of the paravaginal space are carefully incised to gradually expose the space. Once inside the space, the posterior wall of the bladder is pulled toward the ventral side, and the space is expanded by sharp dissection, connecting it with the paravesical space. The tissue between the paravaginal space and the paravesical space is the vesicovaginal ligament. After the vesicovaginal ligament is dissected, the handling of the pelvic sidewall is completed (Figs. 5.3 and 5.4).

S. Han (✉) · J. Wang · J. Na
Department of Gynecology and Obstetrics, Second Affiliated Hospital of Dalian Medical University, Dalian, China

S. Han, J. Wang (eds.), *Open, Laparoscopic, and Robotic Surgery for Cervical Cancer*, https://doi.org/10.1007/978-981-97-7687-0_5

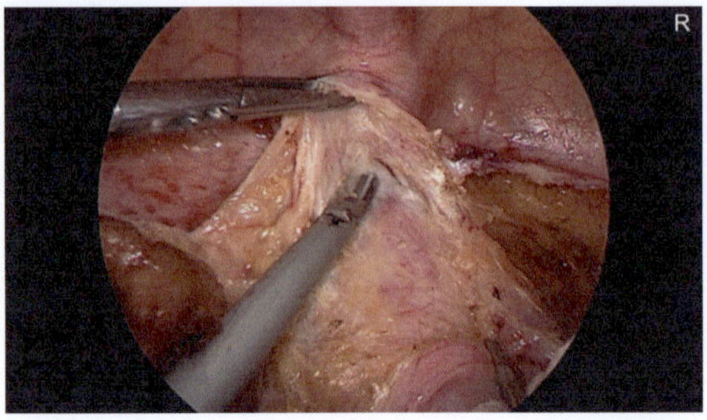

Fig. 5.1 Vesicocervical space

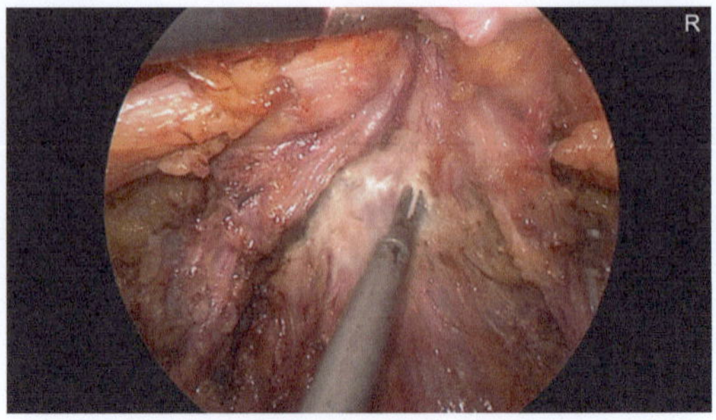

Fig. 5.2 Vesicovaginal space

Fig. 5.3 Paravaginal space

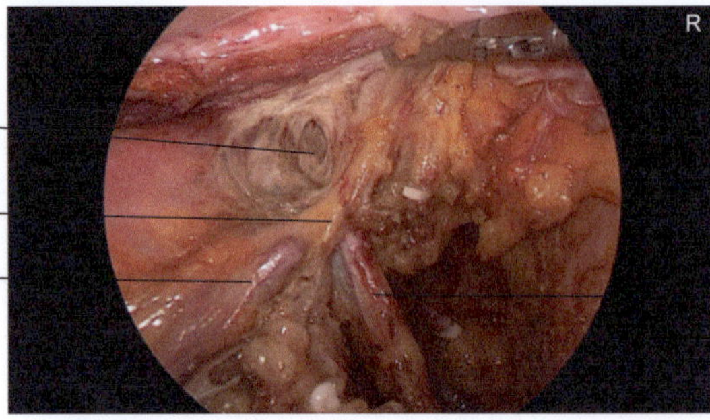

Fig. 5.4 Paravaginal space

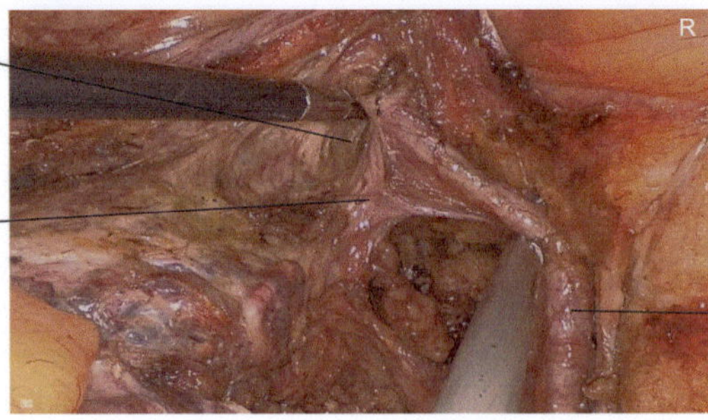

5.2 Lateral Parametrium [1–3]

5.2.1 Paravesical Space

Clinical Significance The paravesical space, situated laterally to the bladder and medial to the external iliac vessels, holds paramount importance in cervical cancer surgery. During surgical procedures for cervical cancer, the paravesical space serves as a critical pathway for accessing and dissecting lymph nodes, especially those located along the external iliac vessels. A precise understanding of the boundaries of the paravesical space allows for safer lymph node dissection without jeopardizing nearby vital structures. It enhances the surgeon's ability to perform accurate lymph node dissections, preserve critical nerves, and achieve successful oncological outcomes.

5.2.2 Pararectal Space

The pararectal space is covered by the peritoneum and contains the ureter below the peritoneum. The ureter, along with its mesentery, divides the pararectal space into the medial Okabayashi's pararectal space and the lateral Latzko's pararectal space.

Clinical Significance The tissue between the paravesical space (Fig. 5.5) and Latzko's lateral rectal space (Figs. 5.6, 5.7, and 5.8) represents the traditional lateral boundary of the cardinal ligament, which serves as the lateral boundary of the lateral parametrium according to the QM-C type requirements. In QM-C type surgery, the lateral parametrial tissue needs to be dissected closely adjacent to the internal iliac vessels, making thorough dissection of these two spaces particularly important. The inferior hypogastric nerve is located within the ureteric mesentery and

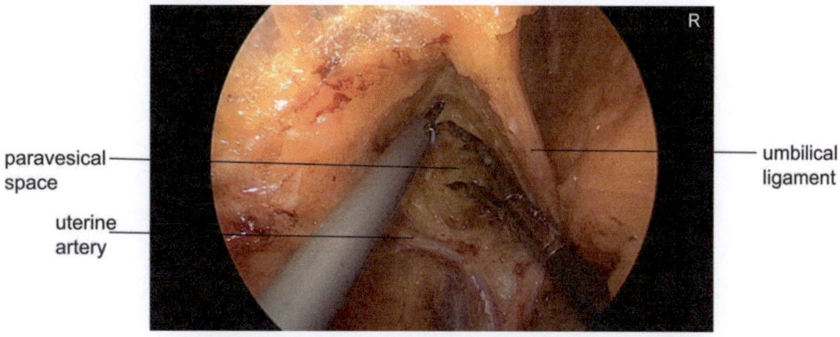

Fig. 5.5 Paravesical space

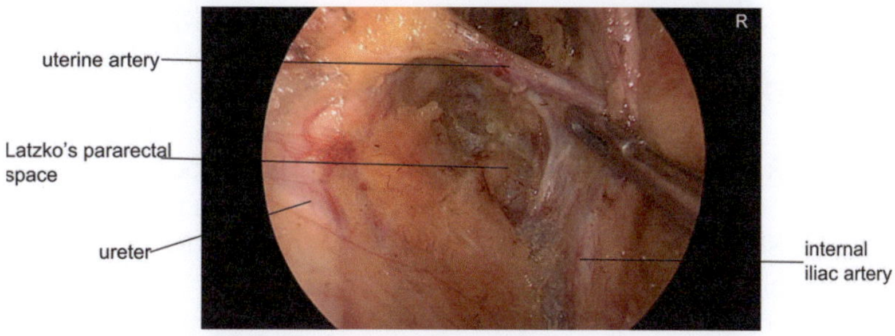

Fig. 5.6 Latzko's pararectal space

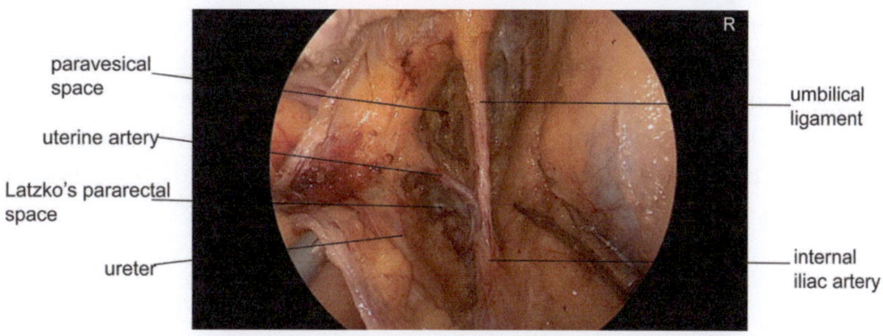

Fig. 5.7 Paravesical space, Latzko's pararectal space (**a**)

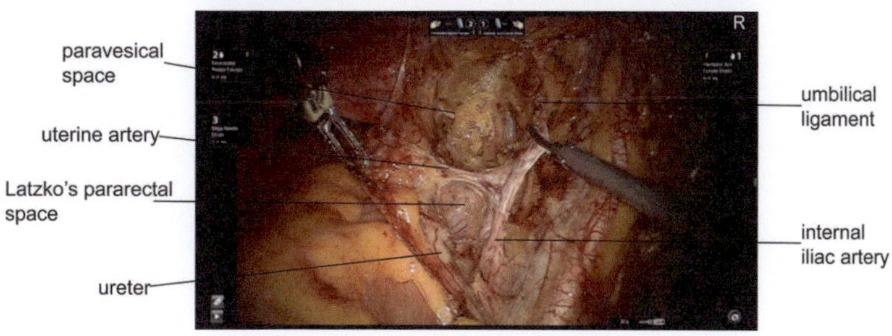

Fig. 5.8 Paravesical space, Latzko's pararectal space (**b**)

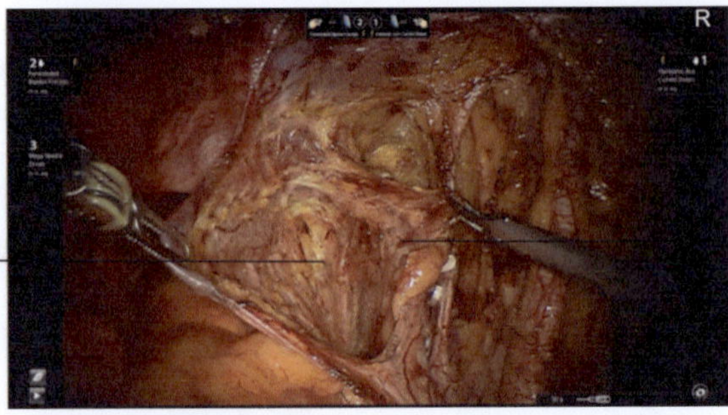

Fig. 5.9 Okabayashi's pararectal space

runs along the outer edge of the rectal mesentery. Adequate exposure of the Okabayashi's pararectal space facilitates identification and preservation of the inferior hypogastric nerve. The caudal boundary of the Okabayashi's pararectal space is formed by the paracolpium. Sufficient exposure of this boundary is beneficial for subsequent visualization and management of the dorsal parametrial uterosacral ligament (Fig. 5.9).

5.3 Dorsal Parametrium [1–3]

5.3.1 Rectovaginal Space

Clinical Significance The exposure and separation of this space can be performed under the guidance of the concept of membrane anatomy, as the exposure of this space involves separating the Müllerian duct primordium unit from the hindgut primordium unit. The exposure of this space requires opening the vaginorectal peritoneum at the "yellow-white" junction, which is actually the connection point between the Müllerian duct primordium unit and the hindgut primordium unit, known as the membrane bridge. After opening the membrane bridge, the vaginal wall is seen to be devoid of fat attachment, appearing white, while the rectum is surrounded by mesentery, appearing yellow. Applying counter-tension to the two embryonic compartments reveals a potential space between them, resembling a white filamentous structure. Separation within this structure allows for a safe and thorough separation of the rectovaginal space. The exposure of the rectovaginal space involves not only separating the space between the vagina and rectum but more importantly, separating the space between the rectal lateral wall mesentery and the inner edge of the uterosacral ligament. As the rectal lateral wall mesentery attaches to the middle segment of the uterosacral ligament, QM-C type surgery requires the excision of the posterior parametrium to the level of the rectum (C1 type) or the sacrum fascia (C2 type, D type). Thus, thorough mobilization of the rectal lateral wall mesentery from the inner segment of the uterosacral ligament is necessary to ensure the safe and adequate removal of the dorsal parametrial tissue (Fig. 5.10).

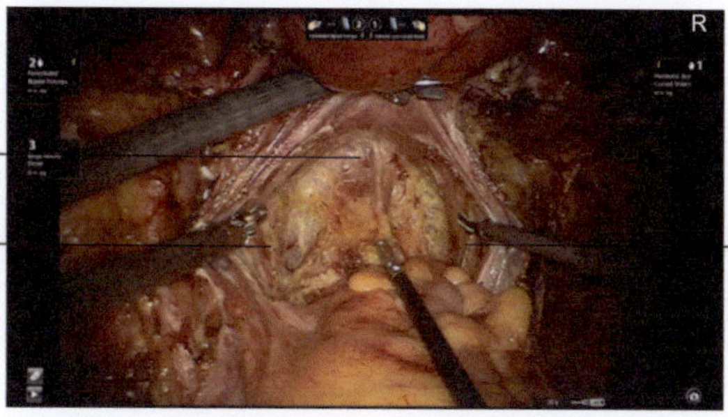

Fig. 5.10 Rectovaginal space

References

1. NCCN. NCCN clinical practice guidelines in oncology—cervical cancer. (2022-12-23) [2023-03-15]. https://www.nccn.org/professionals/physician_gls/pdf/cervical.pdf
2. Querleu D, Cibula D, Abu-Rustum NR. Update on the Querleu-Morrow classification of radical hysterectomy. Ann Surg Oncol. 2017;2017(24):3406–12.
3. Querleu D, Morrow CP. Classification of radical hysterectomy. Lancet Oncol. 2008;9:297–303.

6 Anatomy of Landmark Structures

Jing Na and Ya Li

6.1 Cisterna Chyli

Anatomy The cisterna chyli is an elongated sac-like dilation that is typically located anterior to the first or second lumbar vertebra, behind the right crus of the diaphragm and to the right of the abdominal aorta. It may also be situated at a higher vertebral level. Formed by the convergence of the left and right lumbar trunks and the intestinal trunk, the cisterna chyli is the main collecting vessel for lymph from the pelvis, abdomen, and lower limbs. It serves as the starting point of the thoracic duct [1].

Clinical Significance This anatomical structure is typically involved in lymph node dissection near the upper abdominal aorta. To avoid injury and subsequent chyle leakage, during surgical procedures, excessive dissection and exposure of this structure should be avoided when the left renal vein drains into the inferior vena cava. In cases of postoperative chyle leakage, supportive therapy is generally employed, including a low-fat, high-protein, high-calorie, and high-vitamin diet, along with maintaining unobstructed drainage. After diagnosis, the decision to perform further surgical treatment for chyle leakage is generally based on factors such as daily output, duration, tendency to decrease, and the overall condition of the patient. In cases where the chyle output exceeds 500 ml/day, fasting and total parenteral nutrition (TPN) are required, along with treatment using medium- and long-chain triglyceride emulsions and somatostatin. Surgical intervention is warranted if imaging indicates significant lymphatic vessel rupture and leakage [2].

6.2 Duodenum

Anatomy The duodenum is the initial part of the small intestine, measuring approximately 25 cm in length (equivalent to twelve fingerbreadths). It begins at the pylorus and terminates at the duodenojejunal flexure. Its overall shape resembles a "C," wrapping around the head of the pancreas. With the exception of its proximal and distal ends, most of the duodenum is located posterior to the peritoneum, closely adhering to the posterior abdominal wall between the first and third lumbar vertebrae. It can be divided into four parts: the superior part, descending part, horizontal part, and ascending part [1].

Clinical Significance During high-level para-aortic lymph node dissection, it is crucial to keep the duodenum away from the surgical field to avoid injury (Fig. 6.1).

J. Na (✉) · Y. Li
Department of Gynecology and Obstetrics, Second Affiliated Hospital of Dalian Medical University, Dalian, China

S. Han, J. Wang (eds.), *Open, Laparoscopic, and Robotic Surgery for Cervical Cancer*, https://doi.org/10.1007/978-981-97-7687-0_6

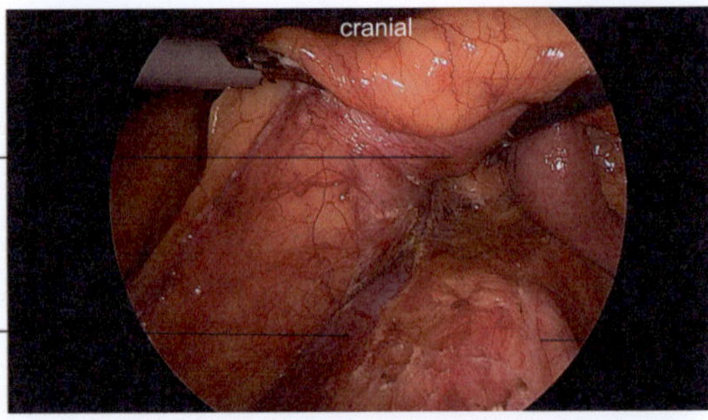

Fig. 6.1 Duodenum

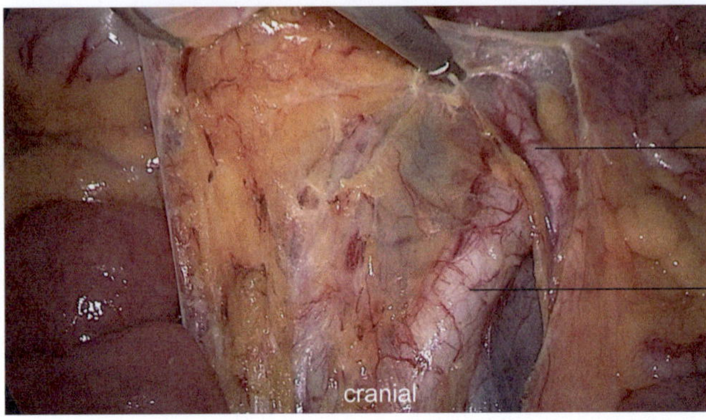

Fig. 6.2 Ureter

6.3 Ureter

Anatomy The ureter measures 25–30 cm in length. It originates from the funnel-shaped renal pelvis, descends anteriorly to the psoas major muscle in the abdominal region, passes medial to the genitofemoral nerve, and transitions into the pelvic part at the pelvic inlet. The pelvic part traverses anterior to the internal iliac vessels, the common iliac artery and vein, and the anterior aspect of the sacroiliac joint. It then continues posteriorly, passing the origin of the umbilical artery and the vessel and nerve of the perineal body, and curves anteriorly and medially to enter the bladder base. The ureter crosses the base of the broad ligament of the uterus about 2 cm lateral to the cervix and is crossed anteriorly by the uterine artery [1].

Clinical Significance The two most vulnerable sites for ureteral injury are the crossing over the iliac vessels and the "tunnel" region of the ureter. By utilizing the retroperitoneal space behind the broad ligament, the crossing over the iliac vessels can be safely exposed. Opening up the paravaginal space allows for sufficient external displacement of the ureter, facilitating the safe manipulation of the vesicocervical ligaments and preventing ureteral injury (Figs. 6.2, 6.3, and 6.4).

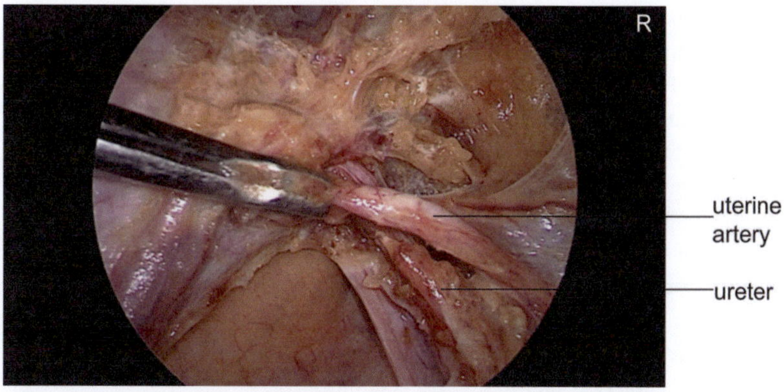

Fig. 6.3 Ureter

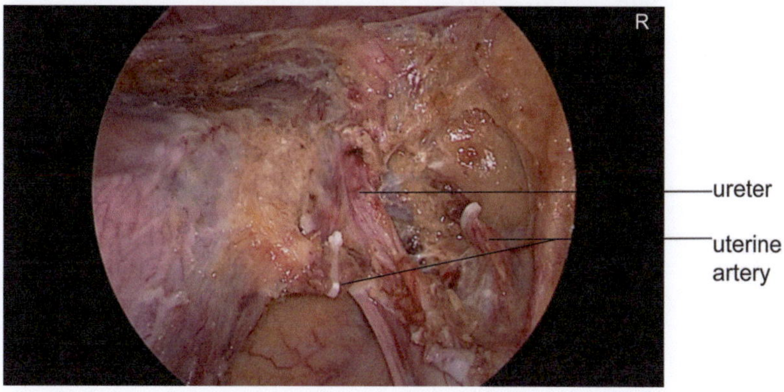

Fig. 6.4 Ureter

6.4 Paracolpium

Anatomy As described in "TE LINDE'S Operative Gynecology," the paracolpium is a connective tissue system extending from the cardinal ligaments above to the levator ani muscle of the pelvic floor below. Positioned along the sides of the vagina, it forms ligaments that connect the vagina to the pelvic sidewalls. It includes tissues from the anterior, posterior, and lateral aspects and serves as an essential support structure for the pelvic floor [3]. According to "New Theroy and Technique for Nerve-Sparing Radical Hysterectomy" authored by Professor Yoshihiko Yabuki from Japan, the term "paracolpium" (paracolpos in Greek) was coined based on Fothergill's (1907) naming convention. It encompasses tissues from the anterior, posterior, and lateral aspects [4, 5].

Clinical Significance Through our surgical experience, our team has determined that the paracolpium's ventral aspect corresponds to a segment of the vesicovaginal ligament, its dorsal aspect corresponds to a portion of the posterior parametrium (including the sacrocardinal ligament and hypogastric nerves), and its lateral aspect corresponds to a portion of the lateral parametrial tissue (including deep uterine veins and adjacent pelvic splanchnic nerves). As a result, the paracolpium can be understood as a composite structure composed of tissues from three different directions. This complex structure can be visualized as a three-dimensional framework centered around the paracolpium and plays a particularly pivotal role in QM-C1 type radical hysterectomy. The hypogastric nerves run along the lateral aspect of the dorsal parametrium, while the pelvic splanchnic nerves traverse through the dorsal part of the lateral parametrial tissue. Consequently, at the point of convergence between the dorsal parametrium and the lateral parametrial tissue, a "crossed intersection" pelvic plexus is formed. Moreover, the composite structure also encompasses the vesicovaginal ligament on its ventral side. In a C1-type surgery, the dissection of the vesicovaginal ligament within the ventral parametrium and the deep uterine veins within the lateral parametrial tissue is conducted as a unified process, followed by lateral elevation. This approach facilitates the separation of the vascular and neural layers within this composite structure, thereby exposing the "crossed intersection" pelvic plexus.

References

1. Standring S. Gray's anatomy, the anatomical basis of clinical practice. 41st ed. New York: Elsevier; 2016.
2. Putu S, Prihastuti R. Diagnosis and management of chylous ascites. Indones J Gastroenterol Hepatol Dig Endosc. 2023;24(1):63–71.
3. John AR, Howard WJ. Te Linde's operative gynecology. 8th ed. Philadelphia: Lippincott Williams & Wilkins; 2003.
4. Yabuki Y. New theory and technique for nerve-sparing radical hysterectomy. 1st ed. Tokyo: Medical View; 2009.
5. Fujii S. Precise neurovascular anatomy for radical hysterectomy. 1st ed. Singapore: Springer; 2020.

7 Re-recognition of Membrane Theory of Ontogenetic Anatomy

Shichao Han and Jun Wang

Based on developmental anatomy, the "compartment" theory emphasizes that the spread of tumor cells is not random and directionless. Instead, tumor cells reside for an extended period within the same embryonic origin (primordial) compartment, also referred to as a morphogenetic compartment, within the tissue. Due to the inhibitory effect of boundaries, tumor cells find it challenging to cross the boundaries of the "compartment" [1]. Then, German gynecologist Dr. Höckel pioneered the complete mesometrial resection (TMMR) for cervical cancer. This procedure involves thorough removal of the entire uterus and proximal vaginal, following the principles of the "Müllerian embryological" origin, with a strong emphasis on achieving complete tissue boundary resection in surgical specimens. This approach differs from the traditional anatomical approach, which primarily focuses on morphological structures [2–4]. Due to the development process in the human embryo, such as the "Müllerian embryonic" development, mesenchyme originating from the lateral mesoderm forms membranes surrounding each "embryonic origin," eventually creating "membrane planes" and "intermembrane spaces." As a result, precise surgical techniques for identifying and dissecting the membrane planes and intermembrane spaces between different embryonic origins have emerged [5]. Membrane anatomy surgery offers a more precise and comprehensive understanding compared to previous approaches such as "space anatomy" or "plane-based structure anatomy." It emphasizes the significance of anatomical landmarks and features, enabling gynecologists to navigate various surgical membrane planes with enhanced precision and accuracy.

Since we are discussing membrane anatomy surgery, it's essential to delve into the terminology related to membrane anatomy. Many terms related to spaces, ligaments, and tissue have been mentioned in the previous text. Here, we will primarily explore how our team, in the practice of membrane anatomy surgery, reinterprets the terminology, structures, and significance of membrane anatomy. We will also discuss how the concept of membrane anatomy can lead to a new understanding of the overall three-dimensional structure when performing QM-C type surgeries.

7.1 Membrane Anatomy Terminology: Membrane Bridge, Primordial Compartment

7.1.1 Membrane Bridges

Gong Jianping [6], in his work "Surgical Membrane Anatomy—A New Basis for Surgery," defines membrane bridges as structures located

S. Han (✉) · J. Wang
Department of Gynecology and Obstetrics, Second Affiliated Hospital of Dalian Medical University, Dalian, China

S. Han, J. Wang (eds.), *Open, Laparoscopic, and Robotic Surgery for Cervical Cancer*,
https://doi.org/10.1007/978-981-97-7687-0_7

between the fascia of various organs. Opening these connections (membrane bridges) allows access to sacred planes resembling angel hair. Coffey [7], on the other hand, considers the peritoneal fold as mesenteric bridges between the parietal and visceral peritoneum.

I would like to express sincere gratitude to these two medical pioneers for their work in the field of membrane anatomy theory and surgical practice. Their contributions have greatly facilitated our application of membrane anatomy concepts in gynecological surgery. However, due to the embryological origin of the female reproductive organs in the pelvic region being distinct from other surgical areas, especially in cases of cervical cancer where the surgical scope often extends beyond the pelvic peritoneum, our team believes that this concept can be further extended to gynecological membrane anatomy surgery. Descriptions regarding "membrane bridges" or "mesenteric bridges" primarily reflect the interconnectedness between embryonic compartments within the peritoneum. For instance, in cases involving the bladder peritoneal reflection, which connects the uterine serosa with the bladder serosa, dissecting the "membrane bridge" between these two structures allows for the separation of two embryonic compartments. Similarly, when exposing the dorsal parametrial sacrouterine ligament, our team typically begins with a lateral approach. We first dissect the "membrane bridge" between the rectal mesentery and the posterior peritoneum, enabling direct access to the space between the rectal mesentery and the sacrouterine ligament. This highlights the significance of the "membrane bridge" in guiding our surgical approach. However, during cervical cancer surgery, numerous anatomical structures are situated outside the peritoneum, and the interconnections between various primordial compartments remain concealed within the abdominal cavity. These encompass the interrelations involving the bladder and the cervix (referred to as the vesicocervical ligament), the bladder and the paracolpium (known as the vesicovaginal ligament), as well as the interconnections between the ureters and the parametrium and paracolpium. How, then, should we employ the principles of membrane anatomy to comprehend these anatomical structures?

If we can define the connections between primordial compartments within the peritoneum as "membrane bridges," then similarly, our team believes that connections between primordial compartments outside the peritoneum can also be referred to as "membrane bridges." So, in cervical cancer surgery, how should we define these membrane bridges? Our team, based on surgical practice, believes that "membrane bridges" are the outermost boundary connecting tissues between primordial compartments' spaces. They serve to enclose the spaces between each primordial compartment. Opening a membrane bridge leads to what can be described as the "Holy plane," akin to an angel's hair [8]. Therefore, we can understand that the vesicocervical ligament serves as a membrane bridge between the Müllerian duct embryonic compartment and the urogenital sinus embryonic compartment; the vesicovaginal ligament also acts as a membrane bridge between the Müllerian duct embryonic compartment and the urogenital sinus embryonic compartment; the connection between the ureters and the parametrium and paracolpium forms a membrane bridge between the ureteric bud primordial compartment and the Müllerian duct embryonic compartment.

7.1.2 Embryonic Compartment

The term "embryonic compartment" is also referred to by some scholars as the "primordial unit" [2]. The understanding of the term "embryonic compartment" may vary among individual doctors. Our team interprets it as a composition of the primordium itself along with its associated supporting structures, including ligaments, blood vessels, nerves, and lymphatic tissue. From this perspective, the Müllerian duct embryonic compartment's embryonic core consists of the uterine body, cervix, and proximal vagina. The supporting structures are formed by the paracolpium, collectively comprising the parametrium laterally, dorsally, and ventrally. Specifically, the lateral support involves the uterine arteries, uterine veins, uterovaginal branches of the pelvic plexus, and the lymphatic fat tissue within. The dorsal support consists of the sacrouterine ligaments, while the ventral support includes the vesicocervical ligaments and vesicovaginal ligaments.

7.2 Reconsideration of Bladder-Level Ventral Parametrial Dissection

7.2.1 Vesicocervical Ligament

The vesicocervical ligament, as the name suggests, is a ligament connecting the bladder and the cervix (Fig. 7.1). It consists of fibrous connective tissue, nerves, blood vessels, and lymphatic tissue. The vesicocervical ligament can be understood as the anterior part of the ureteral tunnel, which doesn't fully reflect the bladder-level resection required in the QM classification [9]. In essence, it serves as the membrane bridge between the embryonic compartments of the urinary and Müllerian systems. We can validate this concept through surgical procedures and, ultimately, by applying the principles of membrane anatomy to guide cervical cancer surgery.

During the surgical procedure, when we are dealing with the ventral parametrium, it is customary to first open the peritoneum covering the bladder (Fig. 7.2) and then proceed to separate the space between the bladder and cervix as well as the space between the bladder and vagina (Fig. 7.3). In the process of separation, we often encounter challenges as we reach a certain point, making it difficult to continue the separation both toward the caudal direction and laterally.

Why does this happen? I believe many surgeons and scholars may encounter this confusion. At this juncture, employing the principles of membrane anatomy for explanation appears most apt.

The management of the ventral parametrium involves three embryonic compartments: the urogenital sinus embryonic compartment, the Müllerian duct embryonic compartment, and the ureteric bud embryonic compartment.

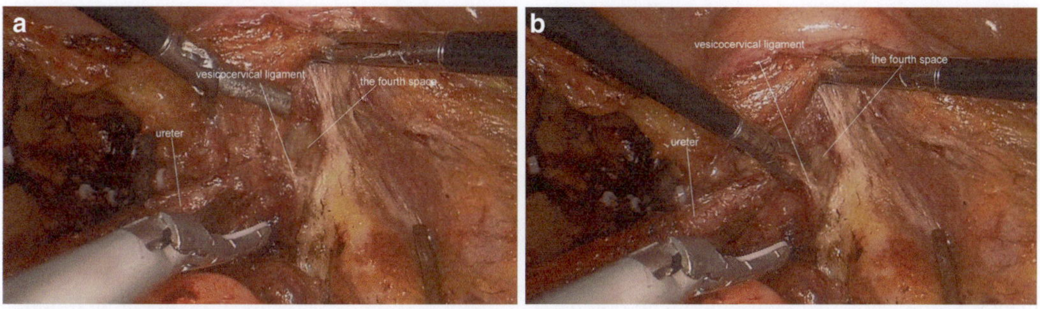

Fig. 7.1 Vesicocervical ligament

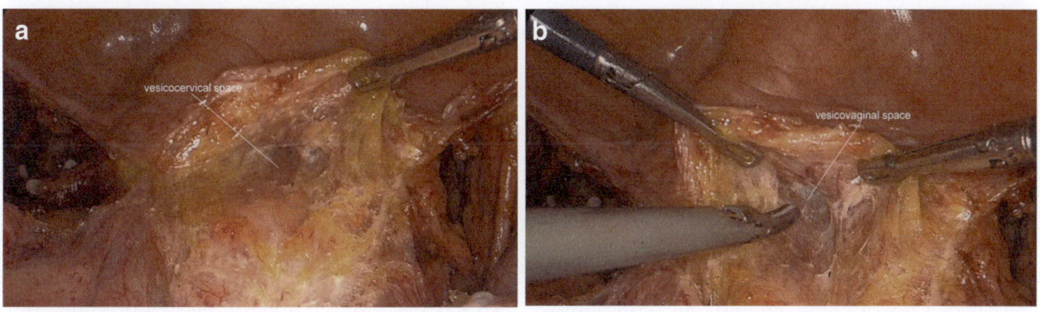

Fig. 7.2 Vesicocervical space and vesicovaginal space

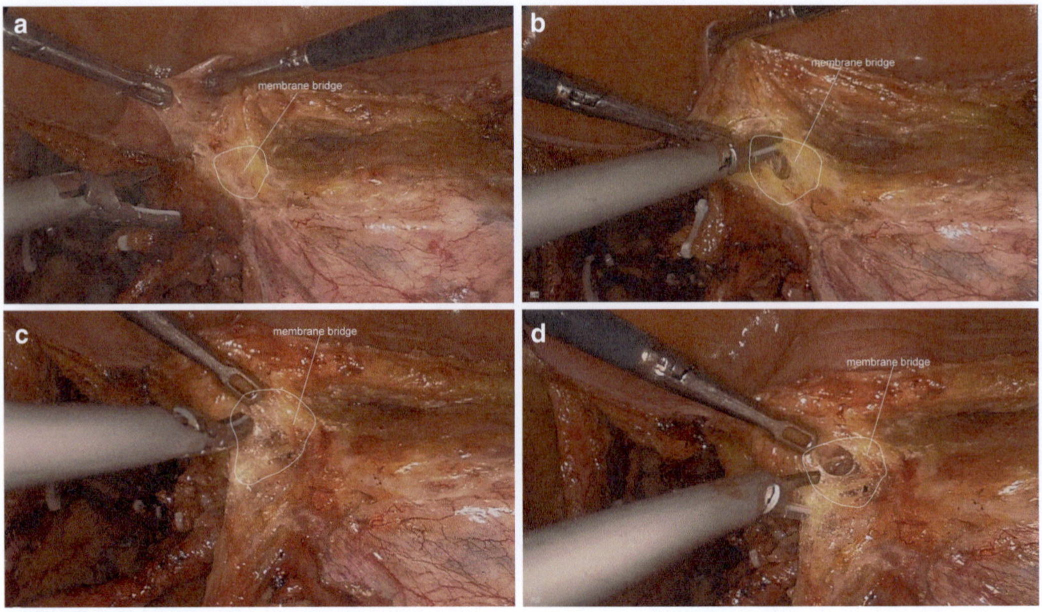

Fig. 7.3 Membrane bridge

We are aware that when different embryonic compartments come into contact, spaces form between them (these spaces are situated within the membranes surrounding each embryonic compartment), and at the junctions and edges of these contacts, there is an enveloping closure similar to an envelope. These closures represent membrane bridges connecting the embryonic compartments, typically composed of dense fibrous connective tissue, often accompanied by vertically oriented blood vessels between the two embryonic compartments.

Theoretically, concerning the connection between the urogenital sinus embryonic compartment and the Müllerian duct embryonic compartment in cervical cancer surgery, this connection occurs at the cranial aspect of the vesicocervical fold peritoneum and at the lateral aspects, where the connective tissues of the bladder sidewalls meet with the paracolpium and parametrium, specifically forming the connection points of the vesicovaginal ligament and the vesicocervical ligament.

If there is no interference from the ureteric bud embryonic compartment, the connection between the bladder sidewall and the parametrium, as well as the connection between the bladder sidewall and the paracolpium, should be continuous. During the separation of the vesicocervical space and the vesicovaginal space, lateral separation is sufficient to reveal the vesicocervical ligament and the vesicovaginal ligament. It can be observed that these ligaments are situated between the vesicocervical space and the bladder sidewall, as well as between the vesicovaginal space and the bladder sidewall. This simplifies the separation between the urogenital sinus embryonic compartment and the Müllerian duct embryonic compartment. The exposure and transection of the vesicocervical ligament and the vesicovaginal ligament only require close proximity to the bladder. It can be understood as the minimal mobilization and preservation of the bladder, which can achieve the bladder-level transection of the vesicocervical ligament and the vesicovaginal ligament as required in the Q-M classification.

However, in practice, the presence of the ureteric bud embryonic compartment makes the separation between the urogenital sinus embryonic compartment and the Müllerian duct embryonic compartment relatively challenging, which is a problem that troubles many gynecologic oncologists.

Due to the interference from the ureteric bud embryonic compartment, the widening of the vesicocervical space and vesicovaginal space during lateral separation becomes challenging. This is because the ureteric bud embryonic compartment traverses between the urogenital sinus embryonic compartment and the Müllerian duct embryonic compartment, turning the separation

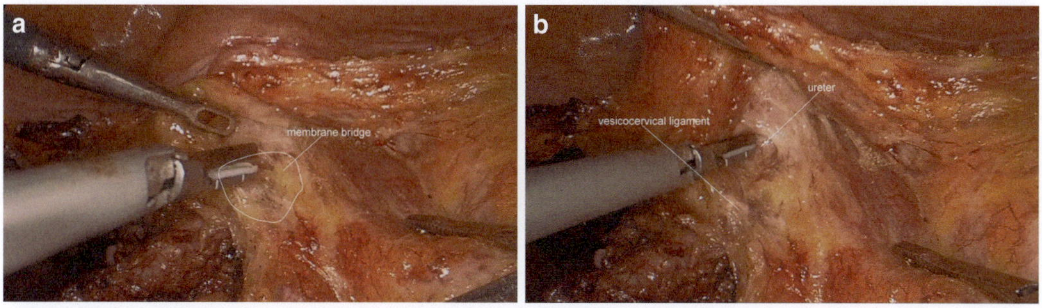

Fig. 7.4 Membrane space between the ureteric bud embryonic compartment and Müllerian duct embryonic compartment

of the two embryonic compartments into the separation of three embryonic compartments.

After the complete separation of the vesicocervical space and vesicovaginal space, the challenge encountered during lateral separation is due to the presence of the ureteric bud embryonic compartment positioned between the urogenital sinus embryonic compartment and the Müllerian duct embryonic compartment, forming a membrane bridge between them. The "exit" segment of the ureter, usually entering the bladder wall, does not have a membrane bridge between the ureteric bud embryonic compartment and the urogenital sinus embryonic compartment. However, a membrane bridge exists between the ureteric bud embryonic compartment and the Müllerian duct embryonic compartment. By using an ultrasonic scalpel to carefully open this membrane bridge, the ureteric bud embryonic compartment can be exposed, allowing further separation into the membrane space between the ureteric bud embryonic compartment and the Müllerian duct embryonic compartment (Fig. 7.4).

At this point, you will notice that there is still a portion of membrane bridge (comprising fibrous connective tissue along with its contained blood vessels, nerves, and lymphatics) connecting the ureteric bud embryonic compartment and the Müllerian duct embryonic compartment, known as the narrow vesicocervical ligament. However, the broad vesicocervical ligament, as discussed earlier, is usually separated by now. To complete the process, our team typically continues with an ultrasonic scalpel to fully disconnect the remaining membrane bridge tissue. This step allows for the complete mobilization and liberation of the ureteric bud embryonic compartment. At this stage, you will observe a dense layer of tissue on the dorsal aspect of the ureteric bud embryonic compartment, which represents the membrane bridge between the urogenital sinus embryonic compartment and the Müllerian duct embryonic compartment. By carefully opening this membrane bridge, the paravaginal space can be exposed, achieving a full separation of the urogenital sinus embryonic compartment and the Müllerian duct embryonic compartment and revealing the vesicovaginal ligament (Fig. 7.5).

7.2.2 Vesicovaginal Ligament

Vesicovaginal Ligament: A ligament comprising fibrous connective tissue, along with associated nerves, blood vessels, and lymphatic tissue, positioned between the outermost edge of the posterior bladder wall and the adjacent paracolpium. Anatomically, it resides within the paravaginal space and the bladder sidewall, forming a membrane bridge connecting the urogenital sinus embryonic compartment and the Müllerian duct embryonic compartment.

This concept seems difficult to understand: we can verify our claims by working backward through the surgical process and ultimately through cervical cancer surgery guided by the concept of membrane anatomy.

After the vesicocervical ligament is detached, many surgeons naturally assume that the next step should be to separate the ureter from the parametrium and paracolpium. However, in practical surgery, we find that even after detaching the vesicocervical ligament, the ureter still remains closely attached to the parametrium and paracol-

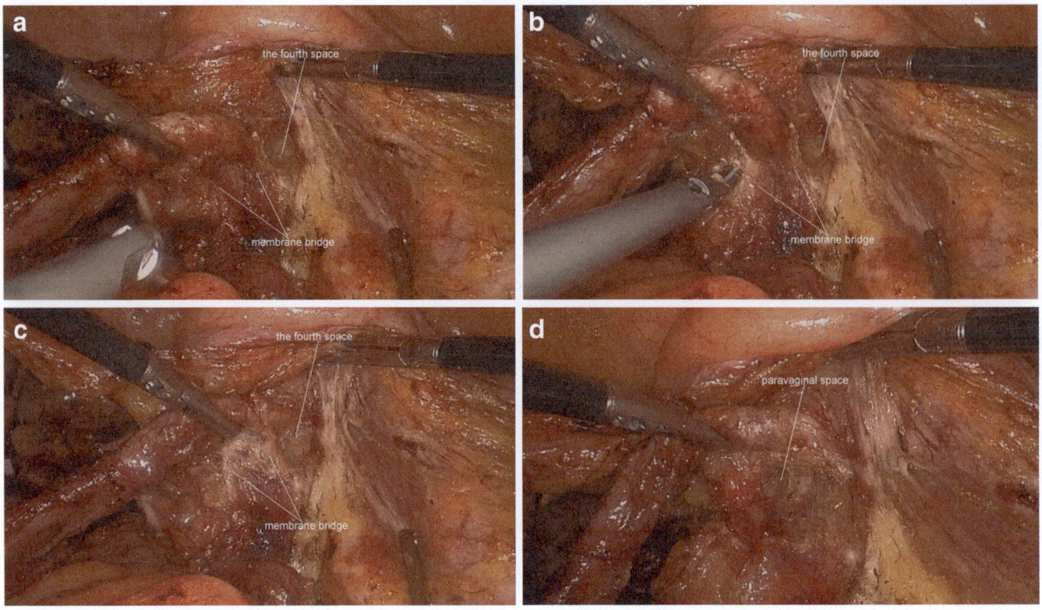

Fig. 7.5 Separation of the urogenital sinus embryonic compartment and Müllerian duct embryonic compartment

pium. This seems challenging to explain and analyze using conventional anatomy. In reality, interpreting this phenomenon through the concept of membrane anatomy appears to be more fitting. The vesicocervical ligament and vesicovaginal ligament both serve as membrane bridges between the urogenital sinus embryonic compartment and the Müllerian duct embryonic compartment. However, due to the interference from the ureteric bud embryonic compartment, these membrane bridges are discontinuous. Therefore, when the vesicocervical ligament is detached, it only reveals the relationship between the ureteric bud embryonic compartment and the Müllerian duct embryonic compartment. There is still a membrane bridge between these two embryonic compartments. At the same time, these two embryonic compartments are connected by membrane bridges. By detaching the connection between these two embryonic compartments, which is the membrane bridge, we can achieve the separation of these two embryonic compartments. This gradually allows the paravaginal spaces on both sides of the membrane bridge to connect, revealing the entire vesicovaginal ligament. What we are about to deal with is the vesicovaginal ligament, which is the essence of the ventral parametrium bladder-level excision in cervical cancer Q-M classification surgery. This area perfectly illustrates the bladder-level excision of the ventral parametrium (Fig. 7.6).

In anatomy, the vesicovaginal ligament is the ligament that connects the outermost edge of the posterior bladder wall to the adjacent paracolpium. It is also the ligament that separates the paravaginal space from the bladder sidewall space. We can still use the concept of membrane anatomy to interpret and understand the vesicovaginal ligament in the ventral parametrium.

The posterior bladder wall belongs to the urogenital sinus embryonic compartment, while the paracolpium belongs to the Müllerian duct embryonic compartment. Therefore, separating these two embryonic compartments reveals the vesicovaginal ligament. Since the vesicovaginal ligament connects the outermost edge of the posterior bladder wall to the paracolpium, this ligament represents the membrane bridge between the urogenital sinus embryonic compartment and the Müllerian duct embryonic compartment on the lateral side.

Typically, the separation between embryonic compartments involves opening membrane bridges and then separating two or more embryonic compartments. The vesicovaginal ligament, considered a membrane bridge, contains the superior vesical veins that drain into the deep

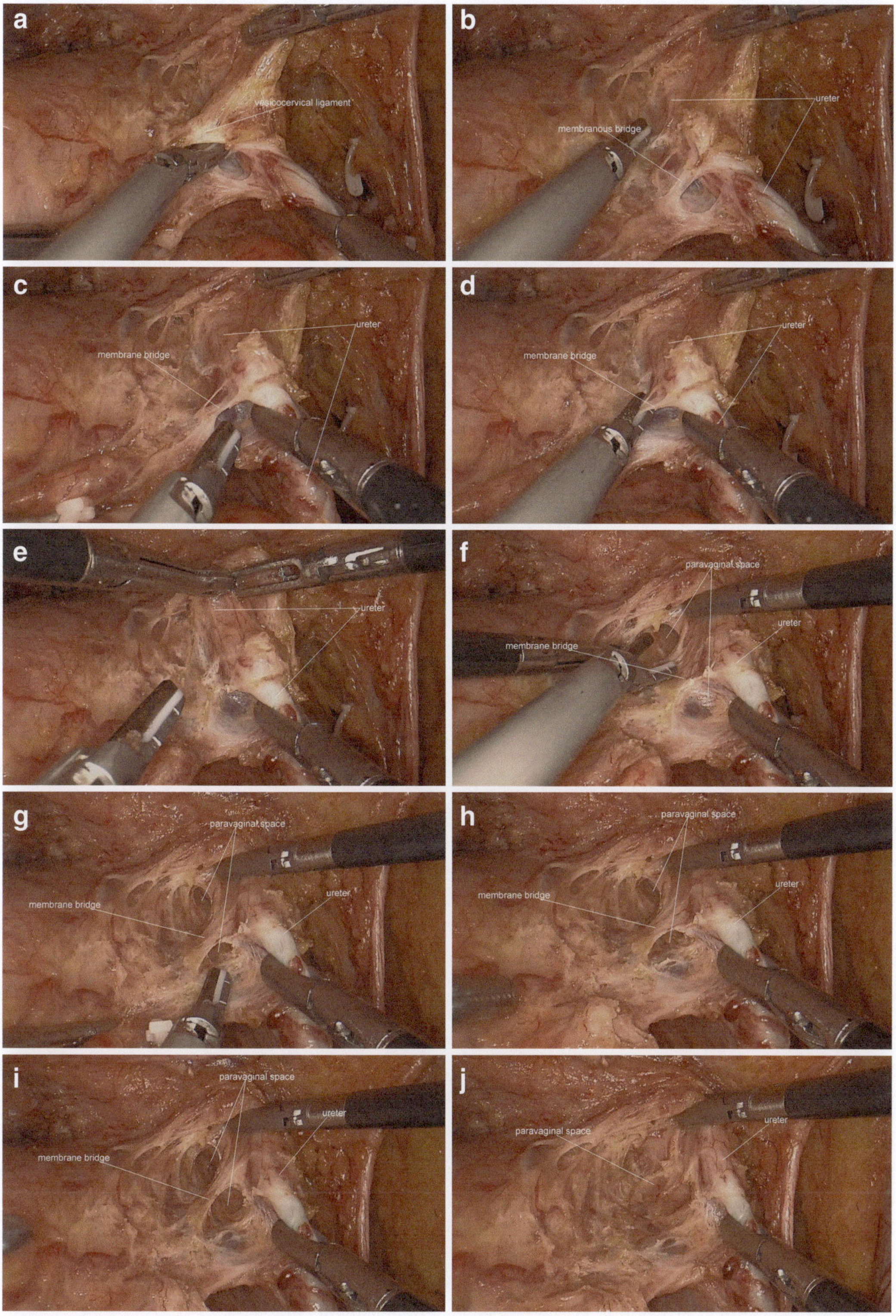

Fig. 7.6 Membrane bridge between the ureteric bud embryonic compartment and Müllerian duct embryonic compartment, and paravaginal space

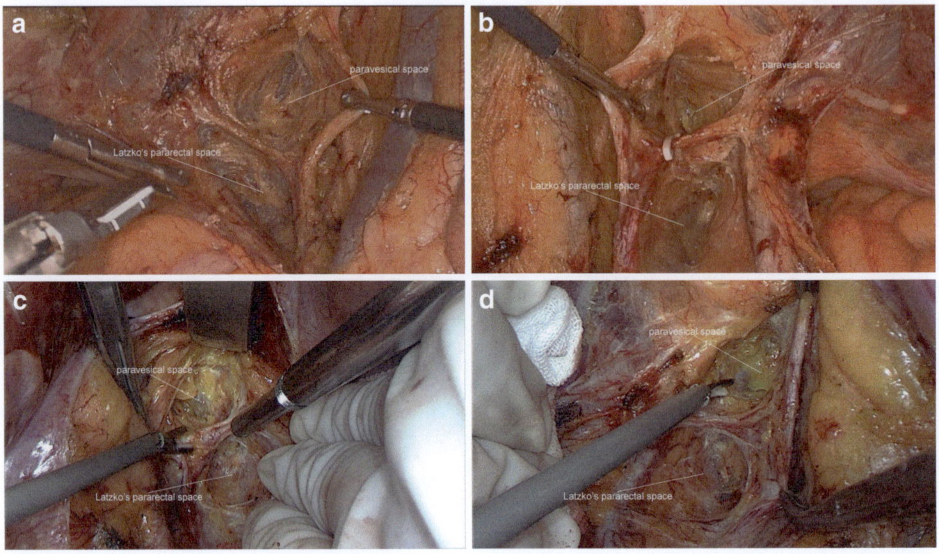

Fig. 7.7 Management of lateral parametrium

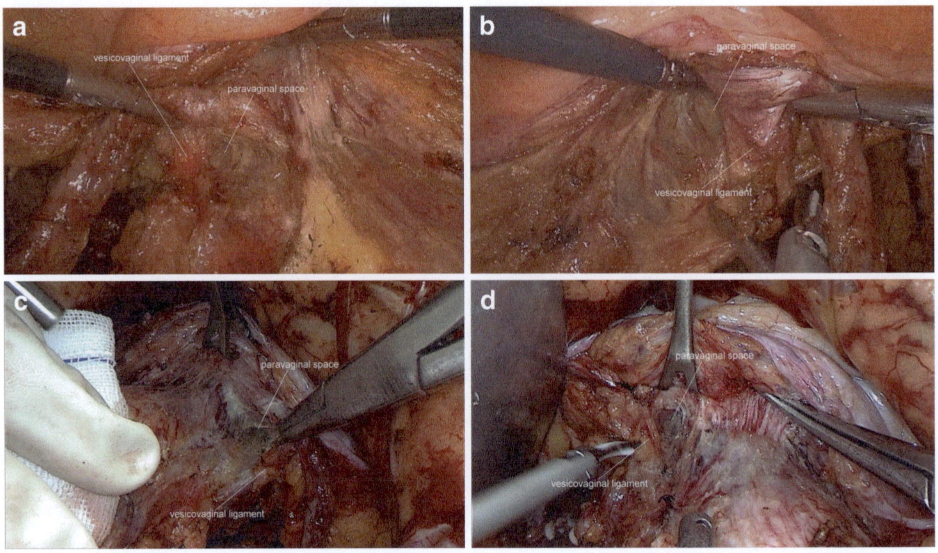

Fig. 7.8 Vesicovaginal ligament and paravaginal space

uterine vein. Therefore, directly detaching this membrane bridge before separating the spaces can lead to uncontrollable bleeding. Understanding this aspect of the surgical procedure through the concept of membrane anatomy can be quite helpful.

During the surgical procedure, as we proceed with lateral parametrial dissection, we have already dissected and freed the paravesical space. This allows for direct visibility of the bladder sidewall and posterior wall (Fig. 7.7).

During the ventral parametrium process, we can easily separate the posterior bladder wall from the paracolpium using membranous dissection. This reveals the paravaginal space, effectively separating the urogenital sinus embryonic compartment from the Müllerian duct embryonic compartment (Fig. 7.8).

To achieve the bladder-level excision of the ventral parametrium, it is sufficient to closely approximate and dissect the vesicovaginal ligament along the posterior bladder wall (Fig. 7.9).

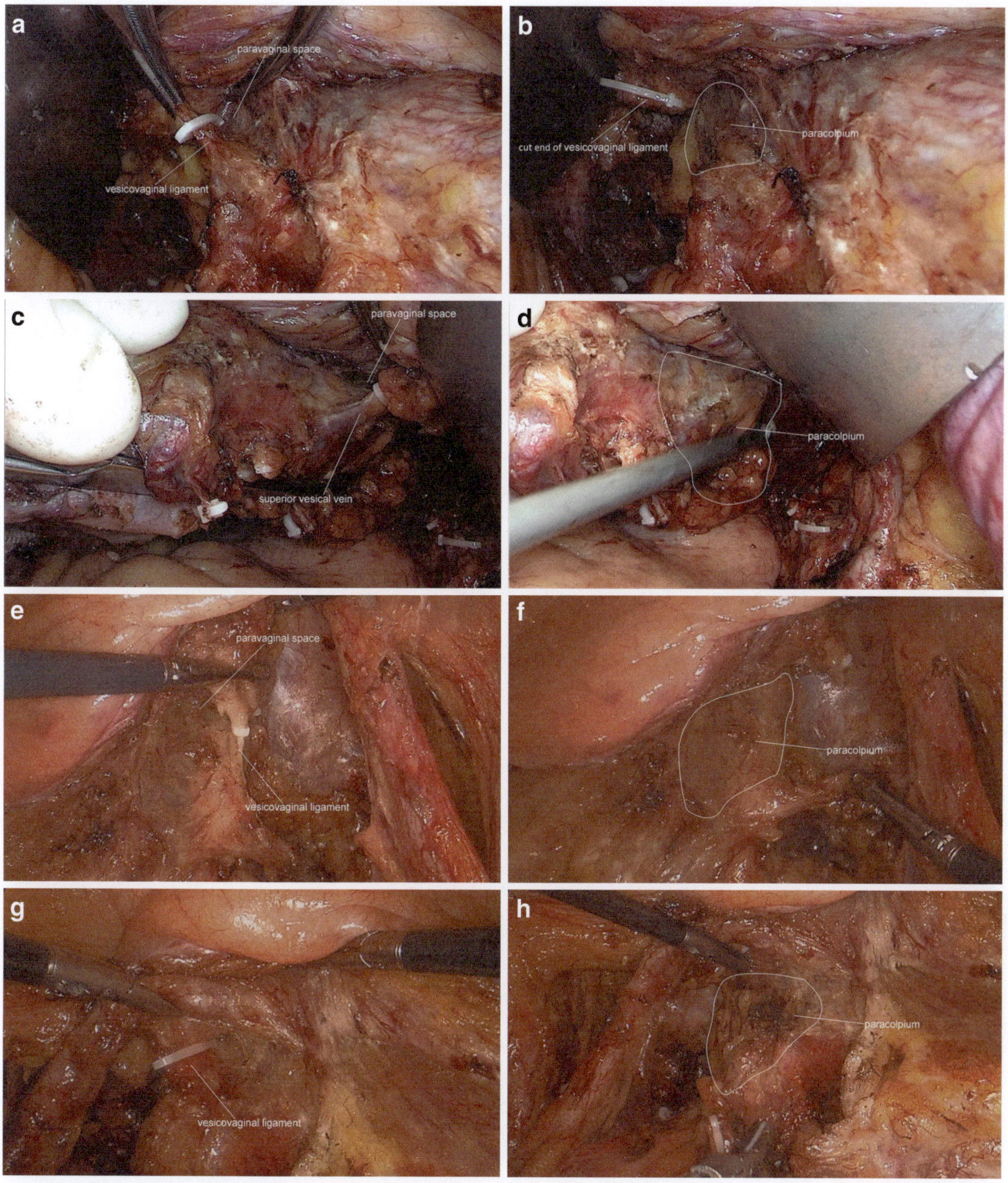

Fig. 7.9 Bladder-level excision of the ventral parametrium

7.3 The Equivalence of "Müllerian Embryological" Total Hysterectomy and QM-C Type Extensive Hysterectomy of Paracolpium and Paracervix

In surgeries guided by the concept of membrane anatomy, it is typically necessary to first open the membrane bridges before proceeding with the separation of embryonic compartments. However, since these membrane bridges often contain large blood vessels, directly detaching them before separating the embryonic compartments can lead to bleeding and even damage to the tissues and organs within the embryonic compartments. Therefore, it is advisable to begin with the separation of embryonic compartments, opening up the potential space between them, and then fully exposing the membrane bridges before detaching them. This approach ensures the complete separation of embryonic compartments.

The vesicocervical ligament and vesicovaginal ligament on the ventral parametrium, the sacrocervical ligament on the dorsal parametrium, and all structures on the lateral parametrium can be considered as accessory supportive structures of the Müllerian duct embryonic compartment. Therefore, C-type radical hysterectomy surgery can be guided by the concept of membrane anatomy to more fully demonstrate what is known as total mesometrial hysterectomy in membrane anatomy surgery.

Therefore, our team believes that understanding parametrium and paracolpium from the perspective of membrane anatomy is more helpful for the progress and growth of readers in the field of surgery.

7.3.1 Ventral Parametrium

Vesicocervical Ligament and Vesicovaginal Ligament: The membrane bridges between the urogenital sinus embryonic compartment and the Müllerian duct embryonic compartment. Vesicocervical ligament (membrane bridge on the ventral side between the urogenital sinus embryonic compartment and the Müllerian duct embryonic compartment): Fibrous connective tissue connecting the bladder to the paracolpium, situated between the vesicocervical space and the paravaginal space. Vesicovaginal ligament (membrane bridge on the dorsal side between the urogenital sinus embryonic compartment and the Müllerian duct embryonic compartment): Fibrous connective tissue connecting the bladder to the paravaginal tissue, ultimately forming the paracolpium along with the lateral and dorsal parametrial tissues, situated between the paravesical space and the paravaginal space (Fig. 7.10).

7.3.2 Lateral Parametrium

The lateral parametrium (Fig. 7.11) consists of the uterine artery, superficial uterine veins, deep uterine veins, the pelvic splanchnic nerve plexus, and the surrounding lymphatic adipose tissue. These structures are located between Latzko's pararectal space and the paravesical space. In C2-type surgery, it is necessary to disconnect

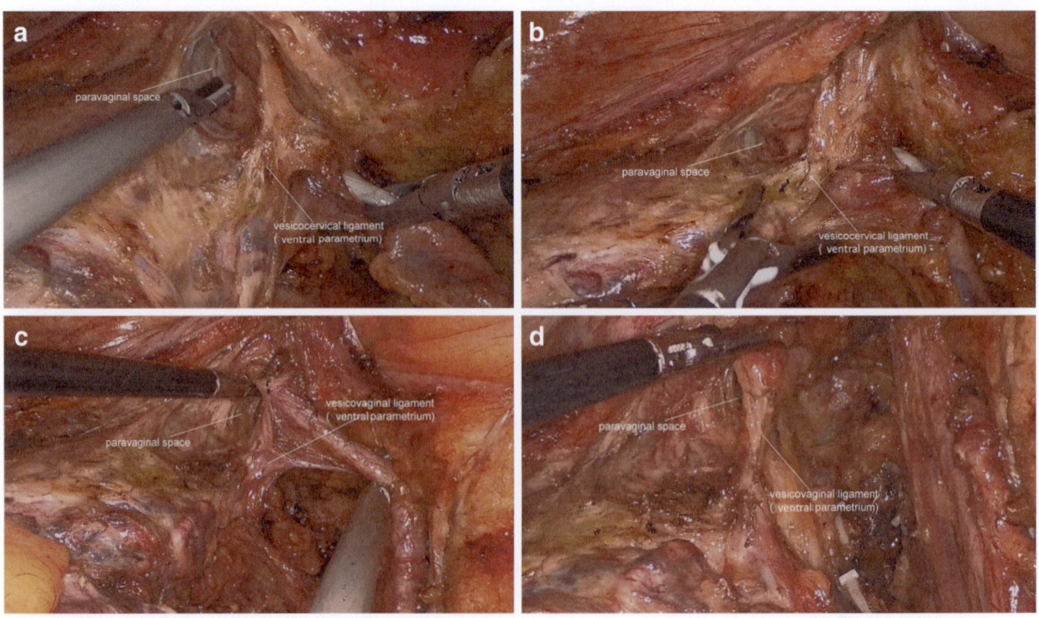

Fig. 7.10 Ventral parametrium

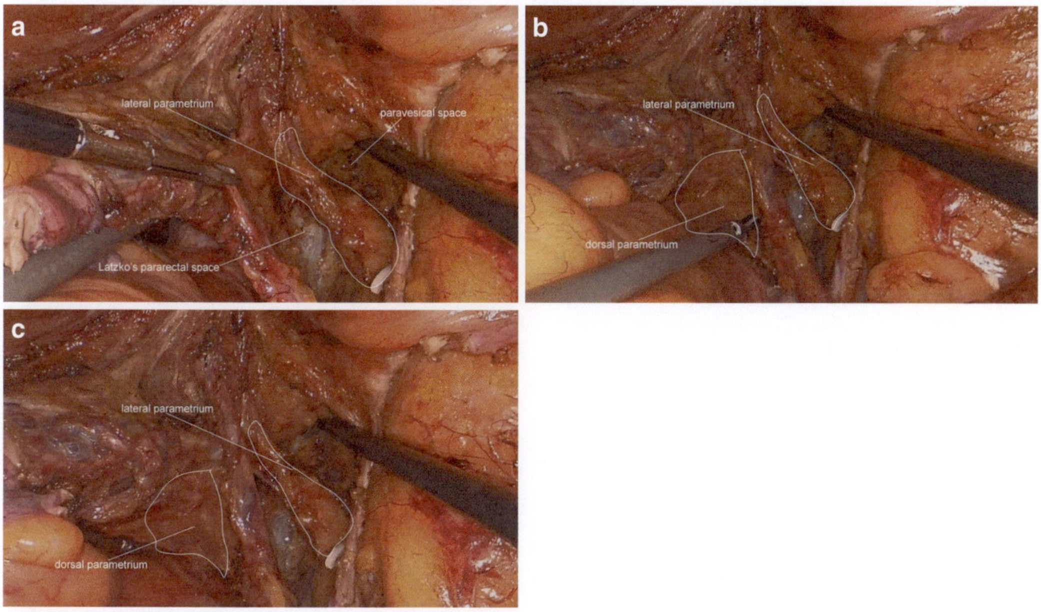

Fig. 7.11 Lateral parametrium and dorsal parametrium

these structures at the inner edge of the internal iliac vessels, which corresponds to the exit point of the vascular portion of the Müllerian duct embryonic compartment. By separating the paravesical space from the vesicovaginal ligament, it ultimately ends at the outermost edge of the paravaginal space, together with the ventral and dorsal parametrium, forming the paracolpium.

Type C1 surgery requires the detachment of the uterine branches, cervical branches, and vaginal branches from the pelvic plexus, while preserving the lateral bladder branches. When viewed from the perspective of embryonic compartments, neither the hypogastric nerve plexus nor the pelvic splanchnic nerve plexus is associated with the Müllerian duct embryonic compartment. However, the branches stemming from the pelvic plexus, which encompass uterine branches, cervical branches, and vaginal branches, are considered constituents of the Müllerian duct embryonic compartment. Therefore, Type C2 surgery goes beyond the embryonic compartment approach. Since Type C2 surgery extends beyond the scope of embryonic compartment-based resection, why does it still have a place? Its existence is justified because Type C1 surgery requires extremely precise procedures. It involves meticulously freeing and dissecting the vascular plane, including the deep uterine veins, superior vesical veins, and inferior vesical veins, located to the outer aspect of the parametrium. This dissection allows for the exposure of the pelvic plexus on the posterior aspect, enabling the preservation of nerves. Any improper handling during this process can lead to bleeding or incomplete resection of embryonic compartments. Therefore, in patients with larger lesions, Type C2 radical hysterectomy may be considered. It involves an extended resection beyond the embryonic compartment boundaries to prevent potential intracavitary tumor spillage.

7.3.3 Dorsal Parametrium

This term refers to the uterosacral ligament, which originates at the cervix or the junction of the cervix and the vagina and terminates at the sacral fascia. During separation, it is necessary to fully separate the mesentery of the hindgut embryonic compartment from the sidewall of the rectum until the level of the levator ani muscle is reached to completely expose the uterosacral ligament. In C1-type surgery, it is located

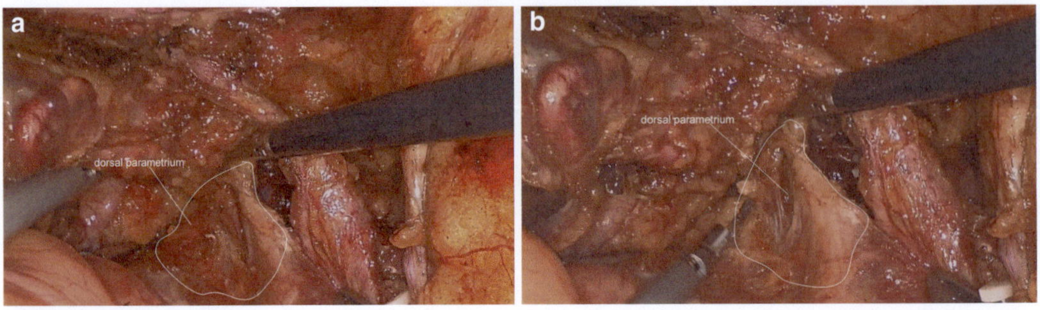

Fig. 7.12 Dorsal parametrium

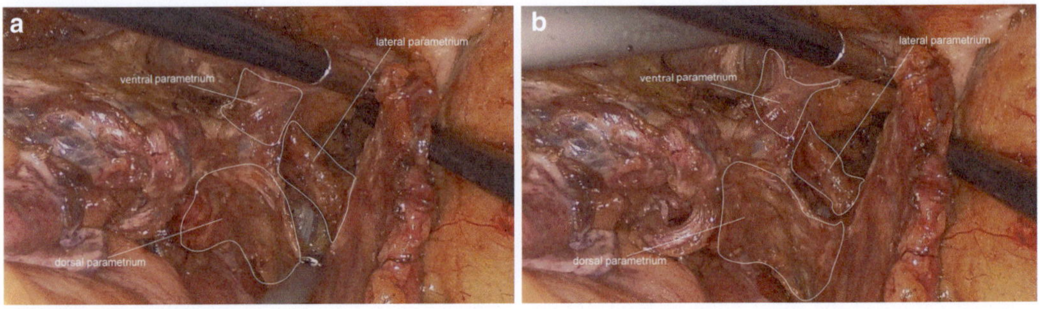

Fig. 7.13 Parametrium

between the Okabayashi's pararectal space and the space formed by the rectal sidewall and the inner side of the sacrocervical ligament In C2-type surgery, it is located between the Latzko's pararectal space and the space between the rectal sidewall and the inner side of the sacrocervical ligament (Fig. 7.12).

7.3.4 Paracolpium

The paracolpium is formed by the convergence of structures from the lateral, ventral, and dorsal aspects of parametrium (Fig.7.13) [10–18].

These include:

The vascular plane is composed of the deep uterine veins from the lateral parametrium, along with the surrounding lymphatic and fatty tissues, as well as the vesical venous plexus located within the vesicovaginal ligament in the anterior parametrium, which drains into the deep uterine vein.

The neural plane consists of the pelvic splanchnic nerve plexus located dorsally in the lateral parametrium and the hypogastric nerve situated laterally in the dorsal parametrium, which together form the inferior hypogastric plexus/pelvic plexus, along with its branches to the uterus, bladder, vagina, and cervix.

The ligamentous plane consists of the sacral ligament of the dorsal parametrium.

These three planes—vascular, neural, and ligament—constitute the paracolpium (Fig. 7.14).

Explained as follows

The superior vesical veins located on the ventral parametrium drain into the deep uterine veins. In certain patients, a section of the middle vesical veins can also be found within the paracolpium, and they drain into the deep uterine veins too. These venous networks are positioned on the surface of the paracolpium, constituting the vascular plane. The pelvic splanchnic nerve

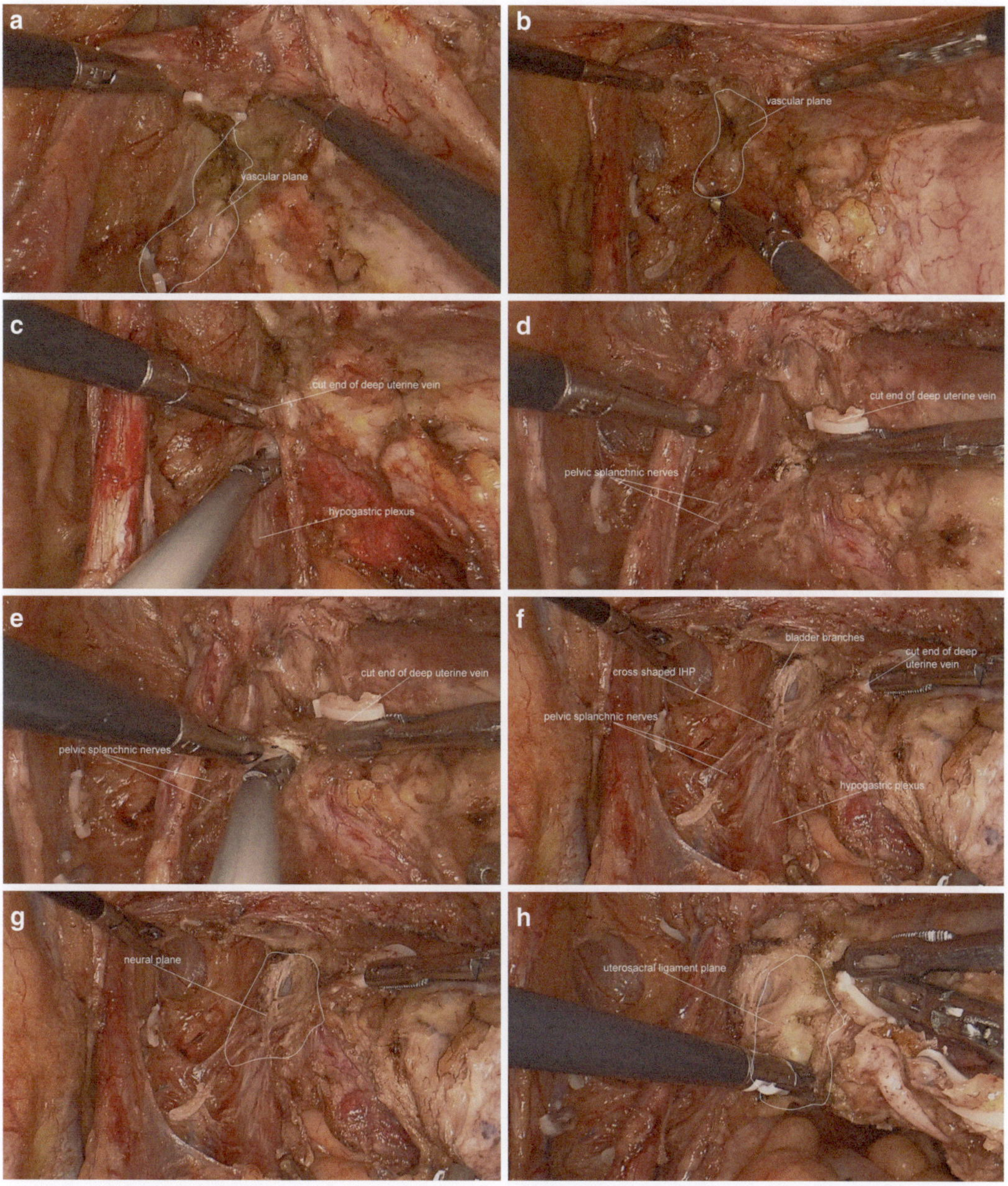

Fig. 7.14 Paracolpium: three planes (vascular, neural and ligament)

plexus is situated dorsally to the deep uterine veins, while the hypogastric nerve plexus is located laterally to the dorsal parametrium. These two nerve plexuses converge on the outer side of the paracolpium, forming a cross intersection, thus creating the neural plane. They are positioned dorsally to the vascular plane, which includes the deep uterine veins, superior vesical veins, and the middle vesical veins. The uterosacral ligament plane is located dorsally to the neural plane.

Therefore, during a C1-type radical hysterectomy, we can use the theory of the three planes to guide the surgical procedure. By mobilizing and lifting the vascular plane consisting of the deep uterine veins, superior vesical veins, and middle vesical veins inward, the neural plane is exposed. Under direct visualization of the nerve intersection, the dissection of inner regional nerves can be performed while preserving the bladder branches of the pelvic plexus [10–18].

7.3.5 The Extent of Vaginal Resection

Because the paracolpium is a three-dimensional structure, as mentioned earlier, when dealing with the caudal aspect in the ventral, dorsal, and lateral parametrium, it is mentioned that it reaches the level of the endopelvic fascia. At this level, the dissection proceeds inwards along the vaginal axis, reaching the circumference of the membrane spaces. The corresponding length of the vagina represents the extent of vaginal resection. Typically, when measuring the specimen ex vivo, this can be around 2–3 cm.

References

1. Manjunath AP, Girija S. Embryologically based resection of cervical cancers: a new concept of surgical radicality. J Obstet Gynaecol India. 2012;62(1):5–14.
2. Höckel M, Horn L, Fritsch H. Association between the mesenchymal compartment of uterovaginal organogenesis and local tumour spread in stage IB-IIB cervical carcinoma: a prospective study. Lancet Oncol. 2005;6:751–6.
3. Höckel M. Ultra-radical compartmentalized surgery in gynaecological oncology. Eur J Surg Oncol. 2006;32:859–65.
4. Höckel M, Horn L, Tetsch E, et al. Pattern analysis of regional spread and therapeutic lymph node dissection in cervical cancer based on ontogenetic anatomy. Gynecol Oncol. 2012;125:168–74.
5. Zhao X, OuYang Y. Demystifying membrane anatomy: toward a new era of abdominopelvic surgery. Innovation (Camb). 2023;4:100370.
6. Gong JP. Rise and mix of membrane anatomy. Zhonghua Wei Chang Wai Ke Za Zhi. 2019;22(5):401–5.
7. Coffey JC. Mesenteric principles of gastrointestinal surgery. 1st ed. Boca Raton: Taylor & Francis Group; 2017. p. 57–68.
8. Heald RJ. The 'Holy Plane' of rectal surgery. J R Soc Med. 1988;81(9):503–8.
9. Querleu D, Morrow CP. Classification of radical hysterectomy. Lancet Oncol. 2008;9:297–303.
10. Wang J, Han S. Cervical cancer surgery illustration. Beijing: People Medical Press, 2022.
11. Wang J, Han S. Practical techniques for cervical cancer surgery. Beijing: People Medical Press, 2023.
12. Han S, Wang J. ovarian cancer surgery illustration. Beijing: People Medical Press, 2024..
13. Han S, Wang J. Practical techniques for ovarian cancer surgery. Beijing: People Medical Press, 2024.
14. Li Y, Na J, Wang X, Song S, Wang J, Han S. Can embrane bridge be used to describe the connective tissue between two different embryonic compartments? An exploratory attempt to standardize the description of embryonic compartment hysterectomy, Intelligent Surgery. 2024;7:80–4. https://doi.org/10.1016/j.isurg.2024.09.002.
15. Han S, Na J, Li Y, Lu J, Wang J. Application and prospect of membrane anatomy in-robot assisted laparoscopic cervical cancer surgery [J]. Journal of Robotic Surgery, 2023;4(05):456–63.
16. Na J, Li Y, Wang X, Song S, Wang J, Han S. Clinical application of embryonic compartment hysterectomy in the treatment of cervical cancer. Chinese Journal of Practical Gynecology and Obstetrics, 2024;40(02):209–14. https://doi.org/10.19538/j.fk2024020116.
17. Han S, Na J, Li Y, Wang J. Surgical procedures and techniques in robot-assisted uterine artery-preserving radical trachelectomy. J Robot Surg. 2024;18:222. https://doi.org/10.1007/s11701-024-01982-y.
18. Li Y, Na J, Wang X, Han S, Wang J. Robot-assisted Müllerian compartment resection for cervical cancer. Front. Oncol. 14:1466921. https://doi.org/10.3389/fonc.2024.1466921.

Part II

Illustration of Radical Hysterectomy for Cervical Cancer Under QM Classification

8 Type QM-A Radical Hysterectomy

Shichao Han and Jing Na

This is a surgical treatment method commonly applied to patients in FIGO stage IA1 without lymphovascular space involvement. Such patients are diagnosed with stage IA1 and have negative margins after "conization" [1].

Type QM-A is a limited radical hysterectomy (i.e., minimal radical surgery) and not a simple extrafascial hysterectomy, which is a smaller operation than the standard modified radical hysterectomy (Type B, described in the next section) but a larger operation than a simple or extrafascial hysterectomy. The goal of the operation is to ensure the complete removal of the cervix down to the vaginal fornix, together with a paracervical margin [2, 3].

As we know, the Laparoscopic Approach to Cervical Cancer (LACC) trial has shown that patients who undergo minimally invasive radical hysterectomy have a poorer prognosis than those who undergo open radical hysterectomy [4]. Uterine manipulators and intracorporeal open colpotomy may be the two main factors responsible for this inferiority [5].

Supplementary Information The online version contains supplementary material available at https://doi.org/10.1007/978-981-97-7687-0_8.

S. Han (✉) · J. Na
Department of Gynecology and Obstetrics, Second Affiliated Hospital of Dalian Medical University, Dalian, China

Our team performs a procedure during minimally invasive surgery to suspend the uterus with absorbable suture stitches. This helps to avoid intraoperative compression of the cervix and tumor spillage. Additionally, for Type QM-A surgery, it is only necessary to resect less than 1 cm of the vaginal cuff, and enclosed colpotomy is difficult to perform. Therefore, our team rinses the vagina repeatedly with 200 ml of sterile distilled water at 42 °C before cuff resection to create a tumor-free environment as much as possible.

8.1 Uterine suspension

The absorbable suture is used to suture the uterine fundus in a figure-eight pattern using 2 stitches (Fig. 8.1a, b). A 0.5-cm incision is made above the pubic symphysis, and a trocar is inserted through the abdominal wall to create a passage for the needle holder of the laparoscope to enter the abdominal cavity and grasp the suture line of the uterine fundus.(Fig. 8.1c–f).

Surgical Experience and Precaution Our team's experience in suturing involves inserting the needle from the posterior wall and exiting at the uterine fundus, which increases the lifting force on the posterior wall and provides good exposure for the dorsal parametrium. The incision above the pubic symphysis does not have a fixed position on the body. Our team's method

S. Han, J. Wang (eds.), *Open, Laparoscopic, and Robotic Surgery for Cervical Cancer*,
https://doi.org/10.1007/978-981-97-7687-0_8

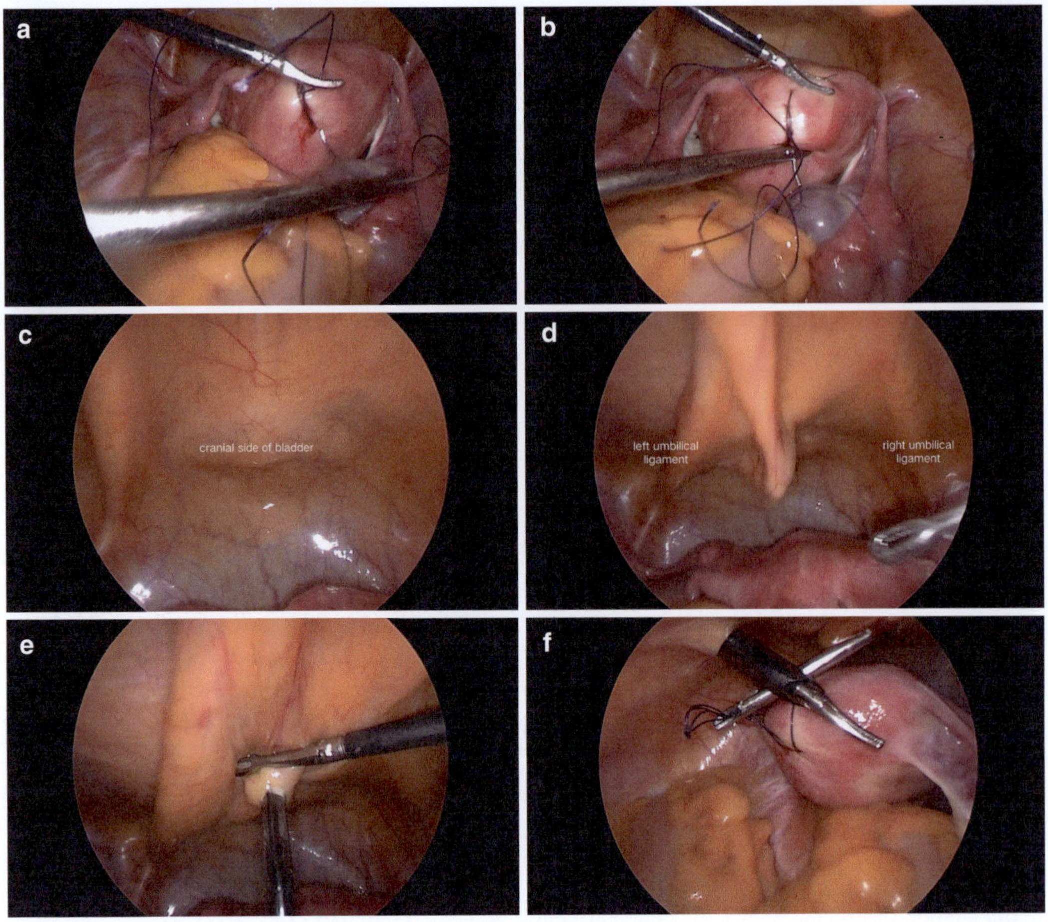

Fig. 8.1 (**a–f**) Uterine suspension

involves determining the position of the bladder in the abdominal cavity under laparoscopy and then identifying the position of the abdominal wall puncture hole by repeatedly pressing the abdominal wall. After penetrating the peritoneal layer, it may be challenging to puncture the peritoneum due to its excessive elasticity. An assistant can use a non-invasive clamp to support the peritoneum at the puncture site to assist in the puncture.

8.2 Exposure of the Lateral Retroperitoneal Space

Pull the uterus to the opposite side, and pull the round ligament toward the ventral and caudal side. Then, pull the suspensory ligament toward the medial side to expose the lateral peritoneum of the pelvic segment (Fig. 8.2a, b).

Surgical Experience and Precautions Pulling the suspensory ligament toward the medial side can improve the visualization of the abdominal aspect of the lateral retroperitoneal space. Use an ultrasonic scalpel to cut the lateral peritoneum at the outer side of the intersection between the ovarian ligament and the common iliac vessel, toward the intersection of the round ligament and the lateral peritoneum (Fig. 8.3a, b).

Surgical Experience and Precautions The suspensory ligament and ureter usually intersect at the surface of the common iliac vessels. By opening the lateral peritoneum at this site, important anatomical structures in the space can

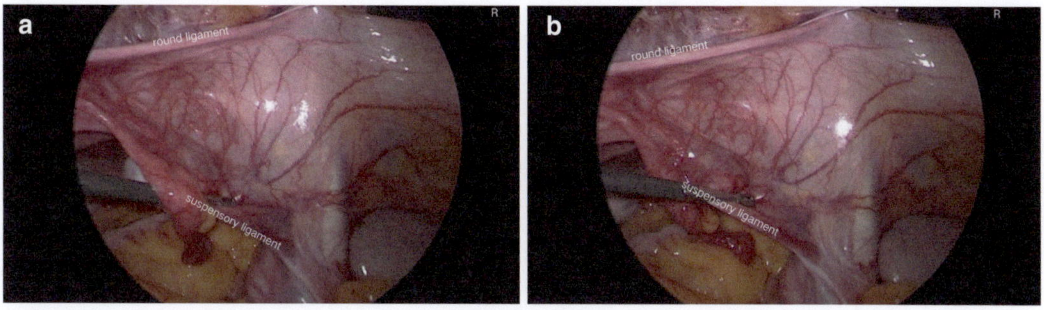

Fig. 8.2 (**a**, **b**) Expose the lateral peritoneum of the pelvic segment

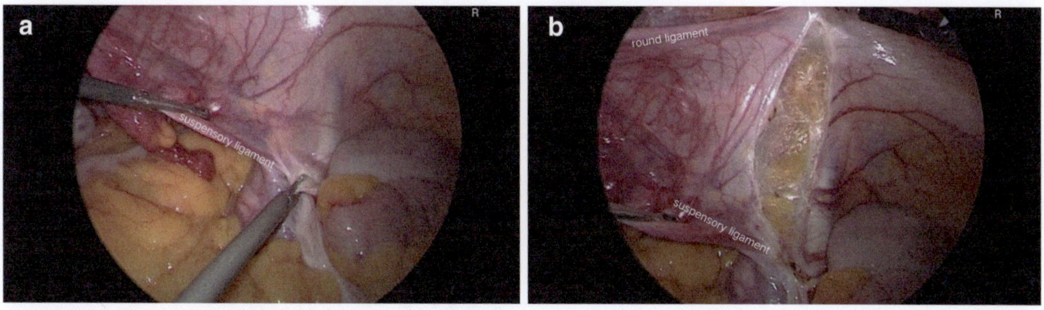

Fig. 8.3 (**a**, **b**) Open the lateral peritoneum along the psoas major

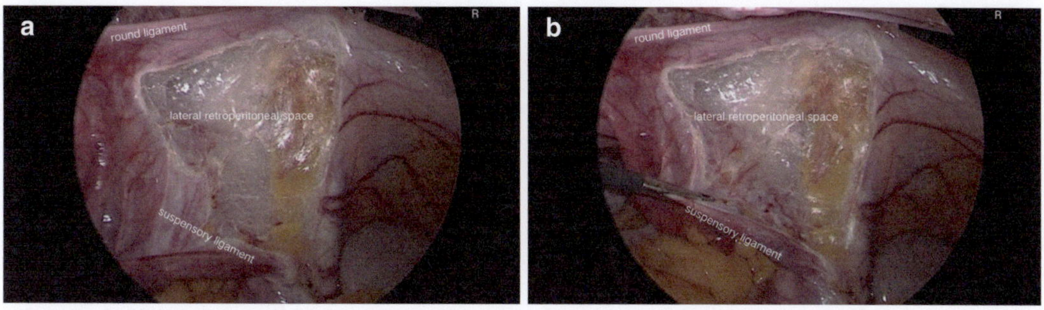

Fig. 8.4 (**a**, **b**) Open the lateral peritoneum along the round ligament

be fully exposed, helping to avoid injuries to the blood vessels and ureters, as well as prevent secondary damage caused by anatomical variations.

At the point where the round ligament intersects with the lateral peritoneum, cut the lateral peritoneum toward the uterine horn along the round ligament. Then, pull the lateral peritoneum inwards to expose the lateral retroperitoneal space (Fig. 8.4a, b).

8.3 Exposure of Important Anatomical Structures in Lateral Retroperitoneal Space

8.3.1 Open the Lateral Retroperitoneal Space

After exposing the lateral retroperitoneal space, it reveals white loose connective tissue, which looks like angel's hair. We can use an ultrasonic

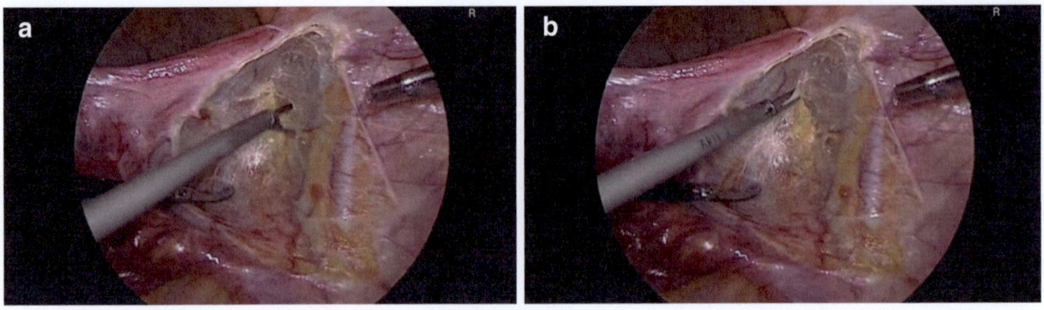

Fig. 8.5 (**a**, **b**) Sharply dissect the lateral retroperitoneal space

scalpel to open the lateral retroperitoneal space and cut the white loose connective tissue (Fig. 8.5a, b).

Surgical Experience and Precautions The ultrasonic scalpel cuts through the white loose connective tissue, while avoiding proximity to blood vessels and the lateral peritoneum. This reduces the risk of thermal damage to the ureter and blood vessels and minimizes bleeding.

8.3.2 Separate the Lateral Retroperitoneal Space

Keep pulling the suspensory ligament and lateral peritoneum toward the medial side while gently pushing the external iliac vessels toward the outer side. Then provide enough tension to separate the lateral retroperitoneal space from the abdominal to dorsal region (Fig. 8.6a–f).

Surgical Experience and Precautions Sharp dissection should be continued until the white loose connective tissue disappears and the yellow fat tissue appears, indicating that the plane of vessels and ureter (i.e., uterine artery, internal iliac artery, and ureter) has been reached. At this plane, it is crucial to avoid any bleeding during surgery. A clear surgical vision can help us easily differentiate important anatomical structures and avoid any adverse injury.

8.3.3 Expose the Origin of the Uterine Artery

By externally pulling the lateral umbilical ligament and internally pulling the suspensory ligament and lateral peritoneum, the internal iliac artery, uterine artery, and ureter can be visualized as important anatomical landmarks. Once this plane is entered, the origin of the uterine artery can be exposed (Fig. 8.7a–d).

Surgical Experience and Precautions If the uterine artery is difficult to expose, we can explore the Latzko's pararectal space and the paravesical space by sharp dissection to expose it.

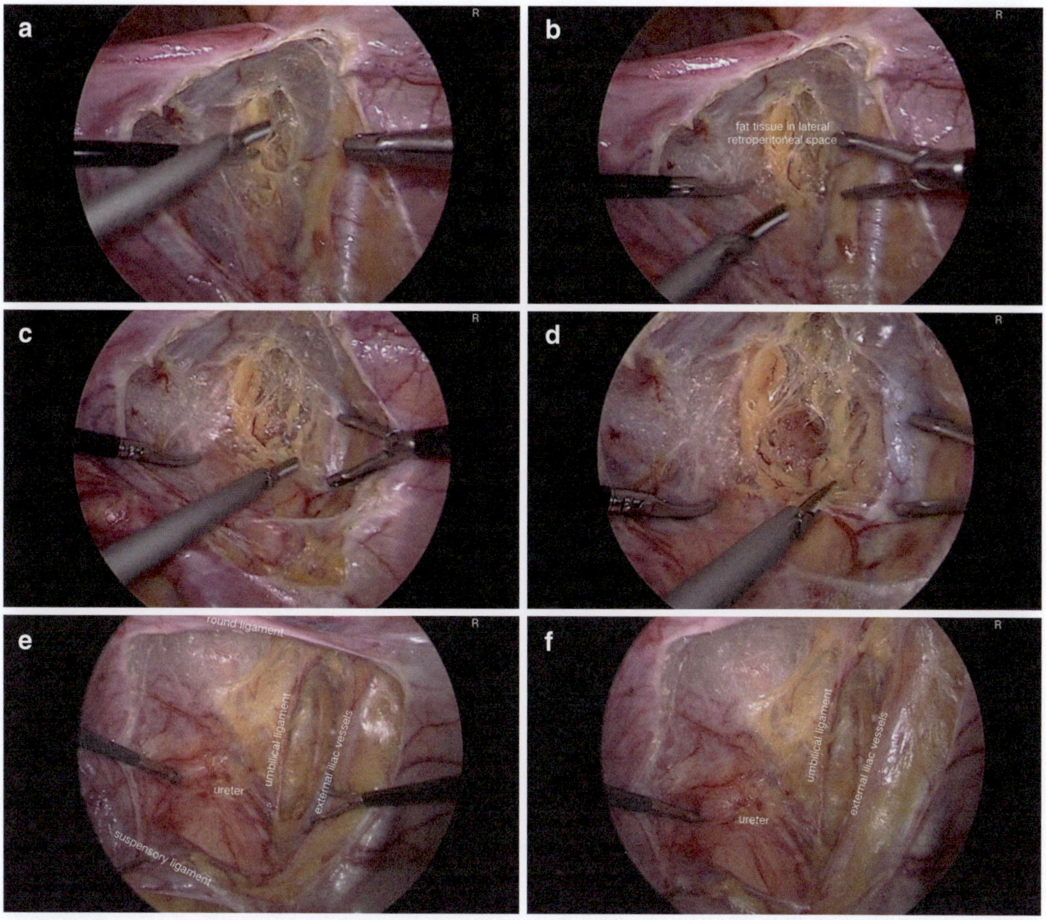

Fig. 8.6 (**a**–**f**) Expose the internal iliac artery

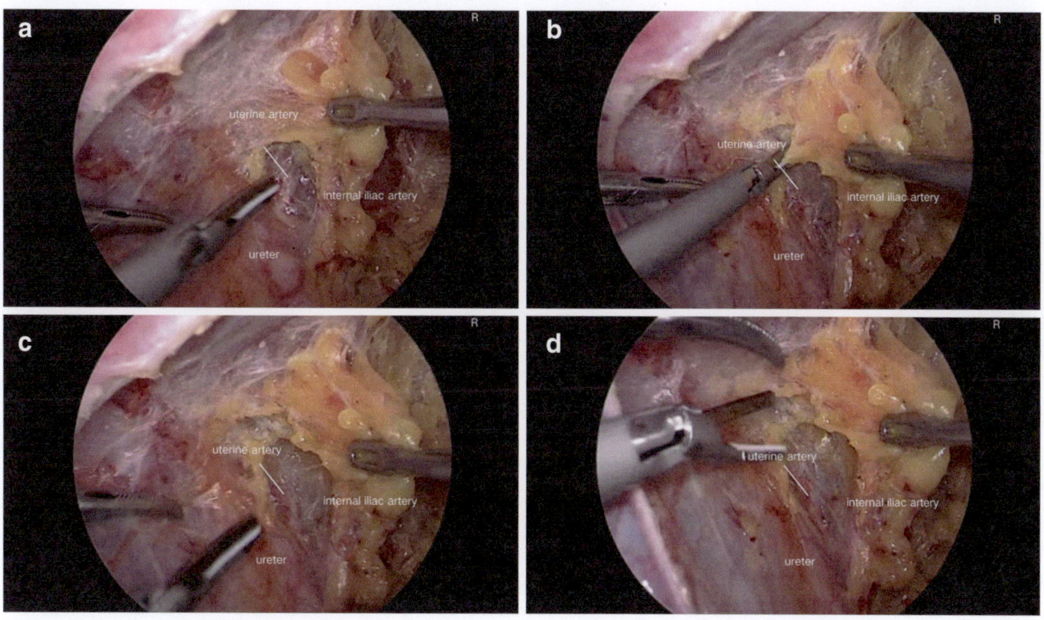

Fig. 8.7 (**a**–**d**) Expose the uterine artery

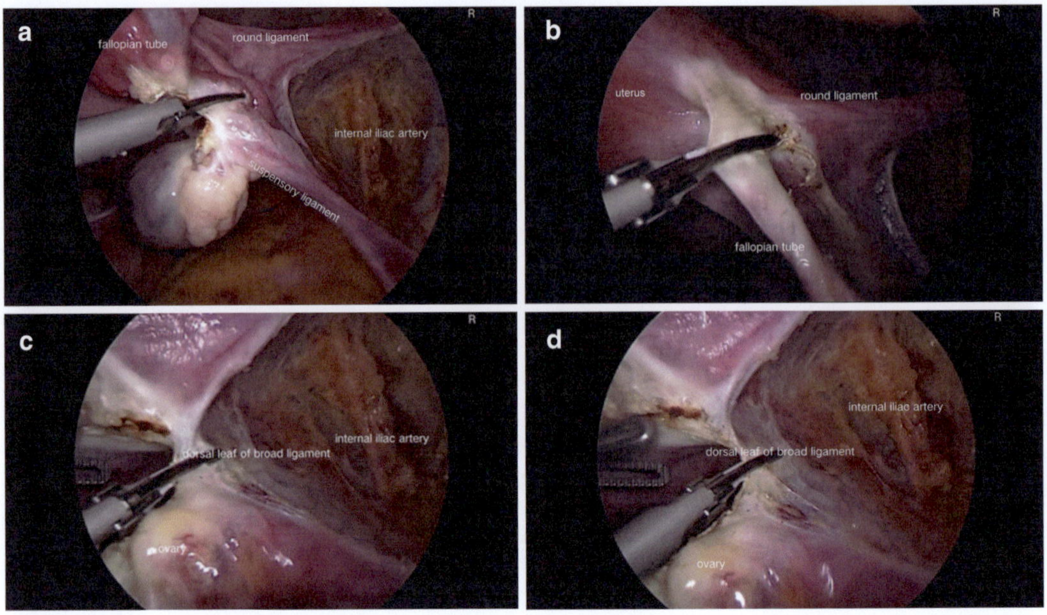

Fig. 8.8 (**a–d**) Salpingectomy

8.4 Salpingectomy or Salpingo-oophorectomy

1. The suspensory ligament is transected, and the fallopian tube and ovary are removed.
2. The fallopian tube and the ovarian ligament can be excised (Fig. 8.8a–d).

Surgical Experience and Precautions The site for transecting the suspensory ligament is at the intersection of the ligament and the iliac vessels, where the three anatomical structures of the ureter, suspensory ligament, and iliac vessels are in closest proximity. It is advisable to fully expose the ligament before transection. Hem-o-lok or bipolar forceps can be used to occlude or coagulate the ligament, respectively, to avoid injuring the ureter. Transecting the suspensory ligament is necessary to create greater tension for subsequent dissection and mobilization of the uterine artery, which requires pulling the lateral peritoneum medially.

8.5 Ventral Parametrium

8.5.1 Open the Vesicouterine Fold

Transect the round ligament and use a sharp dissection method to open the vesicouterine fold (Fig. 8.9a–d).

Surgical Experience and Precautions Pull the peritoneum toward the ventral and caudal side and transect it at the junction of the white and yellow areas.

8.5.2 Expose the Vesicocervical Space and Vesicovaginal Space

Pull the bladder and reflected peritoneum toward the ventral and caudal sides to create tension between the bladder and the cervix/vagina. Then, use sharp dissection techniques to gradually dis-

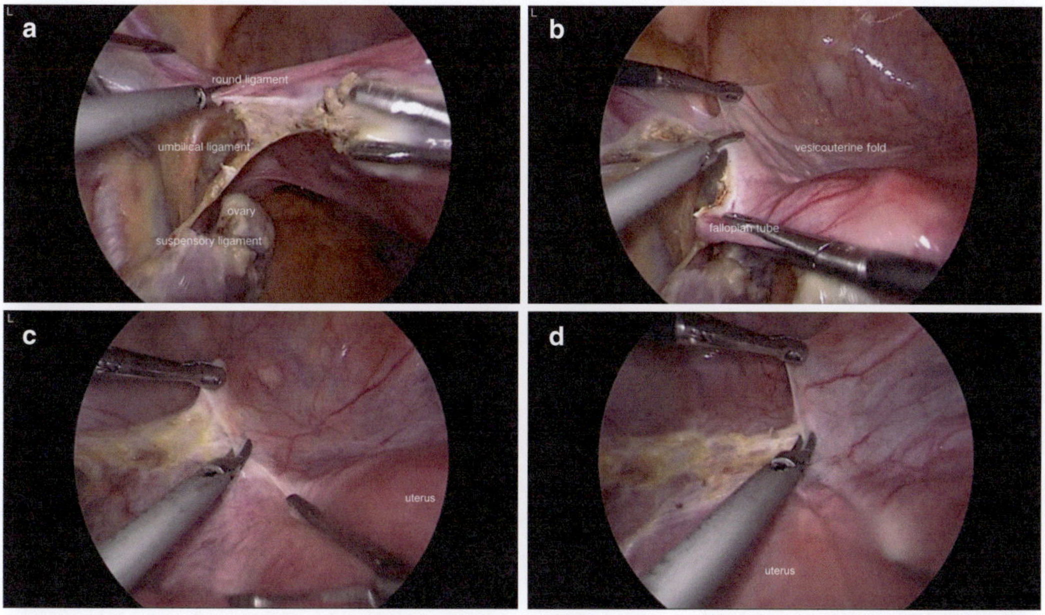

Fig. 8.9 (**a–d**) Open the vesicouterine fold

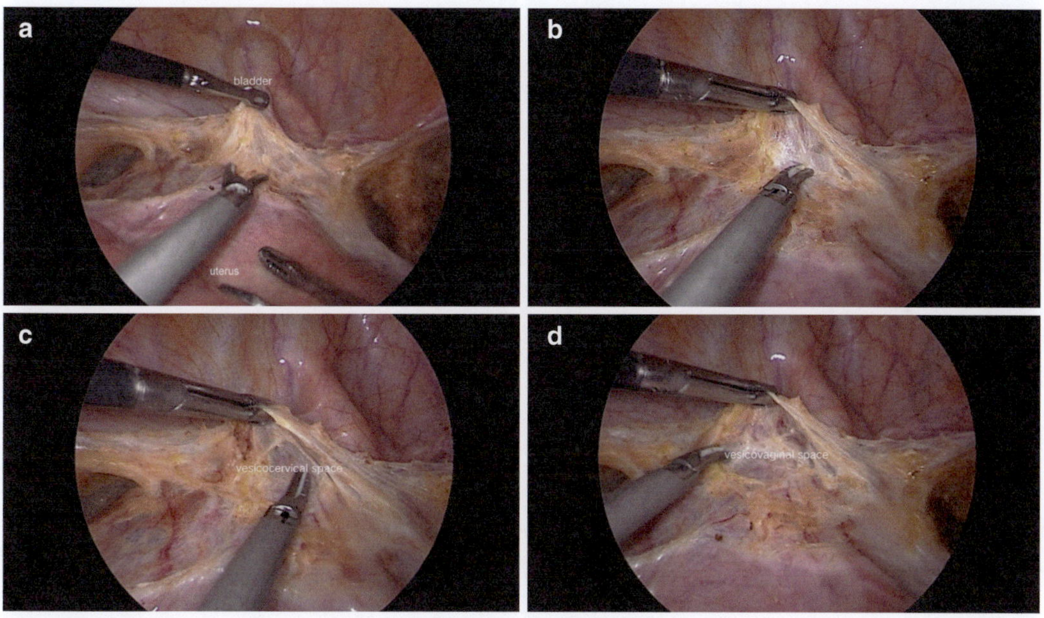

Fig. 8.10 (**a–d**) Expose the vesicocervical space and vesicovaginal space

sect through the white, loose connective tissue until both spaces are fully exposed (Fig. 8.10a–d).

Surgical Experience and Precautions When separating this space, if the separation is biased toward the cervix, bleeding is likely to occur. If the separation enters the area of the cervical fascia, it can cause incomplete cervical membrane structure. From the perspective of embryonic membrane anatomy, this problem can lead to the spread of tumors. If the separation is biased toward the bladder, bladder injury is likely to occur. Type QM-A surgery requires a vaginal resection length of less than 1 cm, so there is no need to expose too much of the vesicovaginal space. Exposing the vaginal wall 1.5 cm below the fornix is sufficient.

8.6 Dissection of the Uterine Artery and Ureter

8.6.1 Separate the Uterine Artery from Its Origin to Its Intersection with the Ureter

Surgical Experience and Precautions During this operation, it is important to maintain adequate tension. During the separation process, pull the lateral peritoneum and ureter medially, and pull the uterine artery to the ventral side. Dissect the dorsal side of the uterine artery to completely expose the proximal segment of the uterine artery.

The transection of the uterine artery should be at the site where it crosses the ureter in type QM-A hysterectomy, due to the very close relationship between the two structures at this point. Directly separating them at the point of crossing can easily lead to bleeding and ureteral injury. Therefore, our team usually prefers to dissect from the origin of the uterine artery.

Continuing to dissect the uterine artery from its origin toward the caudal end, it reaches the intersection of the uterine artery and ureter. At this point, pull the peritoneum and ureter toward the medial and dorsal sides, pull the uterine artery toward the ventral side, and use a combination method of blunt and sharp dissection to free the uterine artery and ureter (Fig. 8.11a–f). At this

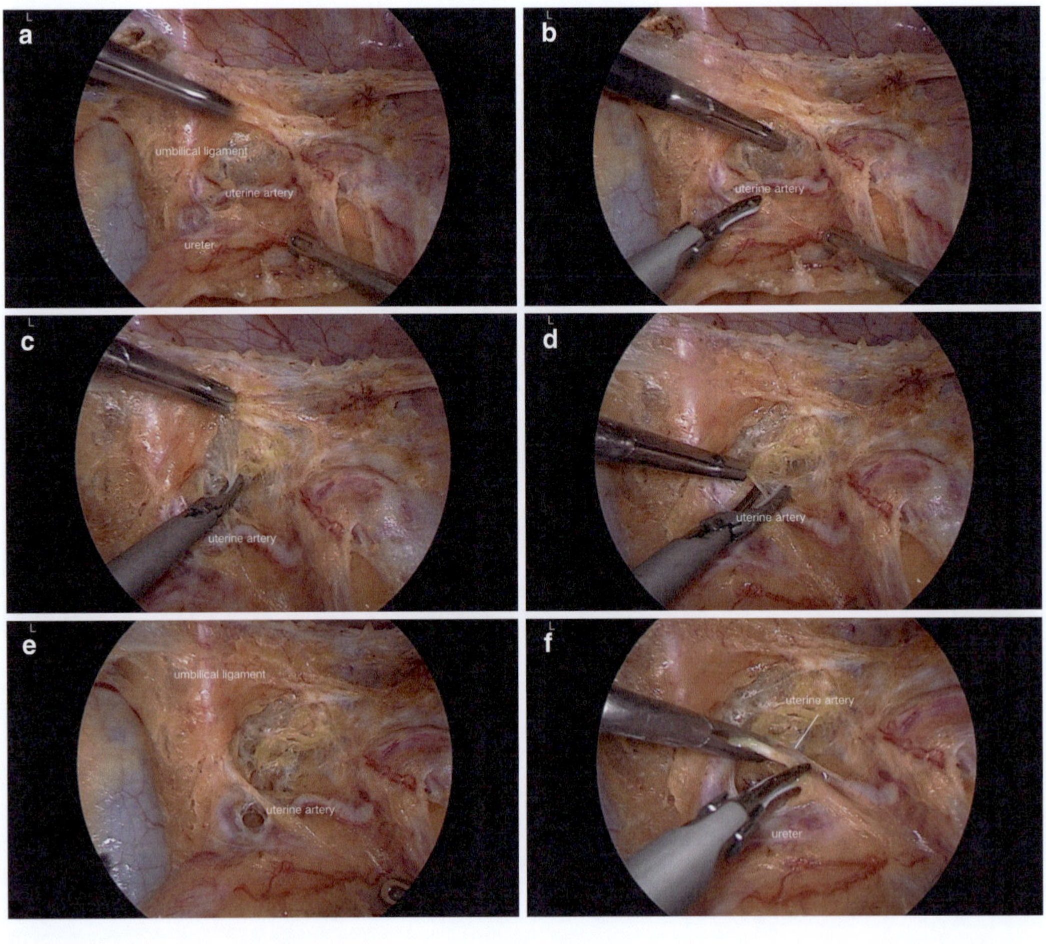

Fig. 8.11 (a–j) Separate the uterine artery

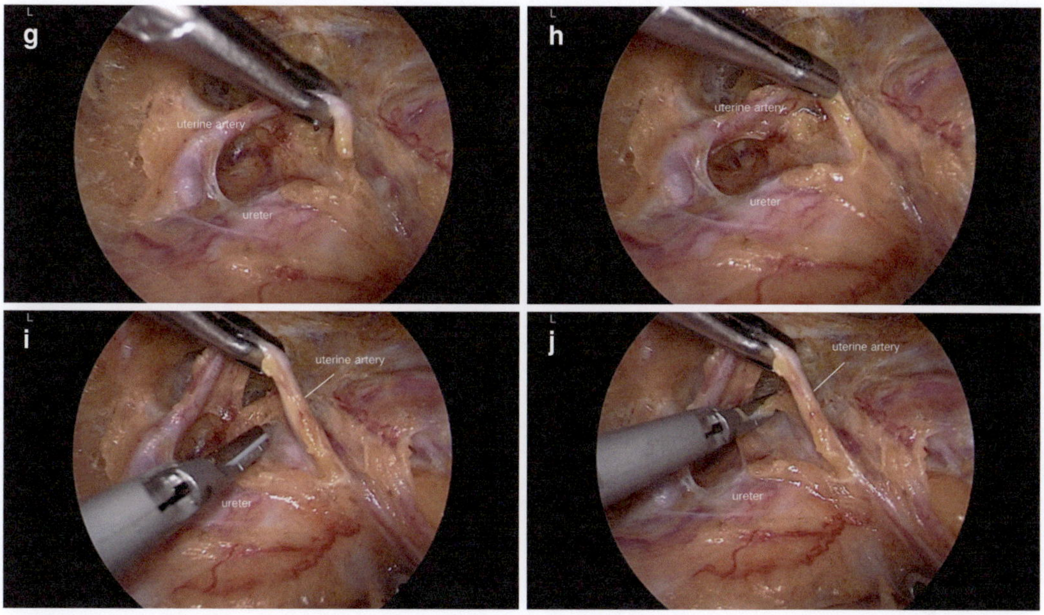

Fig. 8.11 (continued)

point, only the outer part of the ureter is freed, revealing the lateral and ventral sides of the ureter.

Sustainably using sharp dissection, separate the loose connective tissue outside the ureter (Fig. 8.11g–j) to fully separate the space between the ureter and the uterine artery, making subsequent ureteral detachment and vesicocervical ligament processing easier.

8.6.2 Dissection of the Medial Aspect of the Ureter

Surgical Experience and Precautions In Denis Querleu's original article on the Type QM-A classification for radical hysterectomy, he emphasized the importance of opening the "tunnel" for the ureter during surgery. A safe tunnel opening requires adequate exposure of the ureter, which can be achieved by fully exposing it. This facilitates the safe opening of the "tunnel" for the ureter (Fig. 8.12a–d).

8.6.3 Continue Dissecting Along the Ureter Until Reaching the Entrance of the "Tunnel"

To do so, pull the uterine artery ventrally and laterally, and pull the lateral peritoneum and ureter medially and posteriorly using blunt and sharp dissection to separate the ureter and uterine artery. Additionally, pull the ureter laterally, the uterine artery ventrally, and the lateral peritoneum medially and posteriorly toward the entrance of the "tunnel" to free the ureter up to this point (Fig. 8.13a–j).

Surgical Experience and Precautions Our team's experience indicates that to fully release the ureter from the "tunnel," it is necessary to dissect around all sides of the ureter (medial, lateral, ventral, dorsal). However, in Type QM-A surgery, the vesicovaginal ligament does not need to be transected, and therefore, mobilization of the dorsal aspect of the ureter is not necessary.

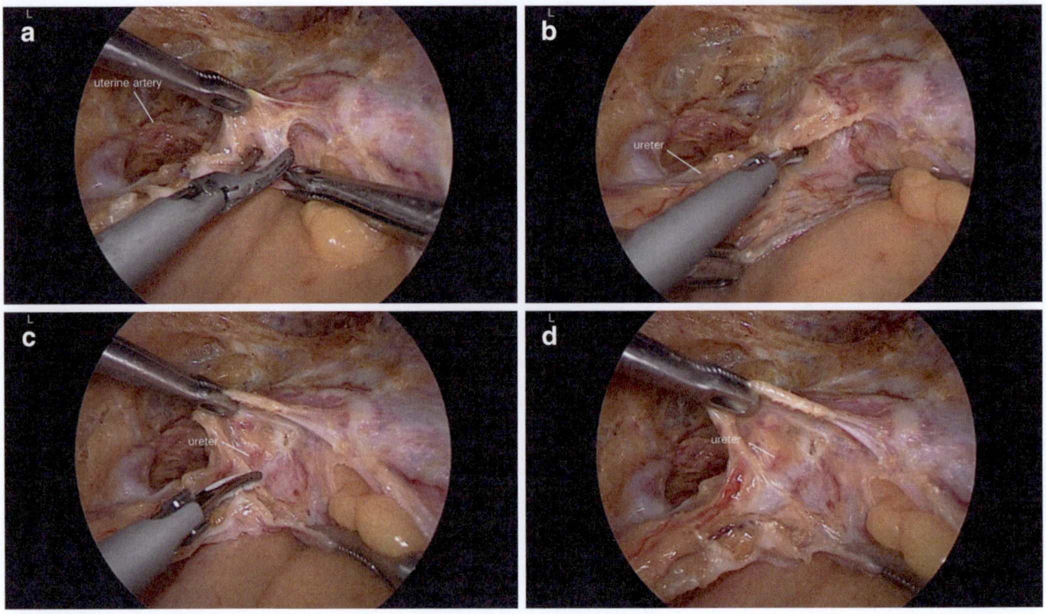

Fig. 8.12 (**a**–**d**) Dissection of the medial aspect of the ureter

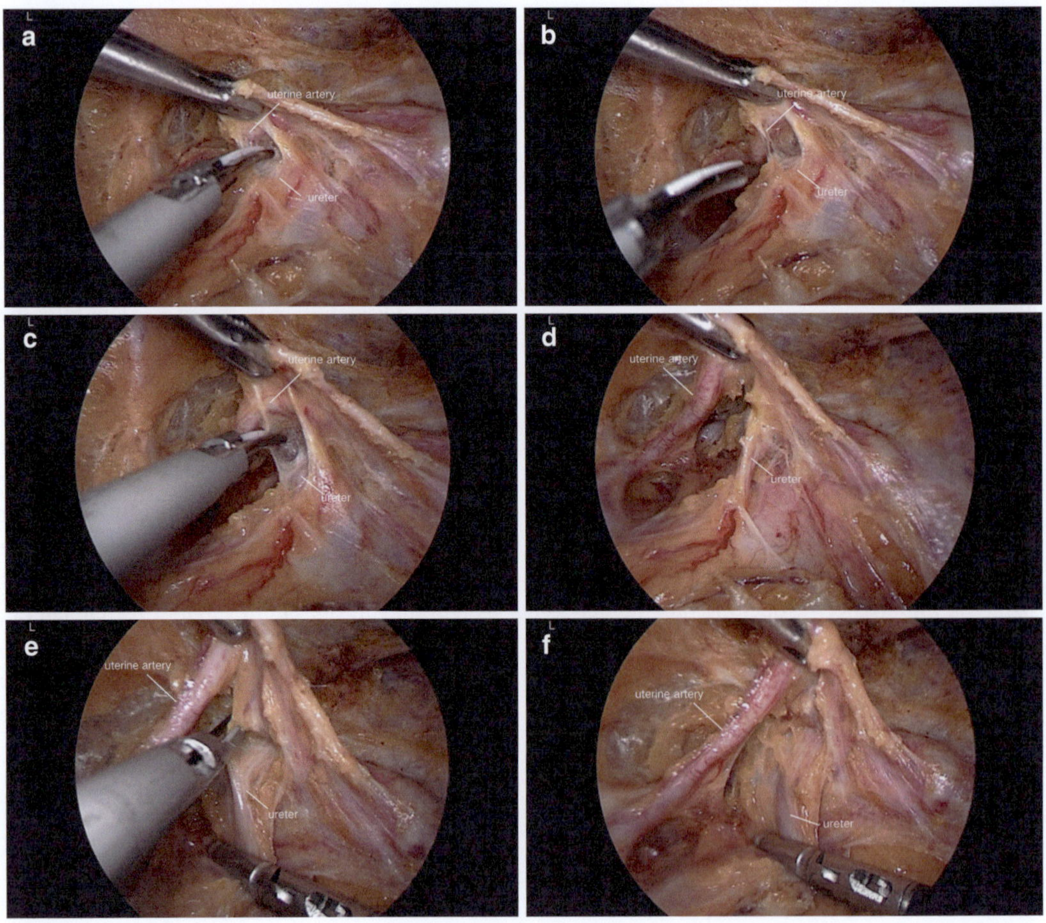

Fig. 8.13 (**a**–**j**) Dissect the ureter until reaching the entrance of the "tunnel"

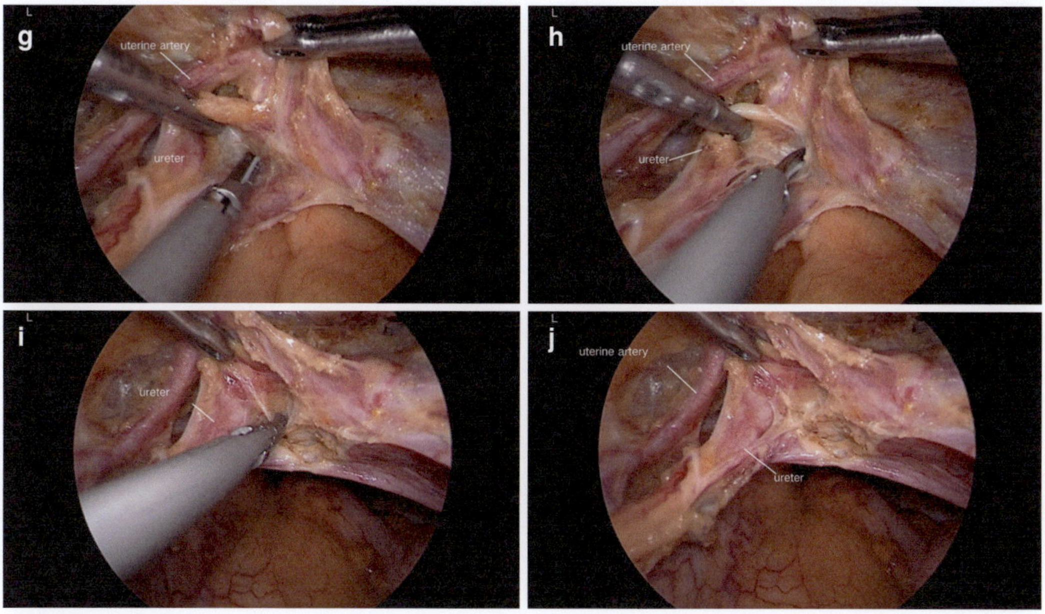

Fig. 8.13 (continued)

8.7 Transection of Uterine Artery

Surgical Experience and Precautions In Type QM-A surgery, it is necessary to transect the uterine artery at the level where it crosses the ureter. Therefore, preoperative dissection and mobilization of the uterine artery and ureter are essential, as they can significantly reduce the risk of ureteral injury during the transection of the uterine artery. However, the steps involved in dissecting the uterine artery and ureter require surgical skills and are not accessible to the general public. As an alternative, after exposing the uterine artery, local dissection and clamping of the artery at the level where it crosses the ureter can be performed, followed by transection of the artery using low-energy instruments. The ureter can then be further dissected.

On the left side, the vesicocervical ligament is transected while preserving the uterine artery, which is applicable for fertility-sparing patients (Fig. 8.14a–c).

On the right side, the uterine artery is transected first, followed by transection of the vesicocervical ligament (Fig. 8.15a–c).

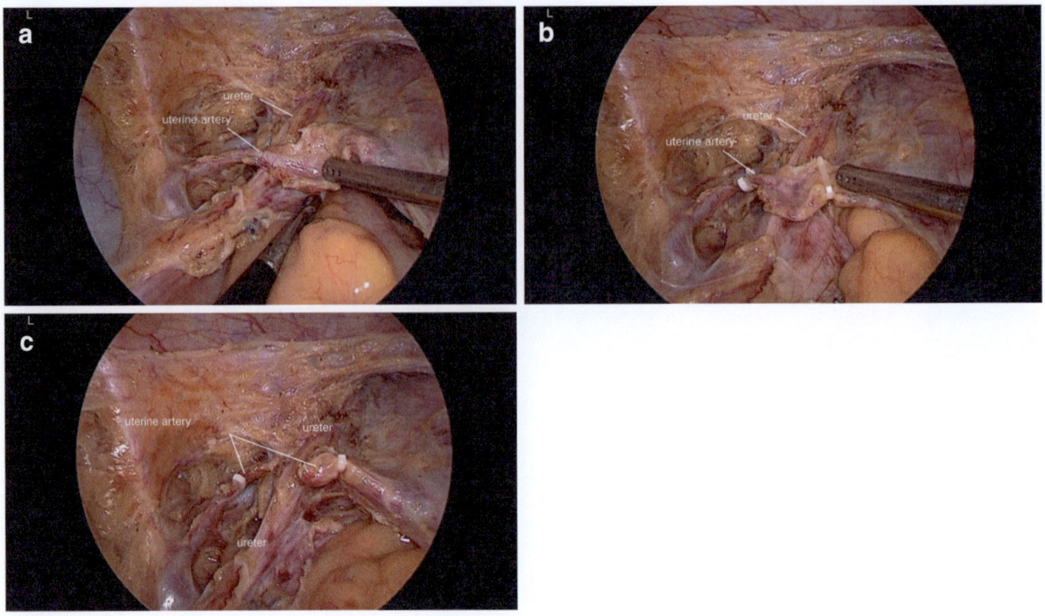

Fig. 8.14 (**a**–**c**) Transect the uterine artery at the level where it crosses the ureter (left side)

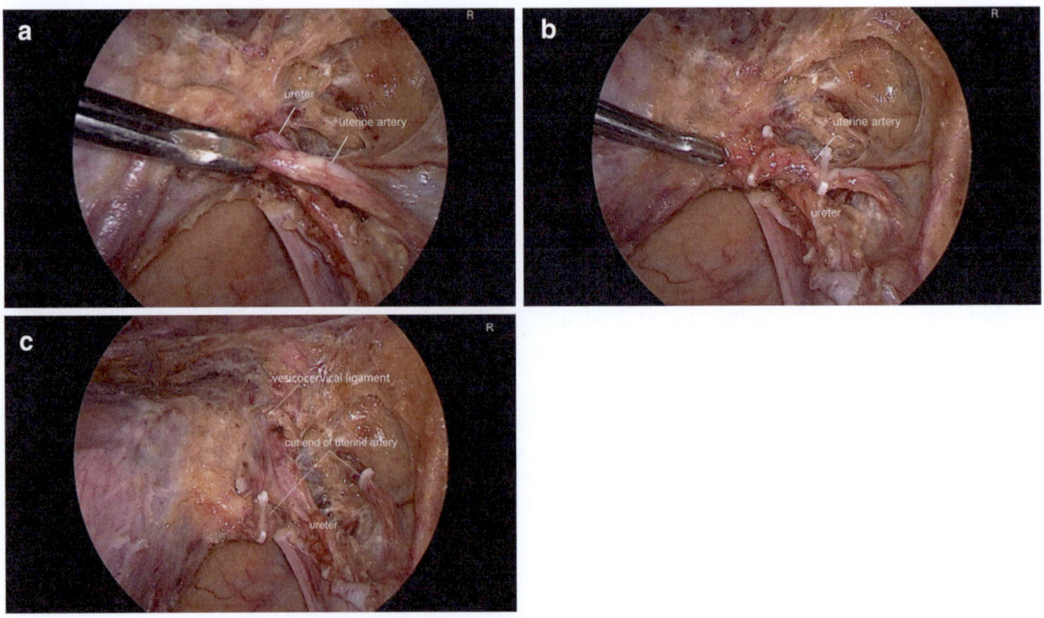

Fig. 8.15 (**a**–**c**) Transect the uterine artery at the level where it crosses the ureter (right side)

8.8 Ventral Parametrium

8.8.1 Exposing the Ureteral "Tunnel" Exit

Enlarge the vesicocervical and vesicovaginal spaces laterally by pulling the bladder in a ventral and lateral direction. Then, use an ultrasonic scalpel to sharply dissect the vesicocervical and vesicovaginal spaces, exposing the ureteral "tunnel" exit (Fig. 8.16a–d).

Surgical Experience and Precautions The vesicocervical ligament is located ventrally to the ureteral tunnel. In Type QM-A surgery, it is necessary to transect the vesicocervical ligament between the ureter and the cervix to open the ureteral "tunnel." Our team's experience has shown that the fourth space is the exit of the tunnel, and therefore, adequate exposure of the fourth space is crucial in managing the vesicocervical ligament.

8.8.2 Transection of Vesicocervical Ligament

The ureteral clamps are placed separately in the exit and entrance of the tunnel to protect the ureter during the transection of the vesicocervical ligament. The vesicocervical ligament is then clamped laterally and ventrally before being transected using an ultrasonic scalpel.

Surgical Experience and Precautions Type QM-A surgery does not require mobilization of the ureter laterally, so there is a concern for kinking or thermal injury to the distal ureter due to en bloc use of heat-generating devices. To avoid ureteral damage, we place ureteral clamps separately at the exit and entrance of the tunnel and transect the vesicocervical ligament between the ureter and cervix (Figs. 8.17a–d and 8.18a–d).

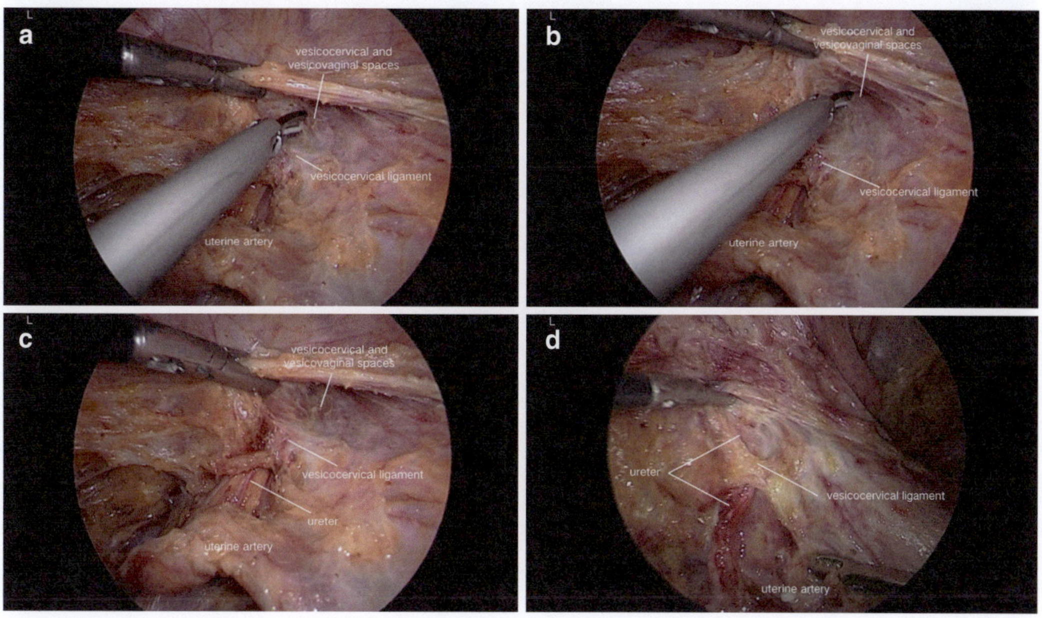

Fig. 8.16 (**a**–**d**) Expose the ureter "tunnel" exit

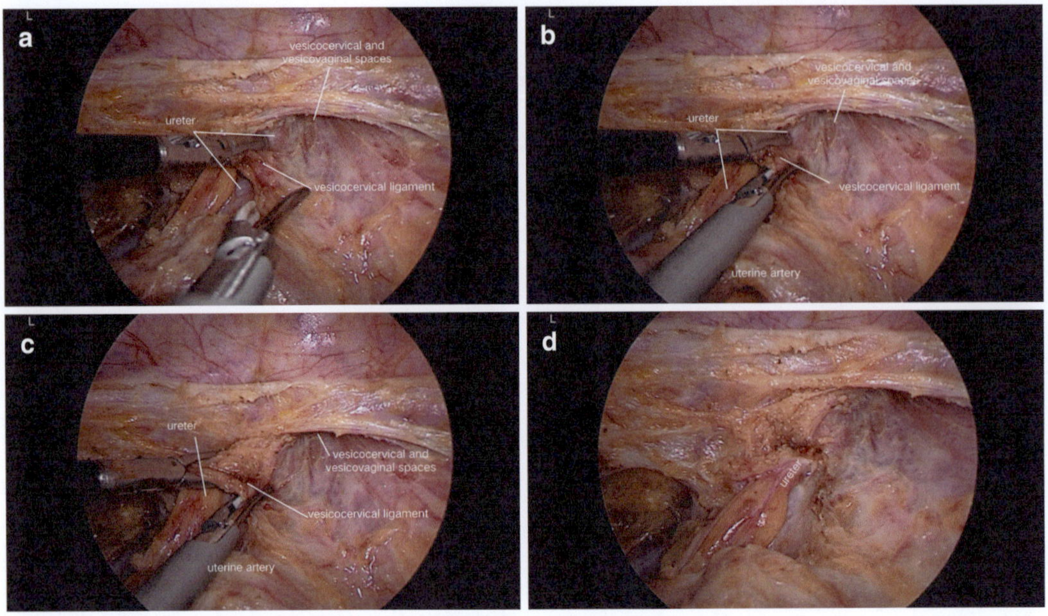

Fig. 8.17 (**a**–**d**) Transect the left vesicocervical ligament

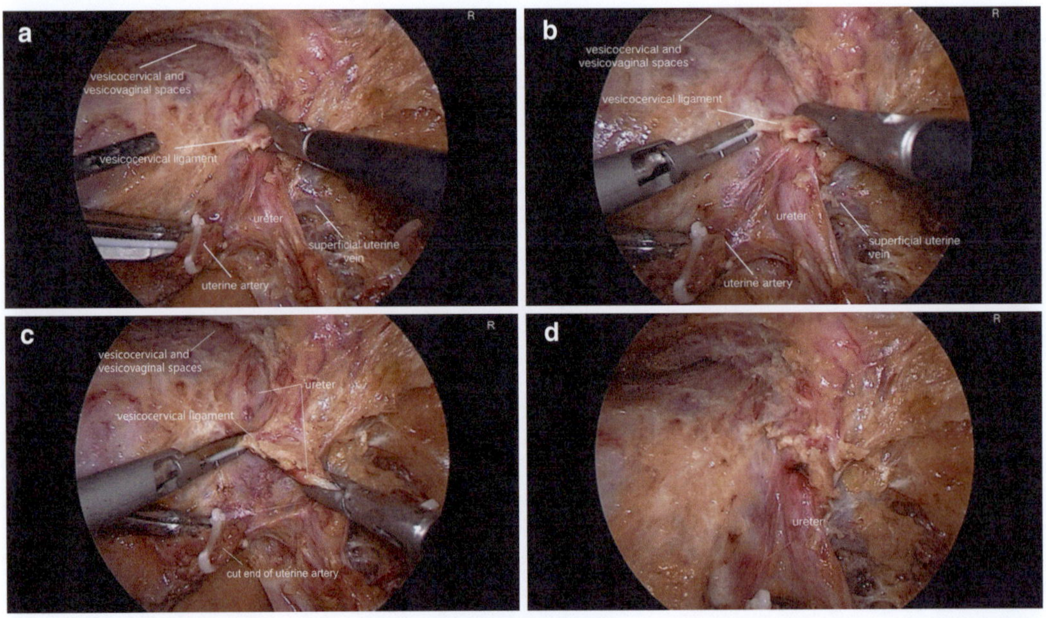

Fig. 8.18 (**a**–**d**) Transect the right vesicocervical ligament

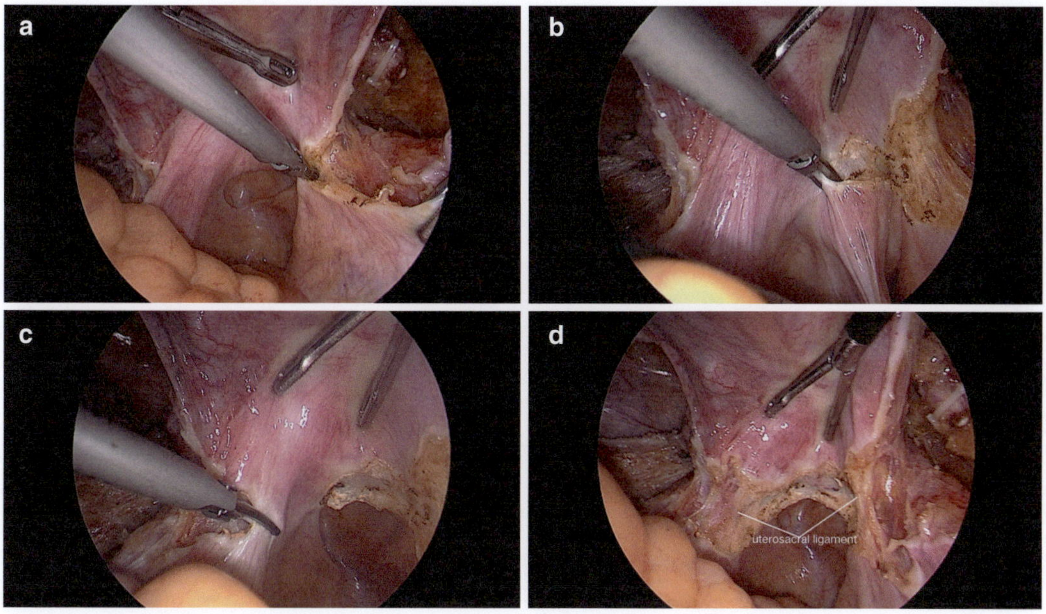

Fig. 8.19 (**a–d**) Divide the peritoneum at the Pouch of Douglas

8.9 Dorsal Parametrium

The peritoneum at the Pouch of Douglas is divided, and the dorsal parametrium is transected at approximately 5 mm. The peritoneum between the uterus and rectum is then lifted from the base of the Pouch of Douglas, and an incision is made on the elevated peritoneum, which is extended with an ultrasonic scalpel across the dorsal side of the cervix (Fig. 8.19a–d).

Surgical Experience and Precautions The Type QM-A surgery requires minimal excision of the dorsal parametrium, approximately 5 mm is sufficient. To avoid injury to the rectum, it is necessary to open the base of the Pouch of Douglas.

8.10 Lateral Parametrium Transection

Bipolar forceps seal the lateral parametrium between ureter and cervix and transect the lateral parametrium using an ultrasonic scalpel.

Surgical Experience and Precautions Type QM-A surgery requires the removal of only the parametrial tissue, without removing the paracolpium. The parametrial tissue is removed between the ureter and the cervix, and there is no need to mobilize the ureter laterally after transecting the vesicocervical ligament. Using ureteral forceps to pull the ureter laterally is safe during lateral parametrial transection (Figs. 8.20a–d and 8.21a–d).

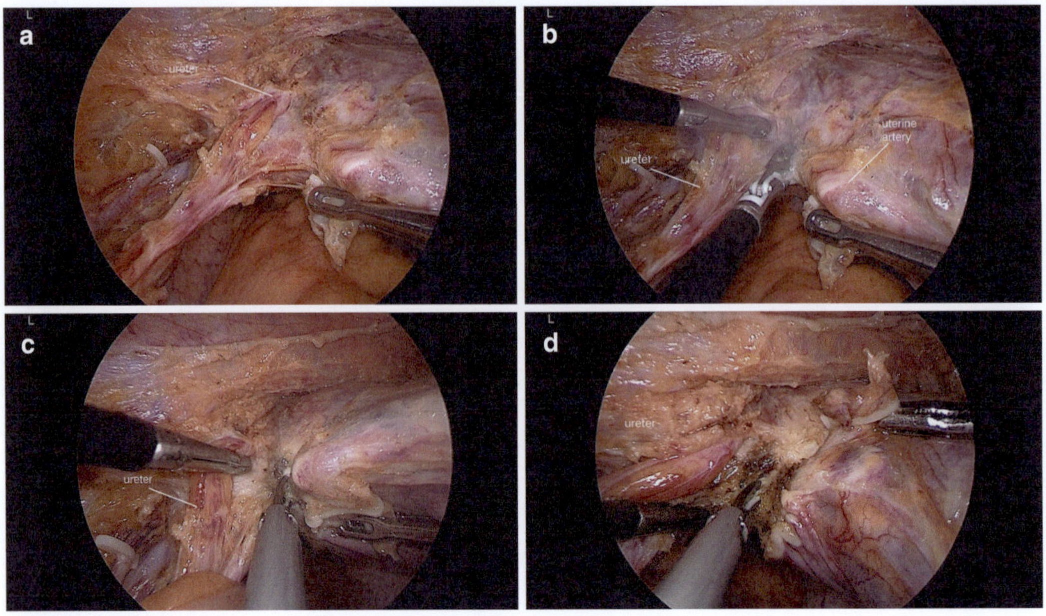

Fig. 8.20 (**a**–**d**) Transect left lateral parametrium

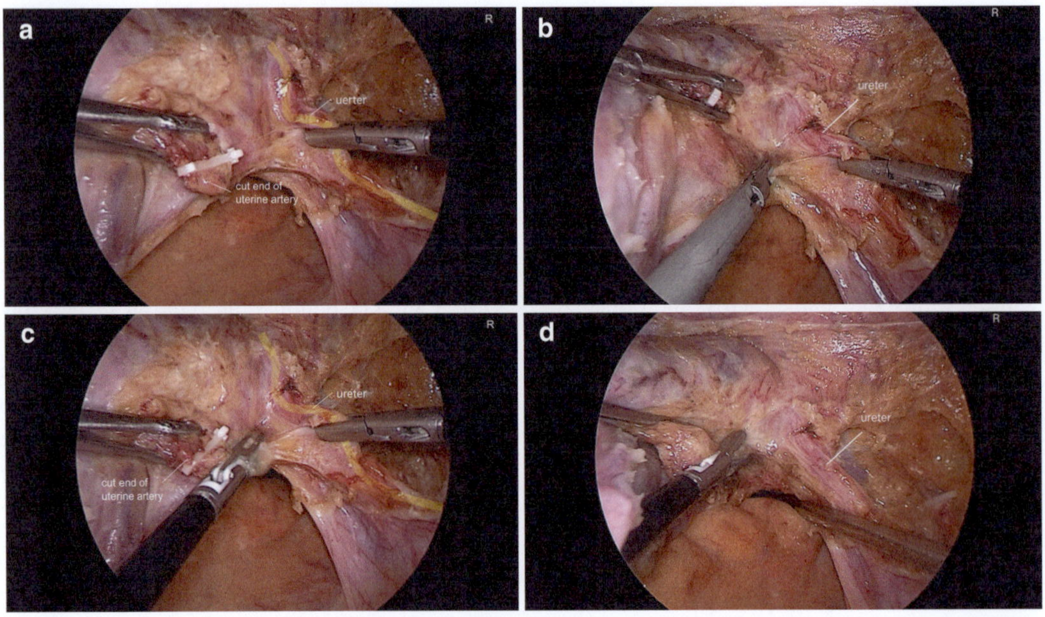

Fig. 8.21 (**a**–**d**) Transect right lateral parametrium

8.11 Amputation of Vaginal Wall

Amputation of vaginal wall with monopolar or ultrasonic scalpel at about 1 cm below the vaginal fornix (Figs. 8.22a–c and 8.23a–c).

Surgical Experience and Precautions Most of these patients experience obvious vaginal congestion after cervical conization. Therefore, to reduce bleeding, bipolar coagulation should be applied to the vaginal wall prior to amputation.

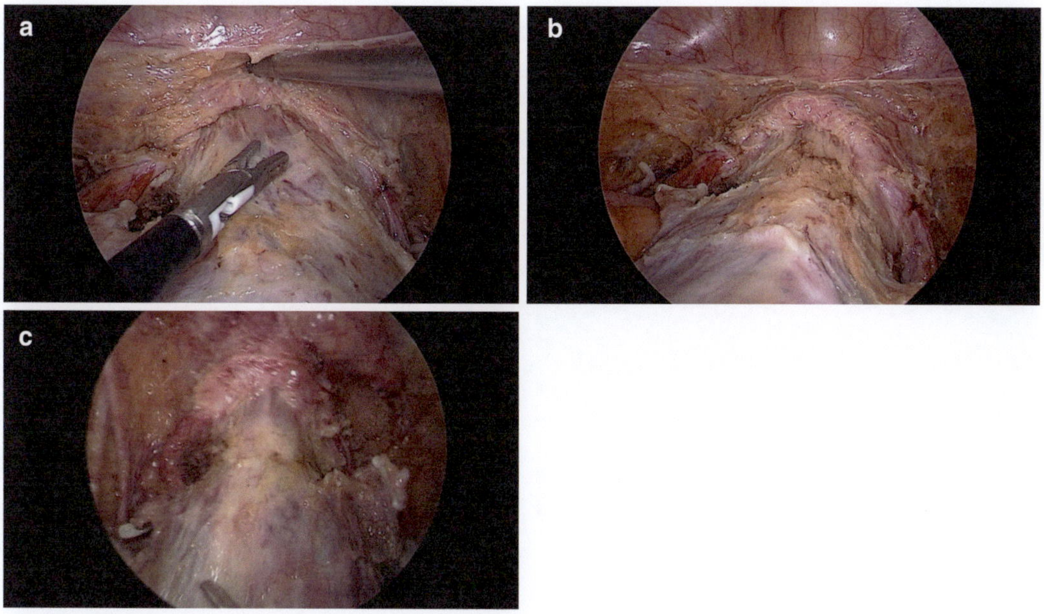

Fig. 8.22 (**a**–**c**) Coagulate the vaginal wall with monopolar

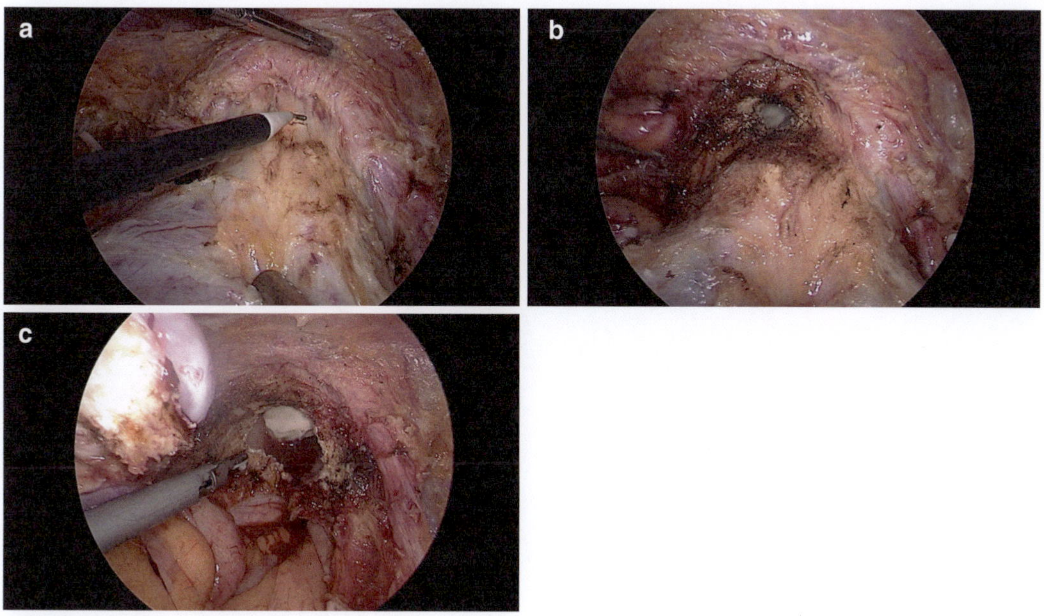

Fig. 8.23 (**a**–**c**) Amputation of vaginal wall

Before the procedure, the vagina should be rinsed repeatedly with 200 ml of sterile distilled water to ensure it is free of tumors.

8.12 Closure of the Vaginal Cuff

Absorbable suture can be used to continuously suture the vaginal cuff (Fig. 8.24).

Careful observation of the pelvic cavity is performed to identify bleeding and ensure hemostasis. The pelvic cavity is then washed with 3000 ml sterile distilled water at 42 °C.

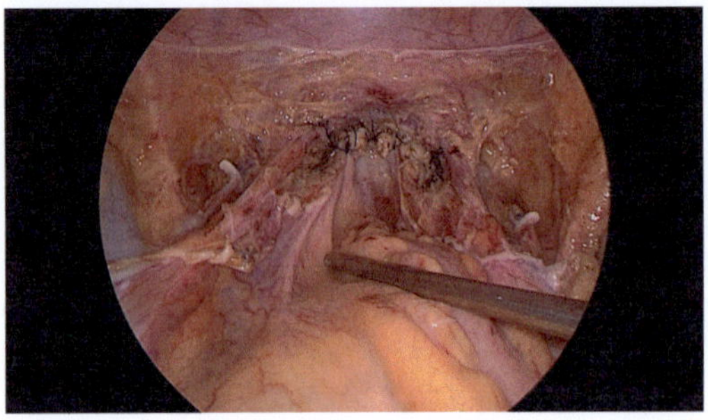

Fig. 8.24 Closure of the vaginal cuff

The QM-A Type Radical Hysterectomy (Laparoscopic) is shown in Video 8.1. The QM-A Type Radical Hysterectomy (Robotic) is shown in Video 8.2.

References

1. NCCN. NCCN clinical practice guidelines in oncology—cervical cancer. (2022-12-23) [2023-03-15]. https://www.nccn.org/professionals/physician_gls/pdf/cervical.pdf
2. Querleu D, Cibula D, Abu-Rustum NR. Update on the Querleu-Morrow classification of radical hysterectomy. Ann Surg Oncol. 2017;2017(24):3406–12.
3. Querleu D, Morrow CP. Classification of radical hysterectomy. Lancet Oncol. 2008;9:297–303.
4. Ramirez PT, Frumovitz M, Pareja R, et al. Minimally invasive versus abdominal radical hysterectomy for cervical cancer. N Engl J Med. 2018;379:1895–904.
5. Dietl A, Klar M, Aumann K. Minimally invasive surgery for early-stage cervical cancer: is the uterine manipulator a risk factor? Am J Obstet Gynecol. 2019;221:537–8.

9 Type QM-B Radical Hysterectomy

Jun Wang and Ya Li

A surgical treatment approach is applicable to patients with Stage IA1 cervical cancer with vascular invasion and Stage IA2 cervical cancer. Most of these patients are diagnosed as Stage IA1 with negative margins after cone biopsy [1–3]. Research has indicated that squamous cell carcinoma of the cervix has a low probability of skip metastasis, whereas cervical adenocarcinoma may have the potential for skip metastasis. Despite negative margins, we cannot be certain that there are no residual cancerous lesions within the cervix. Therefore, our team still performs this surgery using the suspension technique for the uterus, avoiding the potential tumor dissemination that may result from using a uterine manipulator. During the closure of the vaginal cuff, a circular suture is used to close the vagina, and 200 ml of sterile distilled water is repeatedly used to irrigate the vagina. We make every effort to adhere to the principle of en bloc resection to ensure a tumor-free outcome.

9.1 Exposure of the Lateral Retroperitoneal Space

Pull the ovary suspensory ligament medially and make a sharp incision at the intersection of the ovary suspensory ligament, the common iliac vessel, and the ureter to open the lateral peritoneum. Continue the incision along the gap between the iliac vessels and the psoas muscle up to the junction of the round ligament and the lateral peritoneum. From the junction of the round ligament and the lateral peritoneum, make a sharp incision along the round ligament toward the uterine angle, thereby exposing the posterior lateral peritoneal space (Fig. 9.1**a**–**f**).

Supplementary Information The online version contains supplementary material available at https://doi.org/10.1007/978-981-97-7687-0_9.

J. Wang (✉) · Y. Li
Department of Gynecology and Obstetrics, Second Affiliated Hospital of Dalian Medical University, Dalian, China

S. Han, J. Wang (eds.), *Open, Laparoscopic, and Robotic Surgery for Cervical Cancer*,
https://doi.org/10.1007/978-981-97-7687-0_9

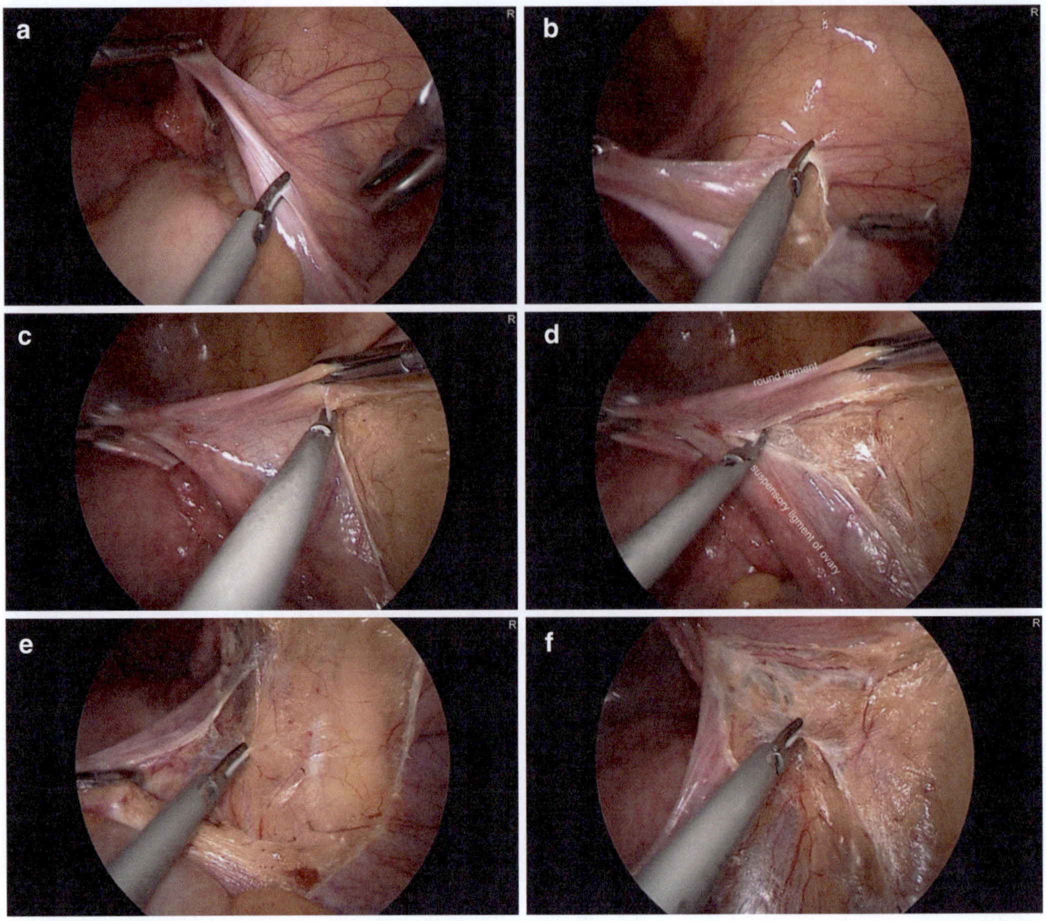

Fig. 9.1 (**a**–**f**) Exposure of the lateral retroperitoneal space

9.2 Management of Adnexa and Uterine Round Ligament

Open the lateral retroperitoneal space and visualize the ureter with a clear view. Gently pull the ovary suspensory ligament ventrally, and then sharply skeletonize and isolate the suspensory ligament. Apply vascular clamps to occlude the ovary suspensory ligament and transect it using an ultrasonic scalpel (Fig. 9.2**a**–**f**).

Continue by closely dissecting the lateral peritoneum along the ovary suspensory ligament toward the uterine angle, and then sharply cut the round ligament near the pelvic wall (Fig. 9.3**a**–**d**) and then sharply separate it toward the uterine angle (Fig. 9.4**a**, **b**).

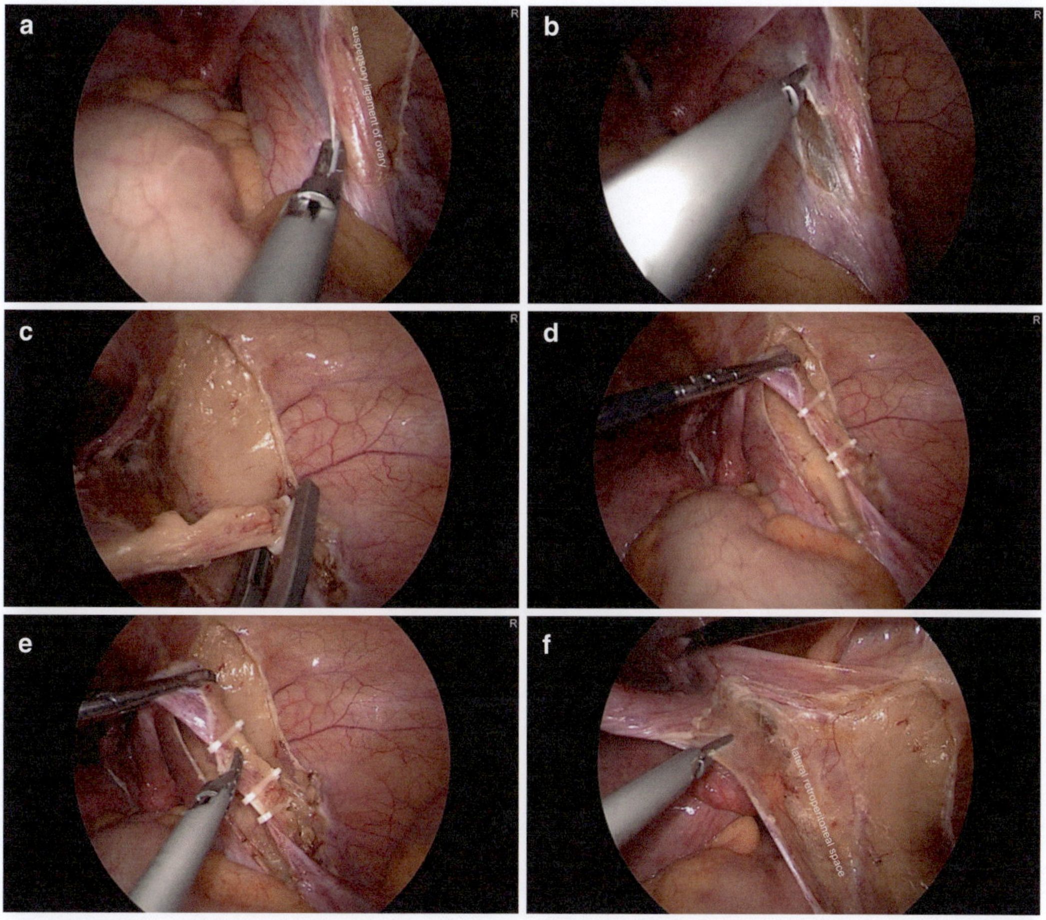

Fig. 9.2 (**a–f**) Transect suspensory ligament

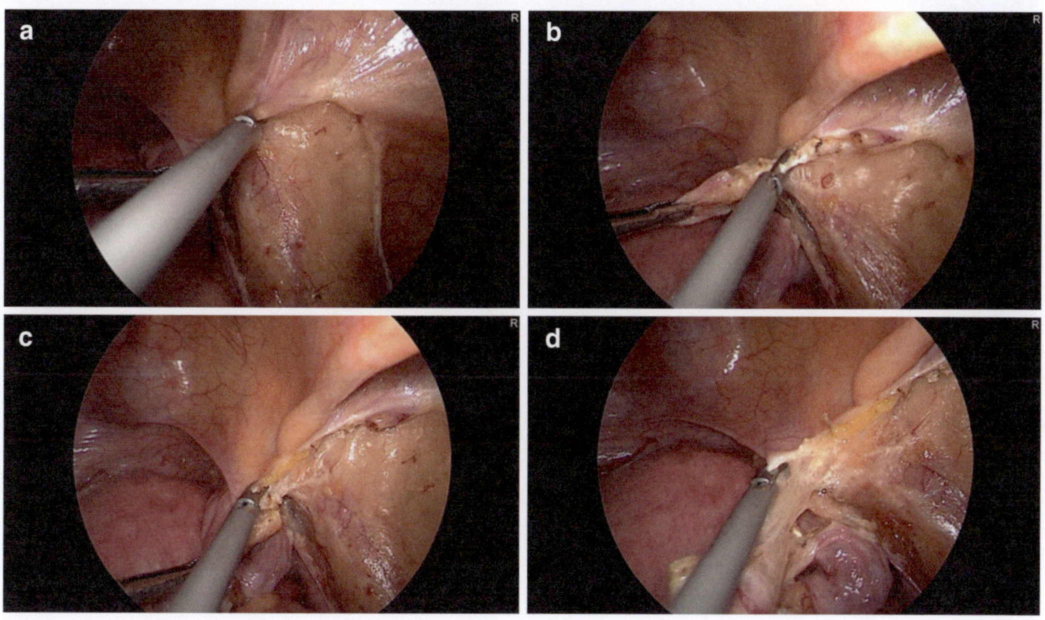

Fig. 9.3 (**a–d**) Sharply cut the round ligament

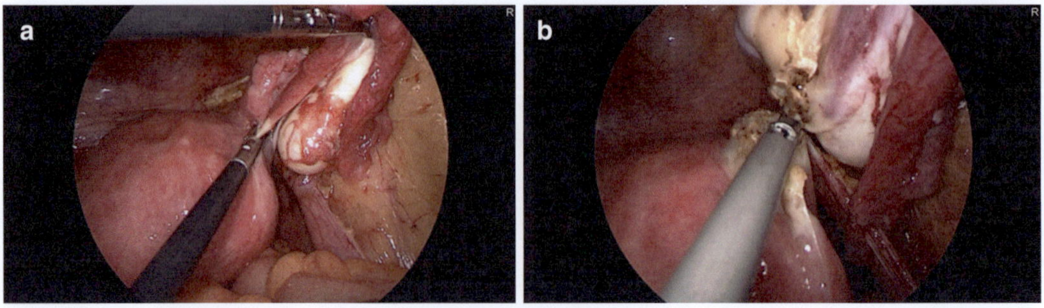

Fig. 9.4 (**a**, **b**) Salpingectomy

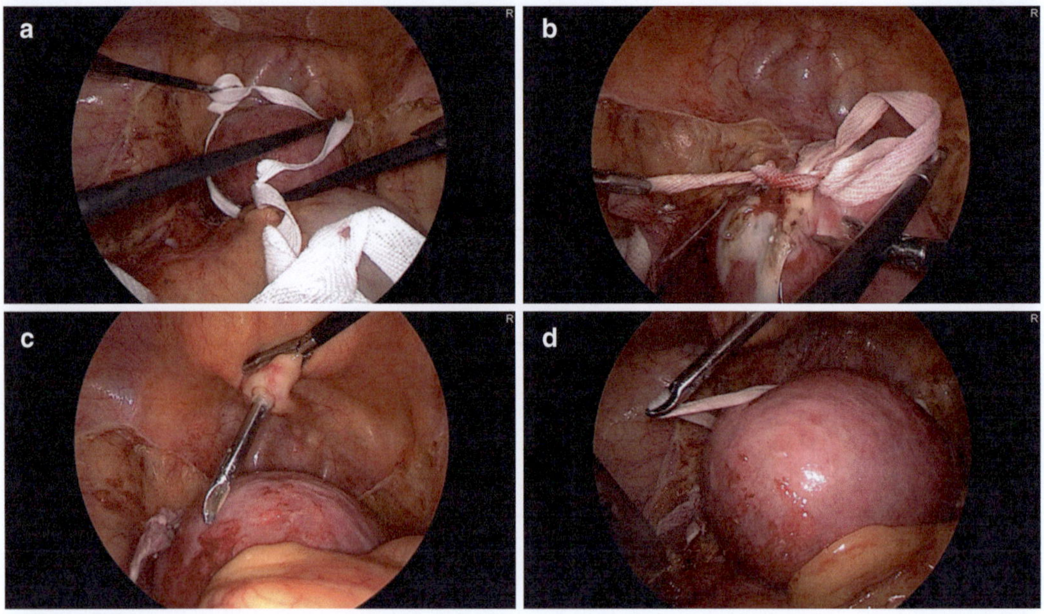

Fig. 9.5 (**a–d**) Suspend uterus

9.3 Uterine Suspension

For cases with relatively large uteri, the tension provided by absorbable sutures at the uterine fundus for suspension may be insufficient, resulting in suboptimal lifting effects. Our team is accustomed to ligating the uterine isthmus with a long tape after excising the bilateral adnexa. Subsequently, a needle holder is inserted through the small incision above the pubic symphysis to lift and suspend the uterus by the ligated tape (Fig. 9.5**a–d**).

9.4 Exposure of the Lateral Parametrium

9.4.1 Exposure of the Obturator Space

Pull the lateral peritoneum medially and use an ultrasonic scalpel to sharply dissect the lateral retroperitoneal space and free the internal iliac artery. First, dissect the obturator space along the outer edge of the internal iliac artery (Fig. 9.6**a**–**f**).

Surgical Experience and Precautions The purpose of freeing the obturator space is to provide sufficient tension for pulling the internal iliac artery laterally, facilitating the subsequent handling of the lateral parametrial tissues.

9.4.2 Exposure of the Uterine Artery

By pulling the internal iliac artery laterally and the lateral peritoneum medially, the course of the uterine artery is exposed. In cases where the uterine artery course is not easily identifiable, a sharp dissection using an ultrasonic scalpel can be performed between the ureter and the internal iliac artery. This approach exposes the course of the uterine artery, including the Latzko's pararectal space on the cranial side and the paravesical space on the caudal side (Figs. 9.7**a**–**d** and 9.8**a**–**d**).

Surgical Experience and Precautions In type B surgery, it is required to resect the lateral parametrial tissues at the level of the ureters. Our

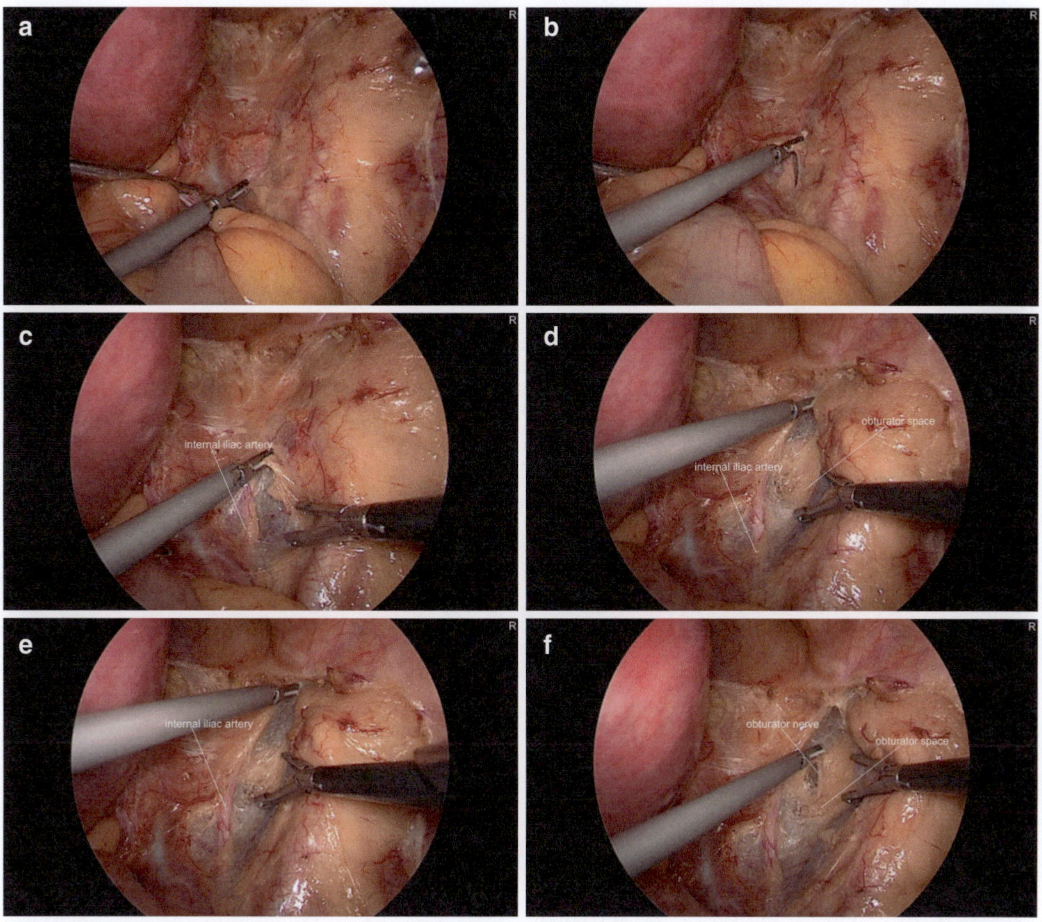

Fig. 9.6 (**a**–**f**) Expose the obturator space

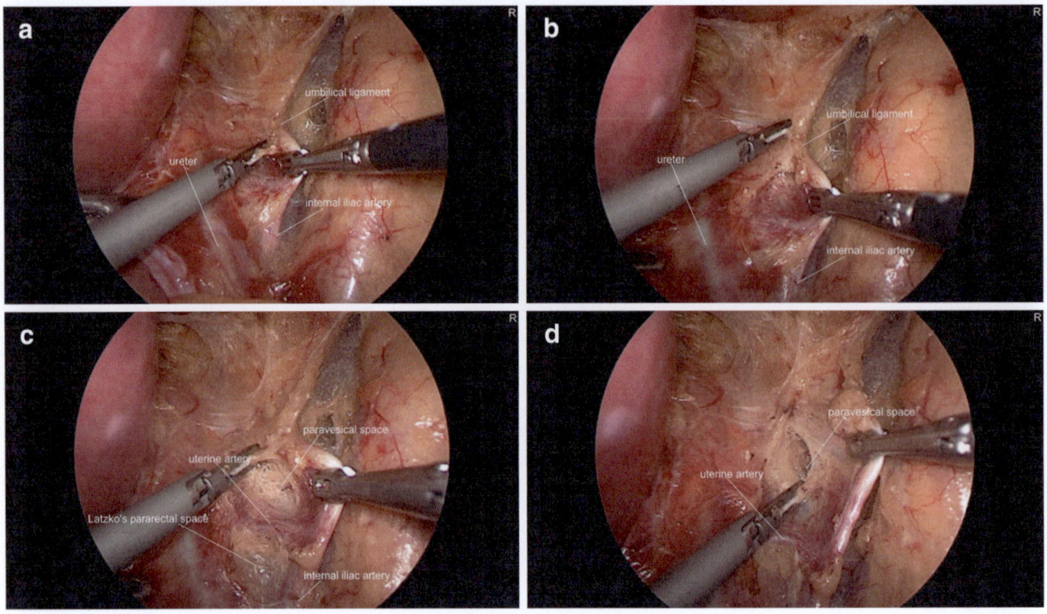

Fig. 9.7 (**a–d**) Expose Latzko's pararectal space

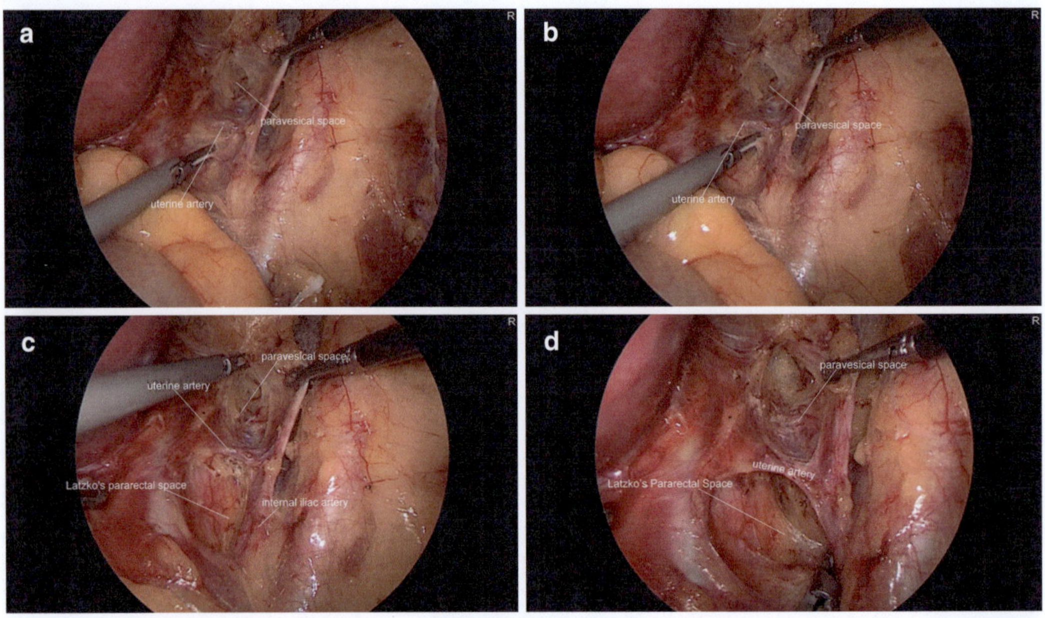

Fig. 9.8 (**a–d**) Expose paravesical space

team believes that directly transecting the uterine artery above the ureters increases the risk of ureteral injury. Therefore, we recommend partially separating the Latzko's pararectal and paravesical spaces to expose a portion of the proximal uterine artery before safely transecting it.

9.4.3 Exposure of Okabayashi's Pararectal Space

Gently pull the lateral peritoneum medially while retracting the ureter laterally. Meticulously dissect the Okabayashi's pararectal space between

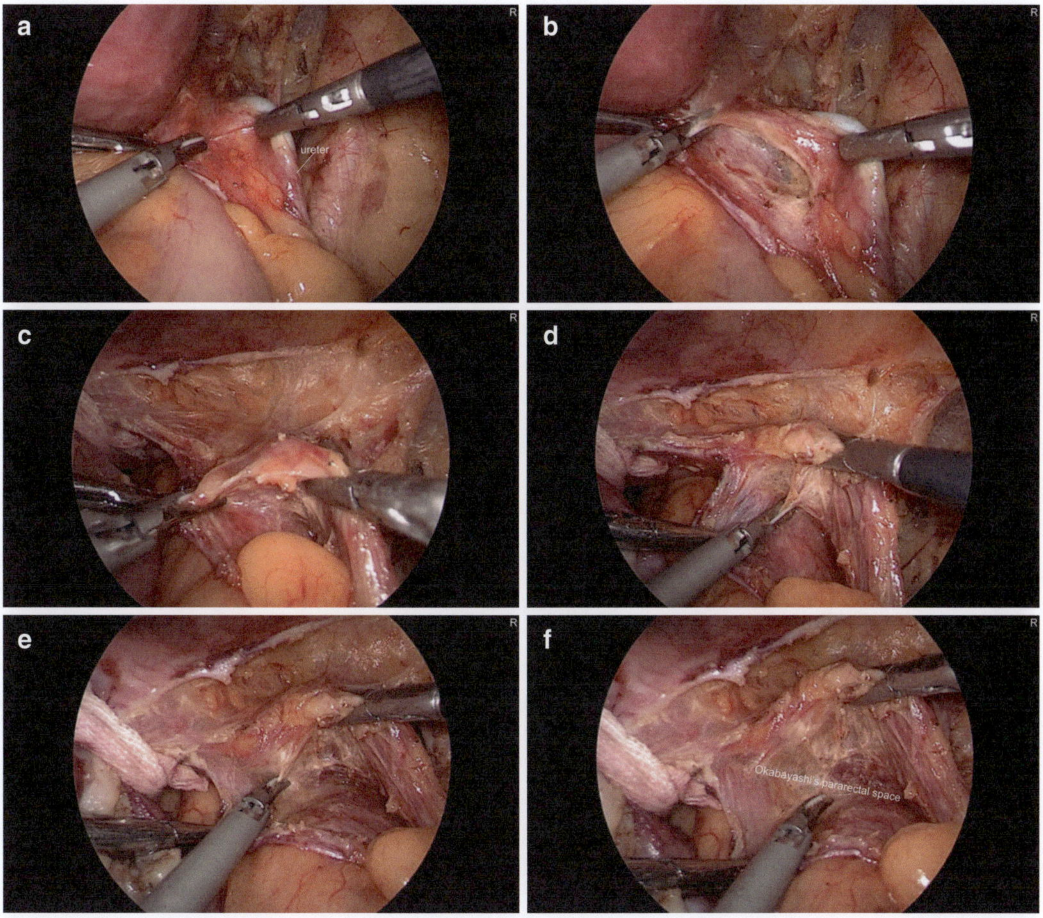

Fig. 9.9 (**a–f**) Expose Okabayashi's pararectal space

the lateral peritoneum and the ureter using an ultrasonic scalpel, gradually extending it toward the dorsal and caudal directions, and continue the dissection until it reaches the vicinity of the parametrium (Fig. 9.9**a**–**f**).

Surgical Experience and Precautions During the opening of Okabayashi's pararectal space, it is crucial to maintain the integrity of the mesoureter. Even if inadvertent perforation of the mesoureter occurs, the dissection should be continued deeper into the retroperitoneal space to separate the hypogastric nerve plexus from the peritoneum of the rectal sidewall. The lateral aspect of Okabayashi's pararectal space includes structures such as the ureter, mesoureter, and the hypogastric nerve plexus.

9.5 Dorsal Parametrial Dissection

In type B surgery, the resection range of the dorsal parametrial uterosacral ligament extends to the level of the rectal peritoneum fold. Our team is accustomed to performing a gentle sharp dissection of the rectal sidewall mesentery from the inner edge of the uterosacral ligament. This approach ensures precise removal of the rectal peritoneum fold while minimizing the risk of injuring the rectum during the transection of the uterosacral ligament. Moreover, it helps avoid inadvertent entry into the wrong plane when opening the rectal peritoneum fold from the midline, which could lead to dissection difficulties. In case of any entry into the wrong plane, the correct planes on both sides can be used to reestablish the correct position between the anterior wall of the rectum and the posterior wall of the vagina. (Figs. 9.10, 9.11, 9.12, 9.13, and 9.14).

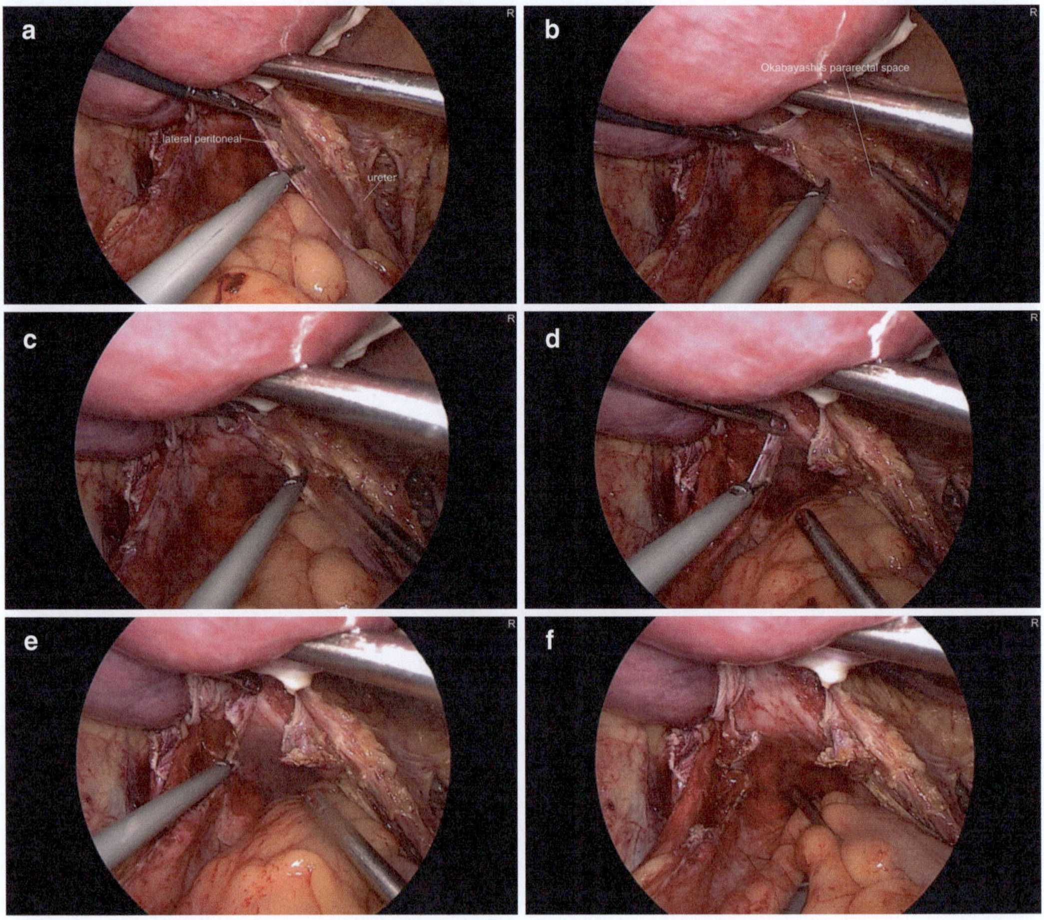

Fig. 9.10 (**a–f**) Open the lateral peritoneum

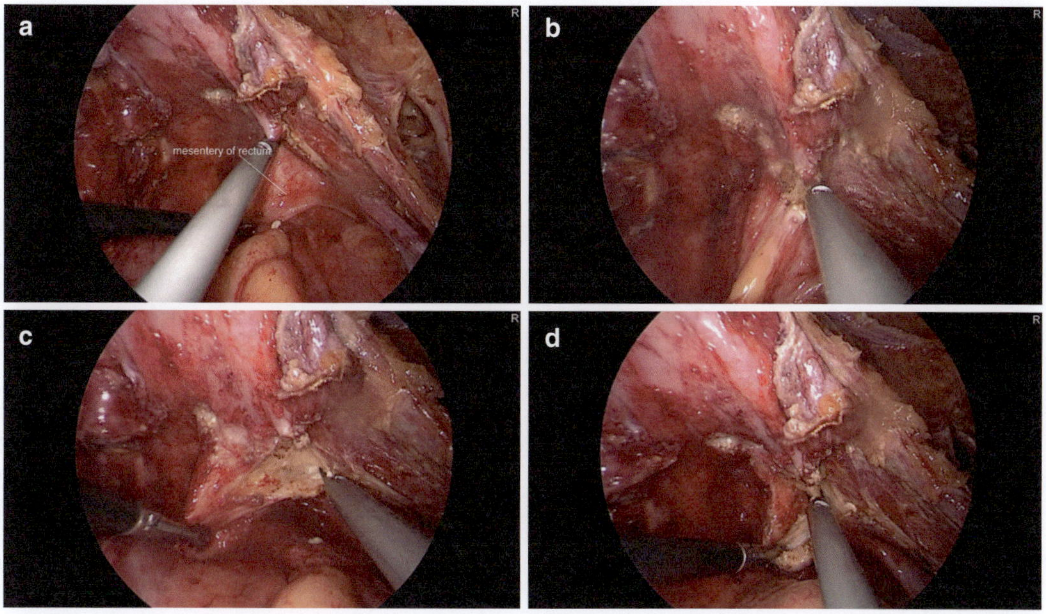

Fig. 9.11 (**a–d**) Sharply dissect the right rectal sidewall mesentery from the inner edge of the uterosacral ligament

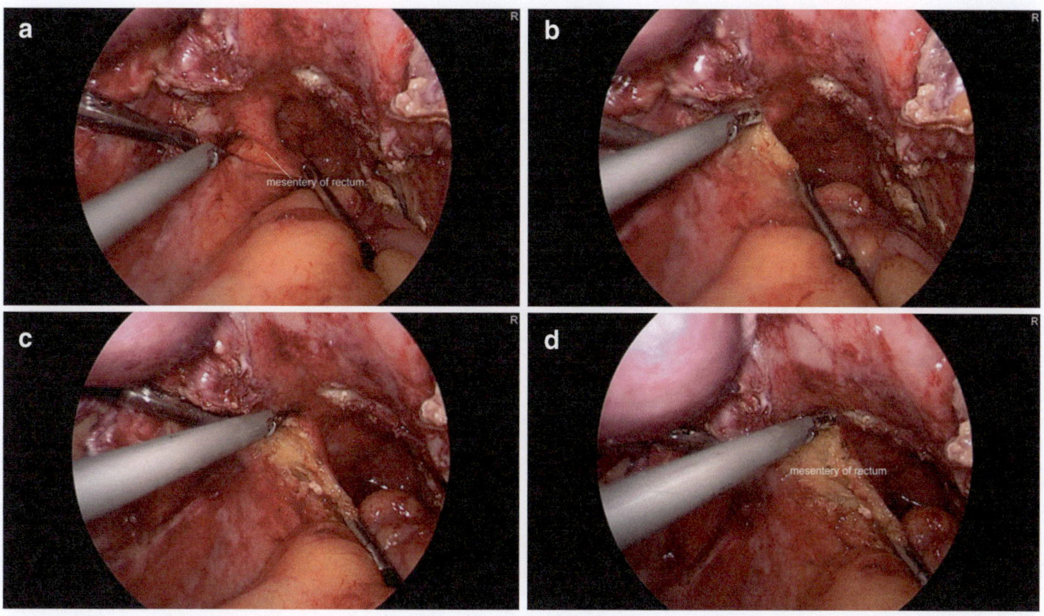

Fig. 9.12 (**a–d**) Sharp dissect the left rectal sidewall mesentery from the inner edge of the uterosacral ligament

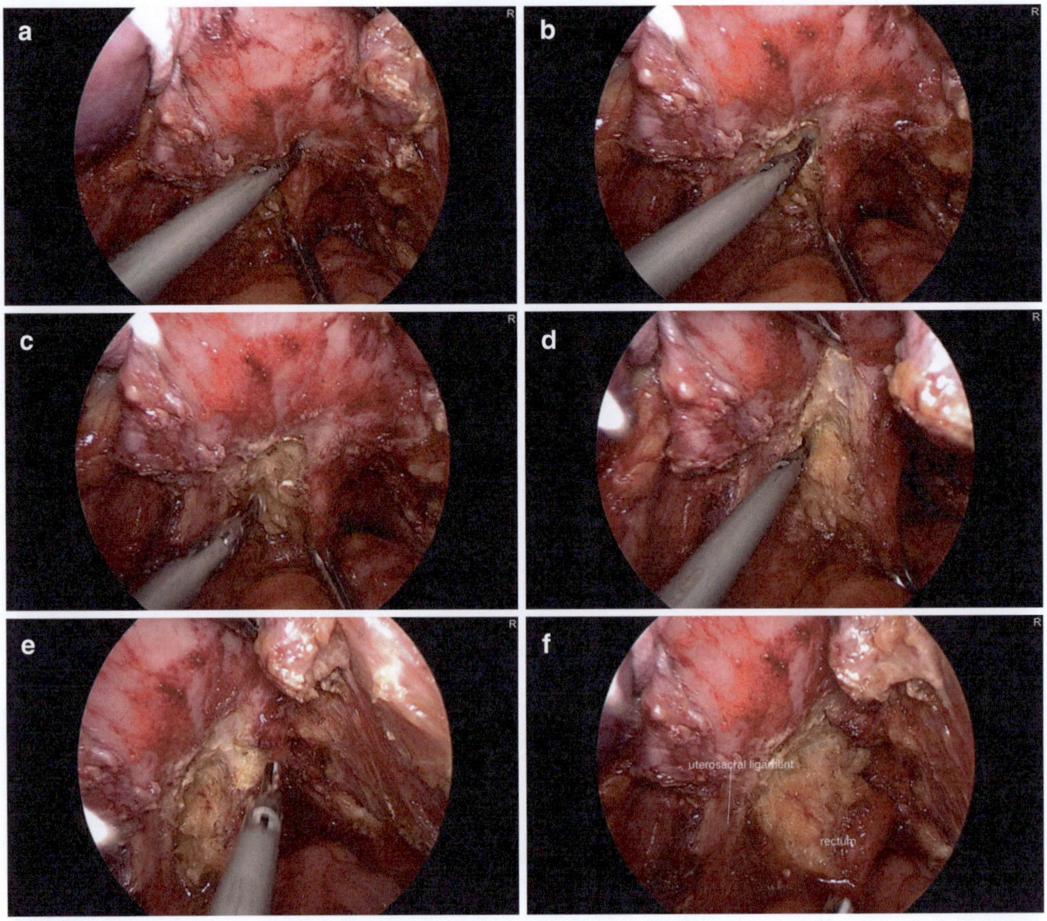

Fig. 9.13 (**a**–**f**) Expose the rectal peritoneum reflection

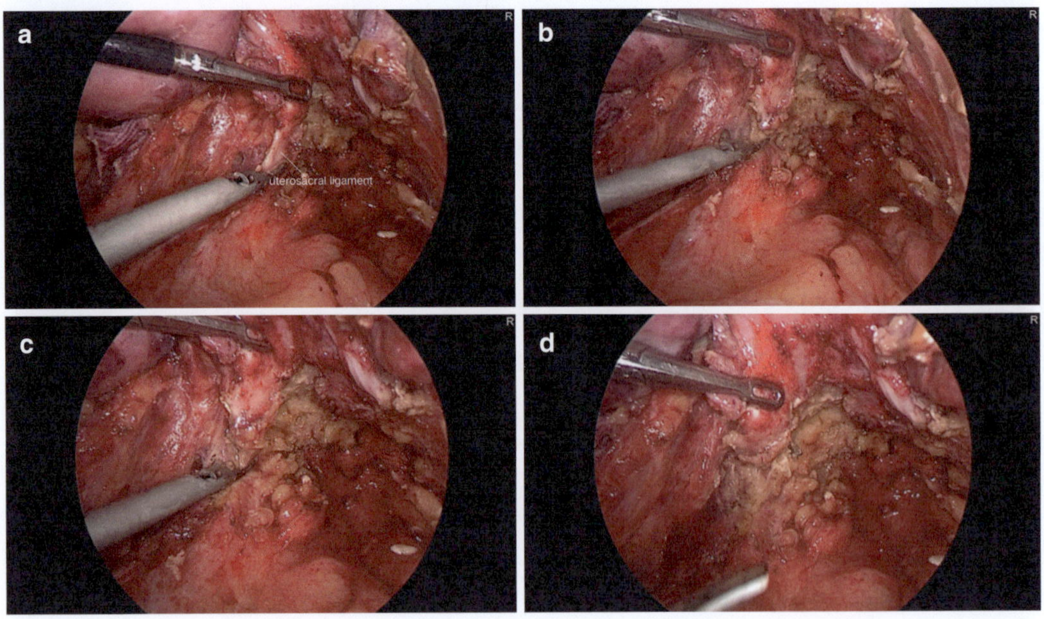

Fig. 9.14 (**a**–**d**) Transect the uterosacral ligament

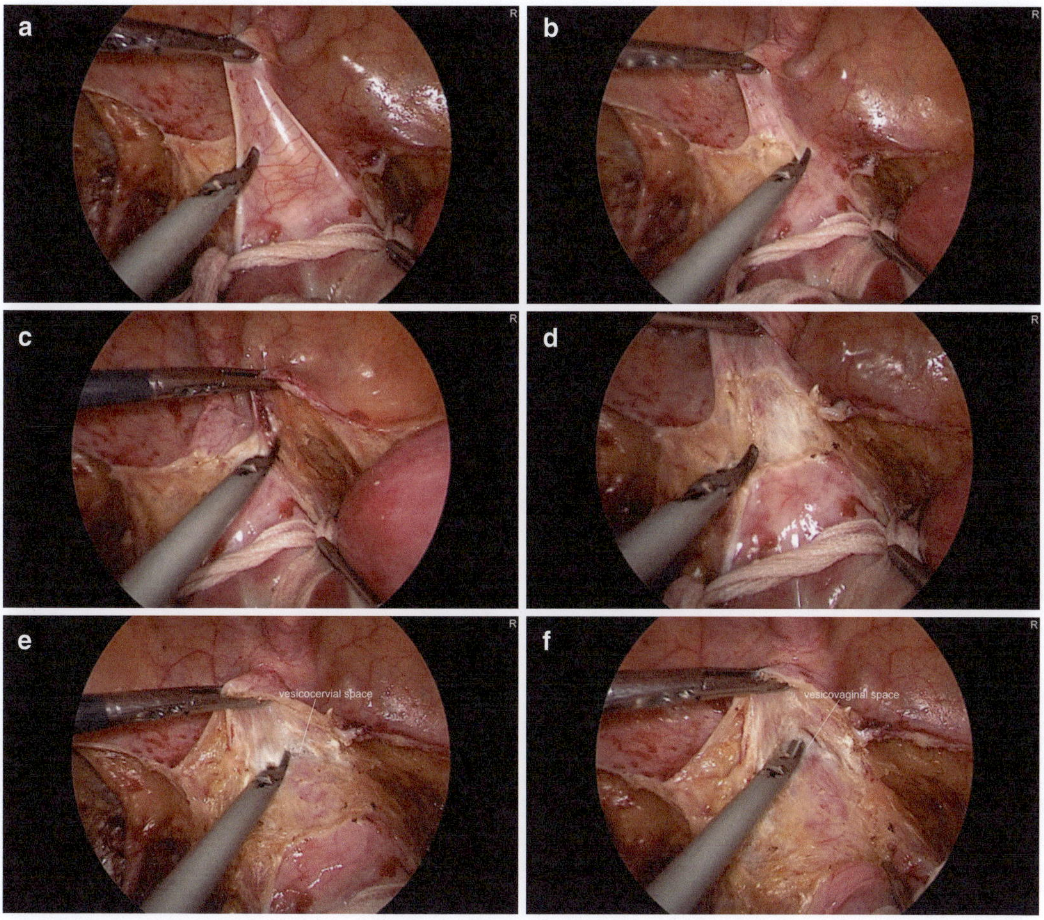

Fig. 9.15 (**a**–**f**) Expose of the vesicocevical space and vesicovaginal space

9.6 Exposure of the Vesicocevical Space and Vesicovaginal Space

Pull the uterus cranially, and gently pull the vesicouterine peritoneum ventrally and caudally. Make a sharp incision at the "yellow-white" junction, and continue pulling the bladder ventrally and caudally. Use an ultrasonic scalpel to dissect and expose the vesicocevical space and vesicovaginal space (Fig. 9.15**a**–**f**).

9.7 Management of the Uterine Artery

Countertraction is applied to the uterine artery and the ureter, and a combination of blunt and sharp dissection is used to fully separate the uterine artery and ureter (Fig. 9.16**a**–**j**). At the point where the uterine artery crosses the ureter, the uterine artery is clamped and occluded with vascular clamps before being transected (Figs. 9.17**a**–**d** and 9.18**a**–**f**).

Surgical Experience and Precautions Directly transecting the uterine artery at the level of the ureter is often unsafe due to the close anatomical relationship between the two structures. It can easily lead to ureteral injury, as this region is rich in vascular supply from the uterine artery to the ureter. In case of bleeding, it may obscure the tissue planes, further increasing the risk of ureteral damage.

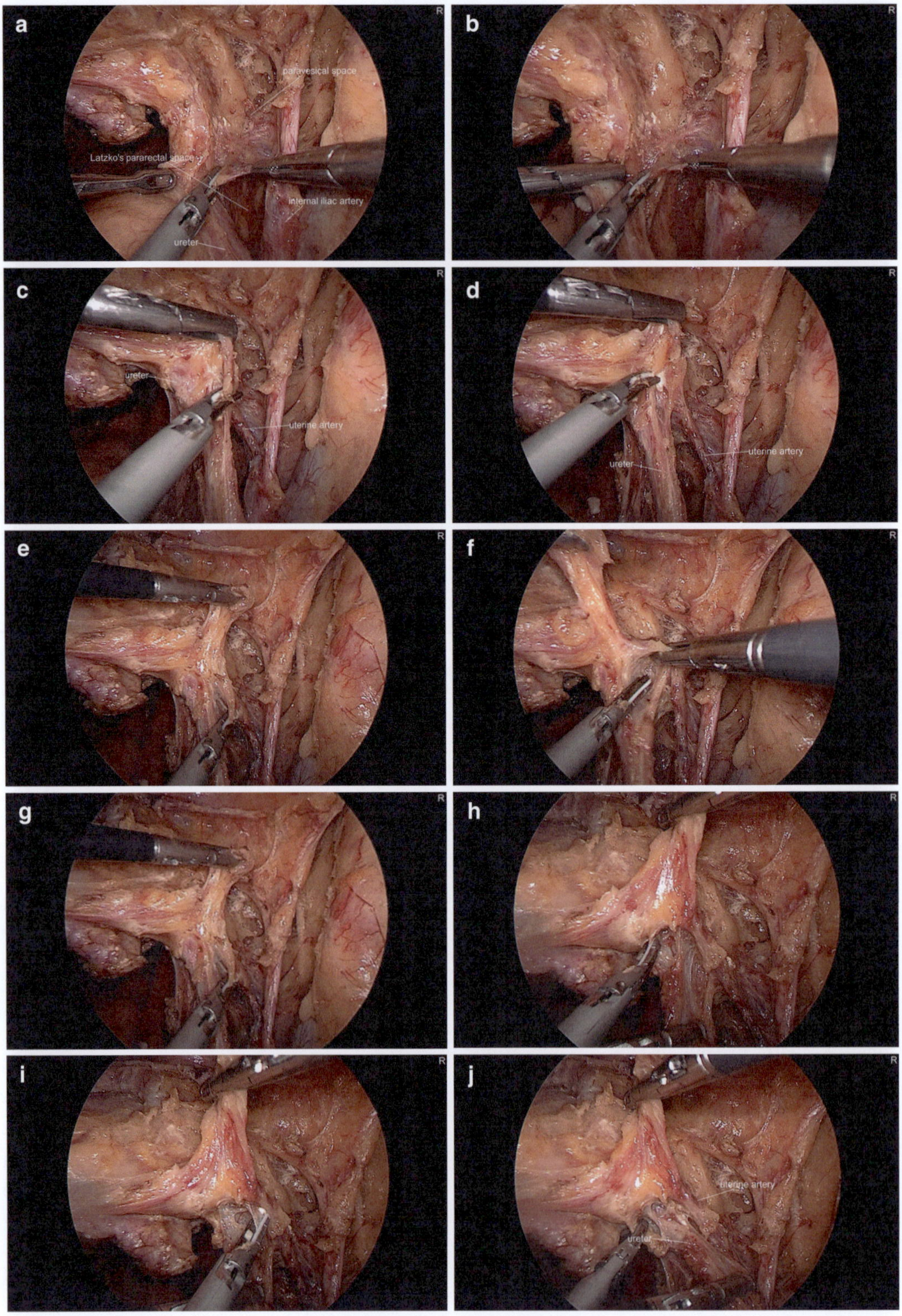

Fig. 9.16 (**a–j**) Separate the uterine artery

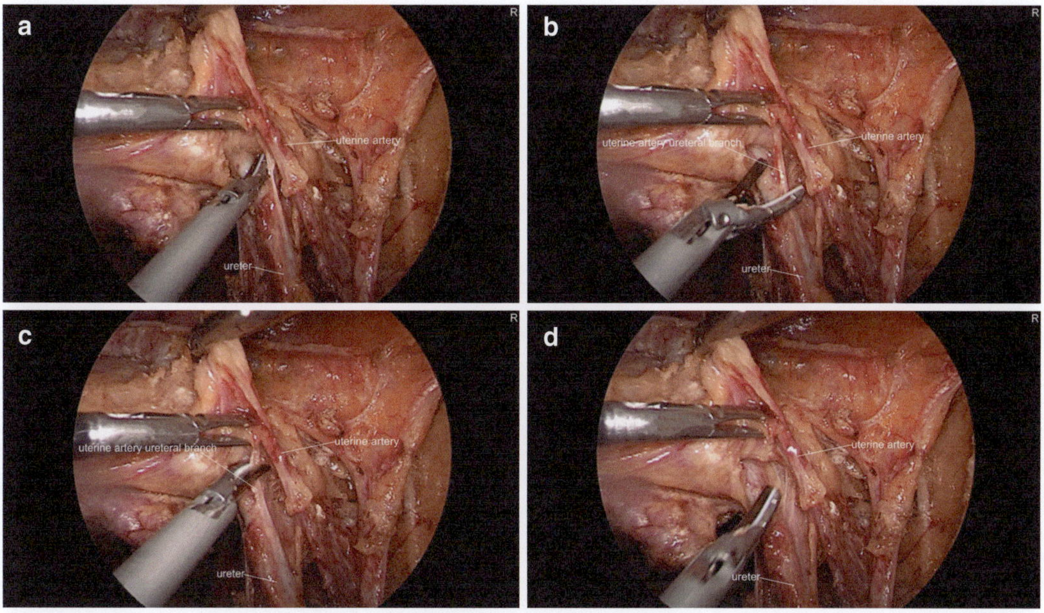

Fig. 9.17 (**a**–**d**) Transect uterine artery ureteral branch

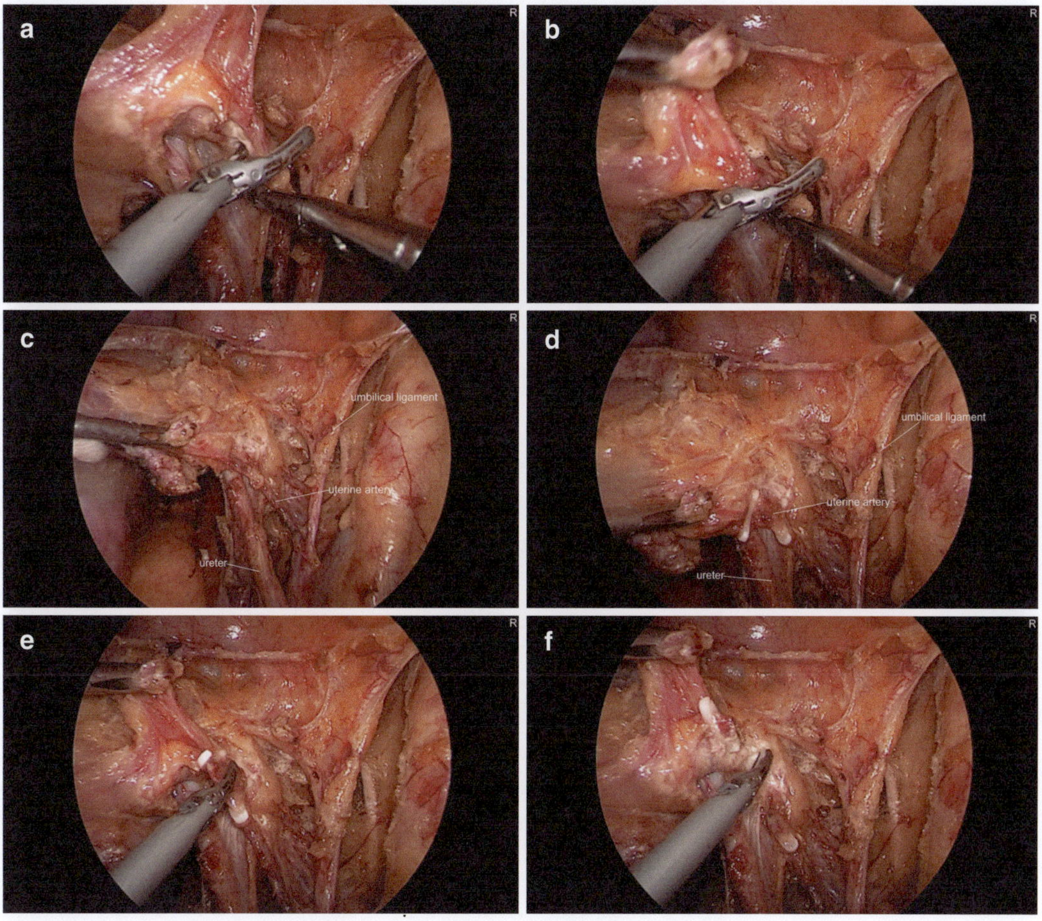

Fig. 9.18 (**a**–**f**) Transect uterine artery

9.8 Exposure of the Fourth Space

Pull the bladder ventrally and caudally, and use the ultrasonic scalpel to sharply and transversely expand the vesicovaginal space, revealing the fourth space (Fig. 9.19**a–l**).

Surgical Experience and Precautions

1. This step is particularly crucial and depends on the safe handling of the vesicocervical ligament and vesicovaginal ligament. Our team prefers to utilize this space to safely transect the vesicocervical ligament and vesicovaginal ligament while maintaining a clear view of the entrances and exits of the ureter "tunnel." Even if bleeding occurs during the transection, it can be managed calmly with suturing and electrocautery to control the bleeding, without concern for injuring the ureter.
2. In type B surgery, the transection of the vesicovaginal ligaments is not necessary. Therefore, the fourth space does not require extensive exposure; it is sufficient to expose it up to the exit of the ureter "tunnel."
3. This area is rich in blood vessels, and making large strides during dissection may lead to bleeding. To minimize the risk of bleeding, a cautious approach is adopted by using the ultrasonic scalpel to make small, incremental cuts and dissections, covering only 1/4 to 1/3 of the scalpel blade's length.

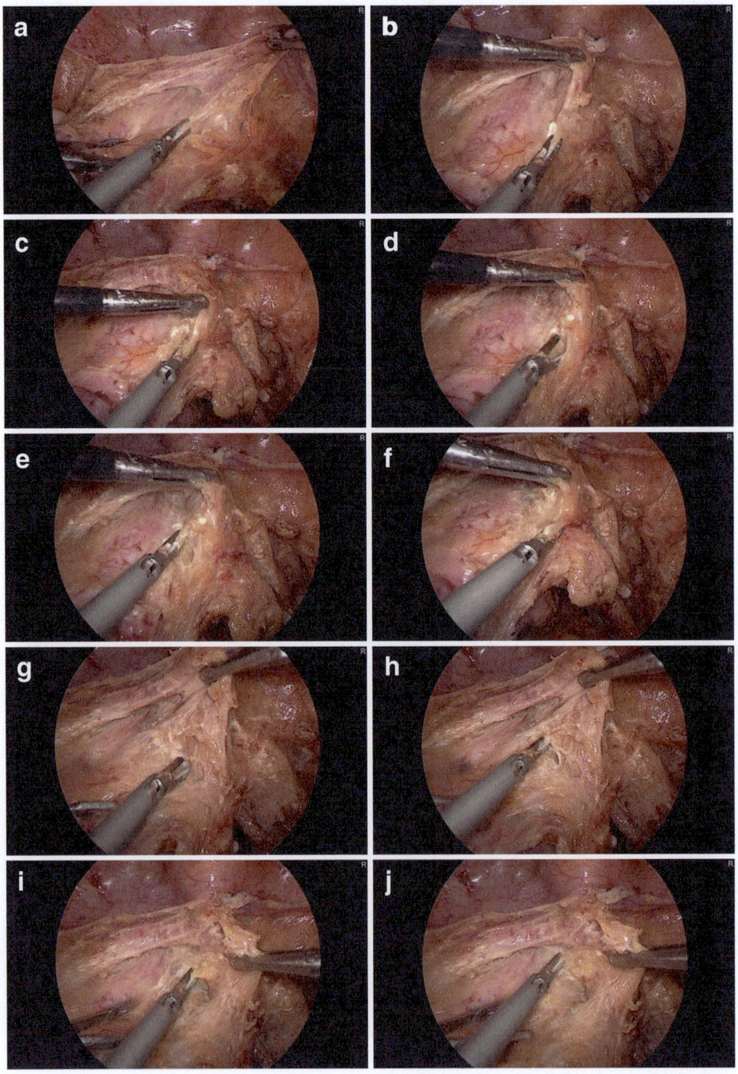

Fig. 9.19 (**a–l**) Expose the fourth space

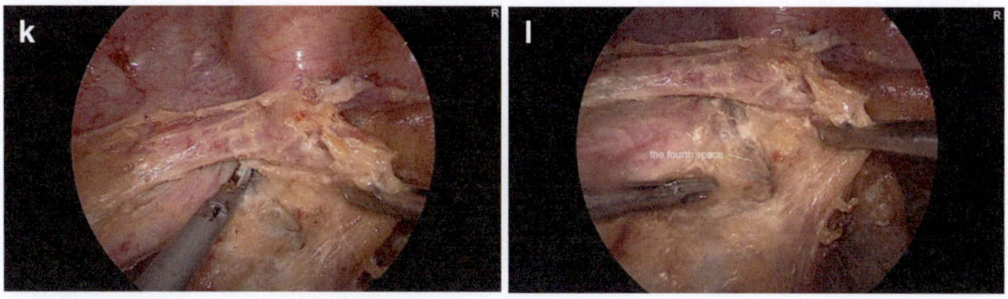

Fig. 9.19 (continued)

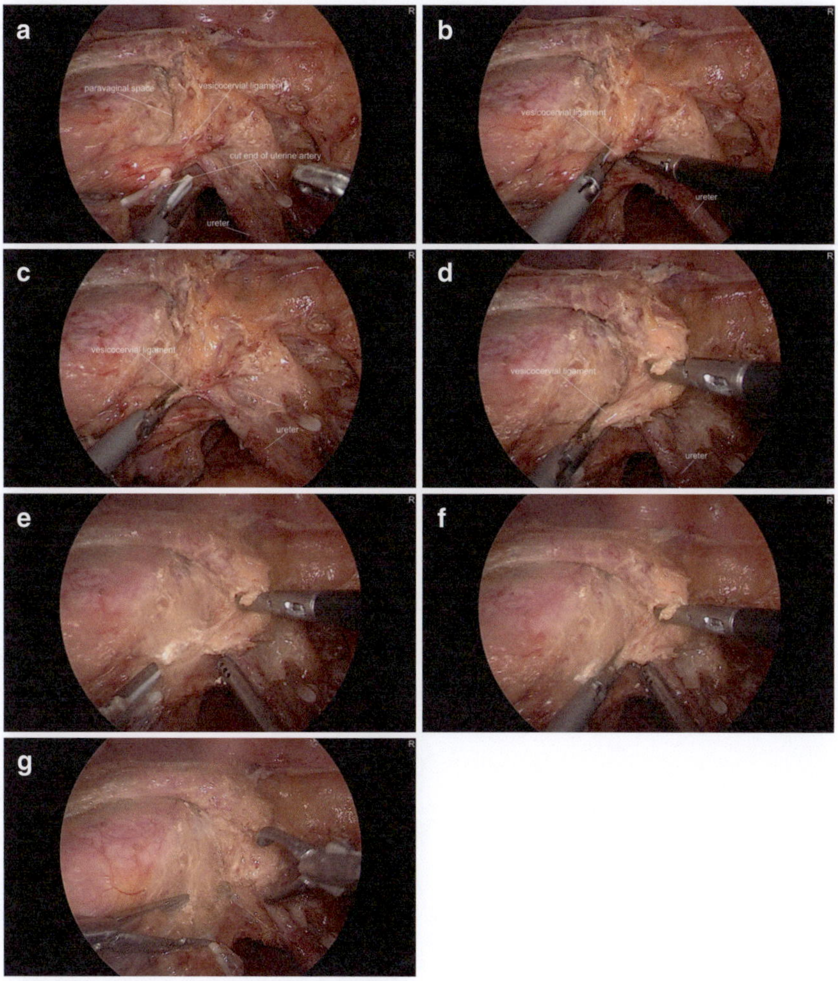

Fig. 9.20 (**a–g**) Transect the vesicocevical ligament on the ventral and medial side of the "knee"

9.9 Ligation of the Vesicocervical Ligaments

Pull the ureter and bladder laterally, and pull the cut end of the uterine artery medially. At this point, the course of the ureter appears to have a bent "knee" shape. Avoiding the ureter, transect the vesicocevical ligament on the ventral and medial side of the "knee" (Fig. 9.20**a–g**).

Surgical Experience and Precautions For a detailed anatomical illustration of the vesicocervical ligament and vesicovaginal ligament, please refer to the specific section on the anatomical dissection of these ligaments in the text.

9.10 Exposure of Partial Parametrial and Paracolpium

Use a clamp to grasp the ureter and pull it laterally. Then, use an ultrasonic scalpel to sharply expand the fourth space, exposing part of the parametrium and paracolpium (Fig. 9.21**a**–**j**).

Surgical Experience and Precautions

1. Expanding the fourth space not only exposes the targeted parametrium for resection but also ensures sufficient lateral displacement of the ureter, effectively moving it away from the ureteral bed, reducing the risk of injury.
2. The resection range of the lateral parametrial tissue is located between the vesicocevical space and Okabayashi's pararectal space, while the resection of the ventral parametrial tissue is located between the transversely expanded vesicovaginal space and Okabayashi's pararectal space.
3. In the QM classification surgery, the resection of paracolpium is not explicitly mentioned. However, our team believes that to achieve a B-type standard resection of the ventral and lateral parametrial tissues, it is necessary to expose and resect a portion of the paracolpium. The resection range of the paracolpium is located between the transversely expanded vesicovaginal space and Okabayashi's pararectal space.
4. During the dissection of the lateral parametrium, ventral parametrium, and paracolpium, their transection occurs in the spaces between each other (as described in Sects. 9.2 and 9.3). Before these structures are transected, it may appear that the spaces between them have "disappeared." This is because the dissection actually reveals the fusion of the paracolpium with the uterosacral ligament complex when exposing these spaces according to the standard protocol.

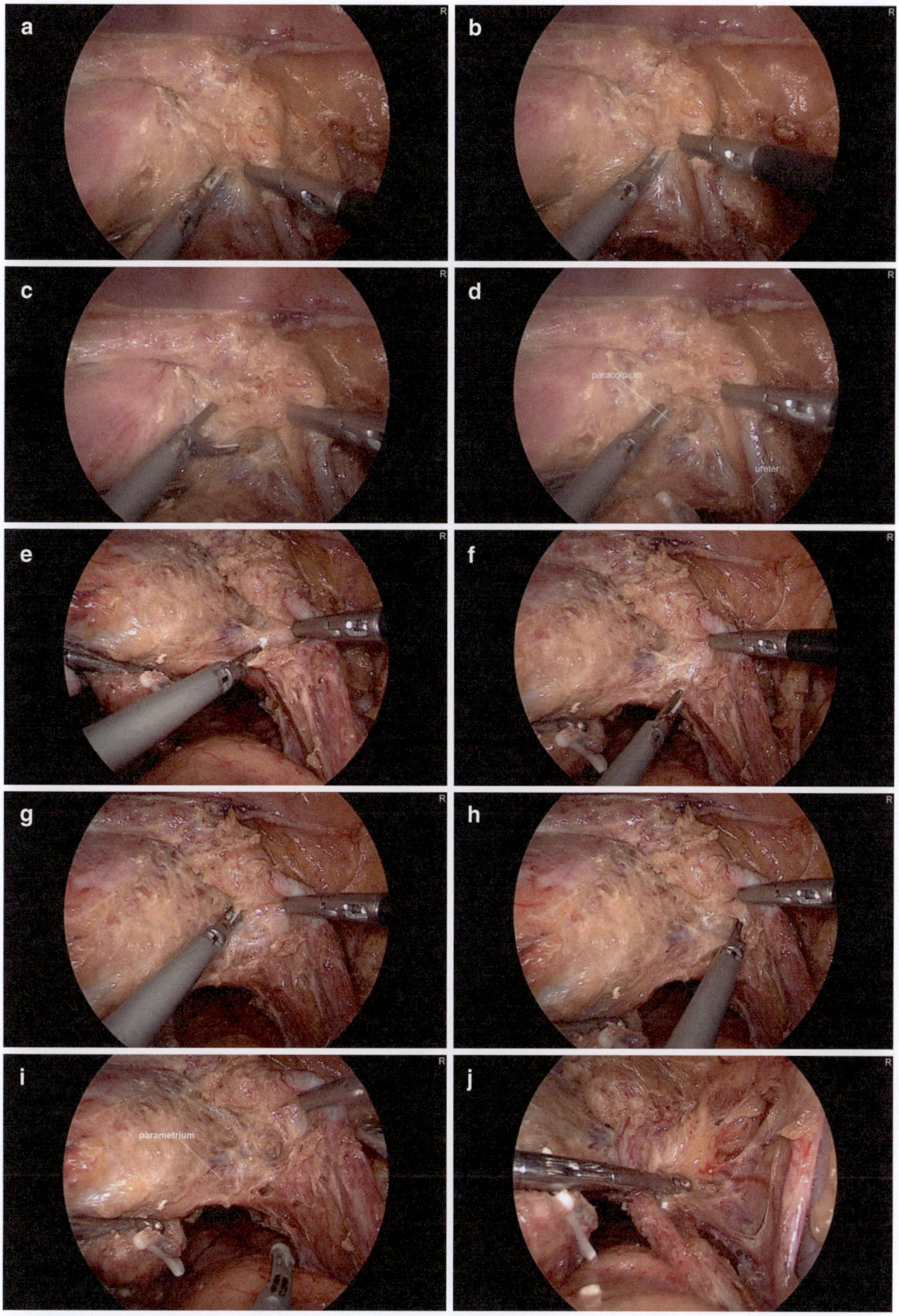

Fig. 9.21 (**a–j**) Expose part of the parametrium and paracolpium

9.11 Transection of Partial Parametrial and Paracolpium

After transecting the lateral parametrial tissue at the midpoint of the ureteral bed, proceed perpendicularly to the lateral parametrial tissue and gradually transect the partial ventral parametrial and paracolpium toward the caudal direction. Whenever possible, make vertical incisions in the direction of the vagina to cut the paracolpium near the vagina (Fig. 9.22**a–j**).

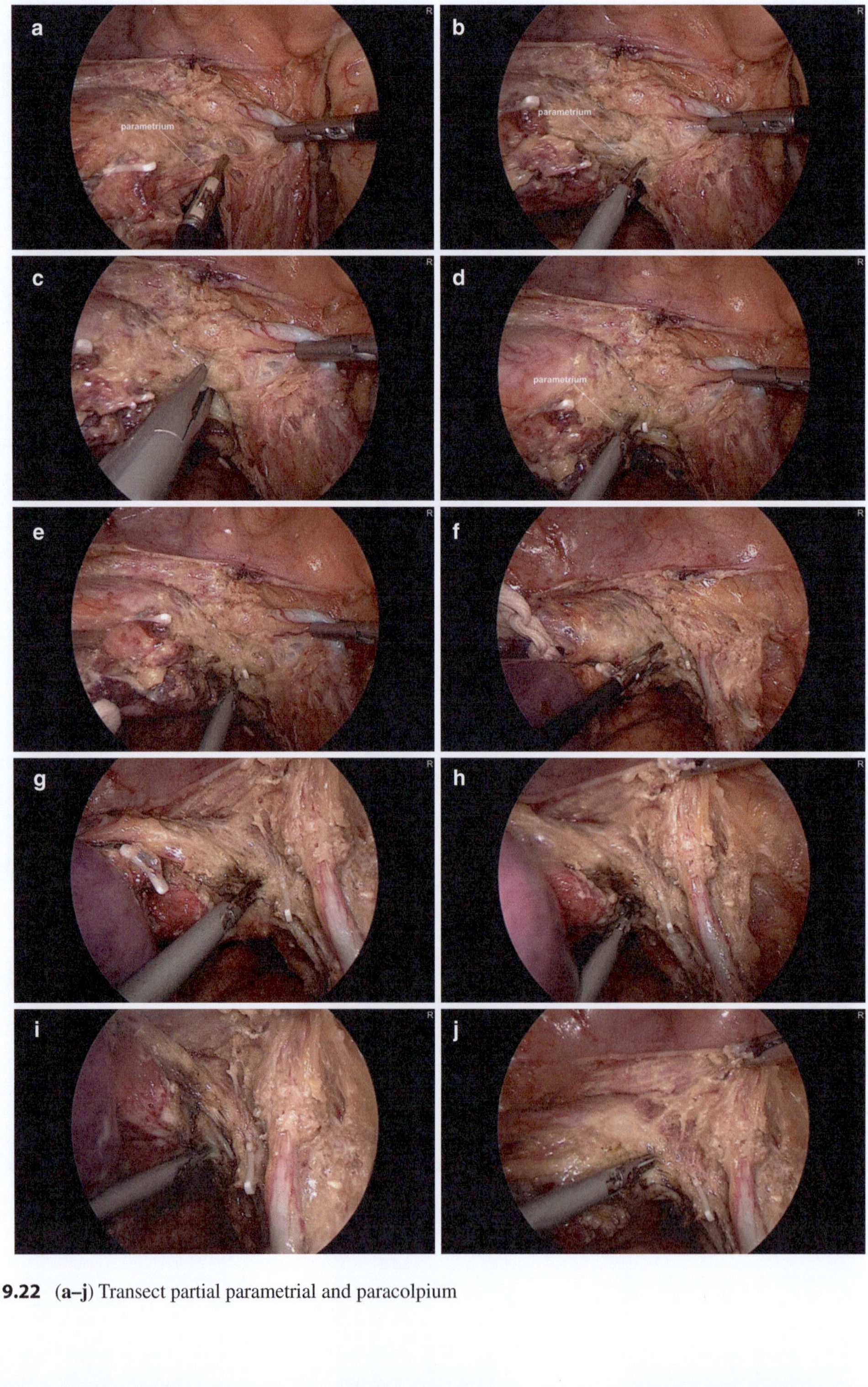

Fig. 9.22 (**a–j**) Transect partial parametrial and paracolpium

9.12 Management of the Vagina

Following the tumor-free principle, a circular closure of the vagina is performed using absorbable sutures (Fig. 9.23**a–c**), and the sealed vagina is irrigated repeatedly with sterilized distilled water (Fig. 9.24**a**, **b**).

A circular incision is made in the vagina approximately 2 cm below the cervix or lesion (Fig. 9.25**a**, **b**). After the circular incision, the uterus is completely removed from the vagina. Finally, the vaginal stump is sutured again.

Surgical Experience and Precautions

1. The vagina is ligated to isolate the cervical cancer lesion. The closed vaginal cavity is thoroughly rinsed with sterile distilled water at 42 °C to ensure a tumor-free environment as much as possible. Subsequently, the vagina is transected, and the uterus is extracted through the vaginal route while ensuring the integrity of the uterus and avoiding any cutting or damage. Finally, the vaginal cuff is sutured.
2. In type B surgery, the vaginal resection length required is 1 cm. However, in patients with an enlarged cervix, the short distance of the detached vagina may not provide enough space for effective circular suturing to achieve complete closure of the vaginal cuff, resulting in ineffective tumor isolation. In such cases, an alternative approach is to perform a trans-

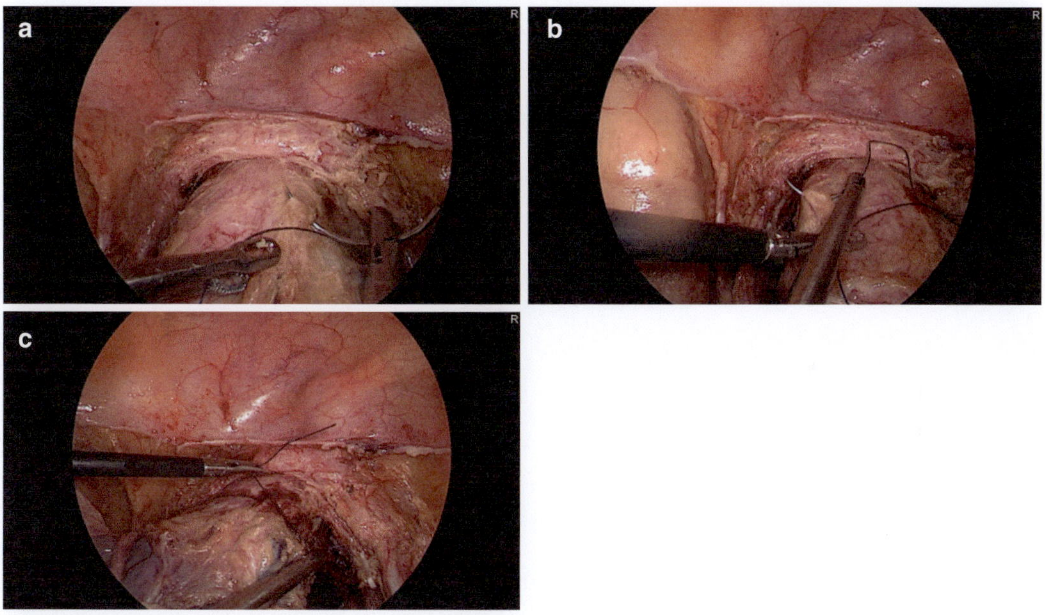

Fig. 9.23 (**a–c**) Close the vagina using absorbable sutures

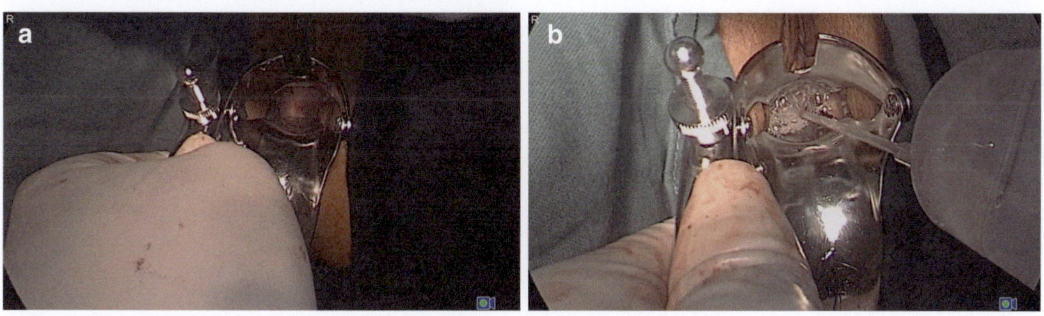

Fig. 9.24 (**a**, **b**) Repeatedly irrigate the sealed vagina with sterilized distilled water

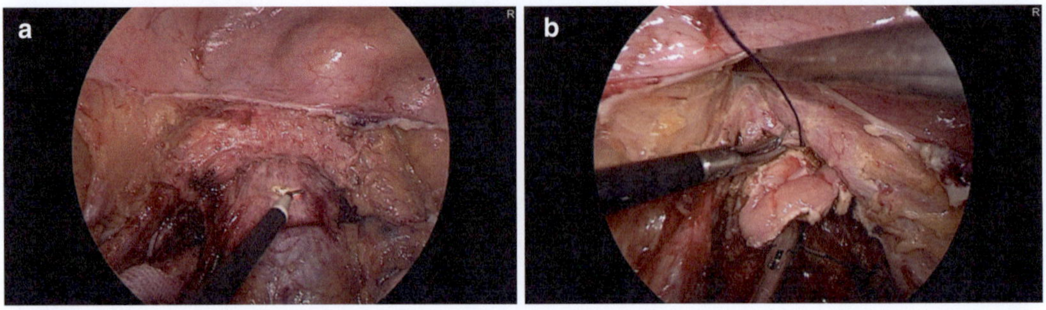

Fig. 9.25 (**a**, **b**) Suture the vaginal stump

vaginal vaginal cuff excision. Throughout the procedure, strict adherence to the tumor-free principle should be maintained to ensure the complete removal of the uterus.

QM-B1 type radical hysterectomy procedure can be found in Video 9.1.

QM-B2 Type Radical Hysterectomy

B2 type radical hysterectomy differs from B1 type radical hysterectomy in that it only requires the individual resection of the paracervical lymph nodes. The technical details and illustrations can be found in Part III, Chap. 15.

References

1. NCCN. NCCN clinical practice guidelines in oncology—cervical cancer. (2022-12-23) [2023-03-15]. https://www.nccn.org/professionals/physician_gls/pdf/cervical.pdf
2. Querleu D, Cibula D, Abu-Rustum NR. Update on the Querleu-Morrow classification of radical hysterectomy. Ann Surg Oncol. 2017;2017(24):3406–12.
3. Querleu D, Morrow CP. Classification of radical hysterectomy. Lancet Oncol. 2008;9:297–303.

10 Type QM-C1 Radical Hysterectomy

Shichao Han, Jun Wang, Jing Na, and Ya Li

Indications for QM-C1 type surgery are cases of localized early-stage disease without evident metastasis, including: Stage IB1–IB2, Selected stage IB3-IIA1 [1–3].

10.1 Suspending the Uterus

Place two absorbable sutures in a figure-eight pattern at the uterine fundus (Fig. 10.1a, b). Make a 0.5 cm incision above the pubic symphysis on the abdominal wall, and establish a channel with an abdominal wall puncture device. Use a laparoscopic needle holder to enter the abdominal cavity through this channel and clamp the sutures at the uterine fundus to lift the uterus (Fig. 10.1c–f).

Surgical Experience and Precautions Our team has found that it is helpful to insert the needle more toward the posterior wall and exit at the uterine fundus during suturing. This technique increases the lifting force on the posterior wall, creating better exposure for subsequent management of the dorsal parametrium.

There is no fixed projection position for the incision above the pubic symphysis on the body surface. Our team's approach is to determine the location of the bladder under laparoscopic visualization, then repeatedly press the abdominal wall to identify the abdominal wall puncture hole position. After the puncture device penetrates the peritoneum, it may be difficult to pass through due to the high elasticity of the peritoneum. An assistant can use atraumatic forceps to support the peritoneum at the puncture site, facilitating the puncture process.

Supplementary Information The online version contains supplementary material available at https://doi.org/10.1007/978-981-97-7687-0_10.

S. Han (✉) · J. Wang · J. Na · Y. Li
Department of Gynecology and Obstetrics, Second Affiliated Hospital of Dalian Medical University, Dalian, China

S. Han, J. Wang (eds.), *Open, Laparoscopic, and Robotic Surgery for Cervical Cancer*, https://doi.org/10.1007/978-981-97-7687-0_10

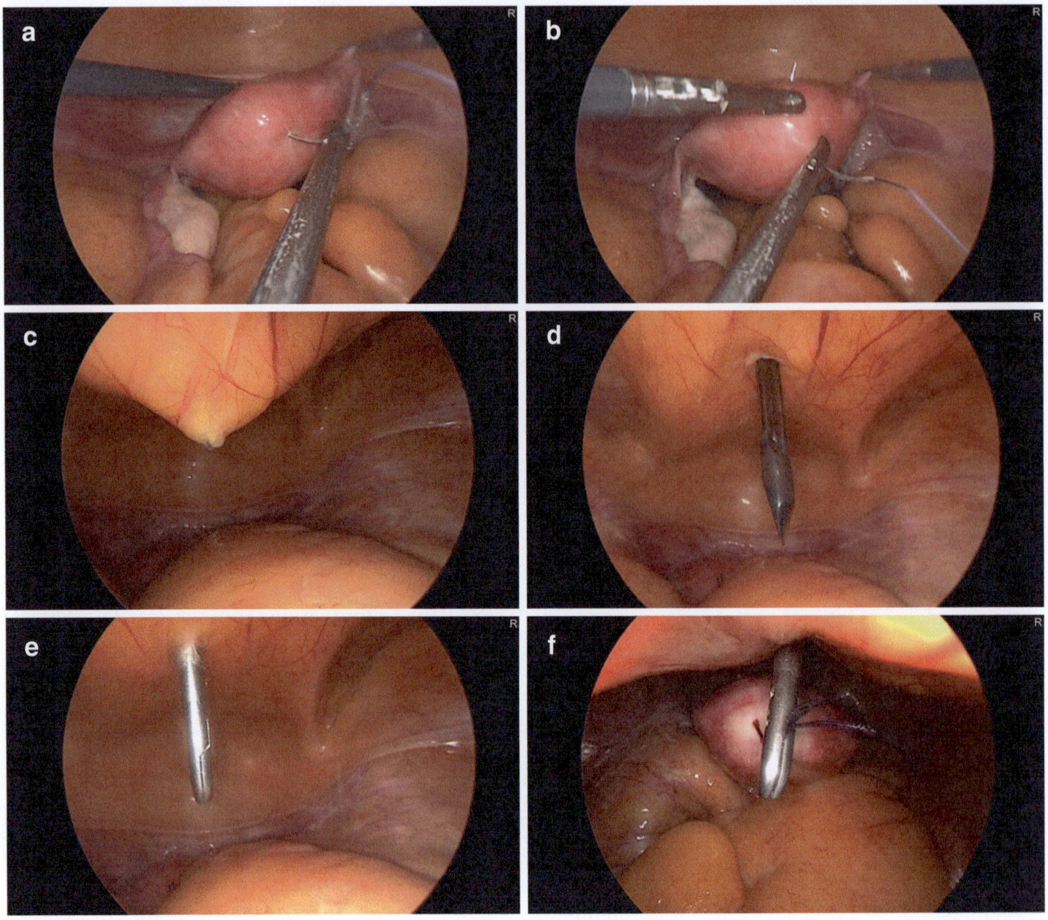

Fig. 10.1 (a–f) Suspend uterus

10.2 Exposure of the Lateral Retroperitoneal Space

Unlike QM-A and B surgeries, extensive hysterectomy in QM-C requires full exposure of the lateral retroperitoneal space to lay the foundation for subsequent resection of the parametrium and pelvic lymph nodes.

Pulling the ovary suspensory ligament medially and the round ligament laterally and caudally can expose the lateral peritoneum on the ventral side of the lateral retroperitoneal space.

Sharp opening of the lateral retroperitoneal space is achieved by opening the peritoneum at the junction of the ovary suspensory ligament and the iliac vessels, and then sharply cutting along the surface of the psoas major muscle toward the tail end, reaching the junction of the round ligament and the lateral retroperitoneal space. At the same time, the peritoneal incision is enlarged toward the head side to lay the foundation for subsequent lymph node dissection and adnexal handling.

Incising the lateral peritoneum along the round ligament toward the uterine angle reveals the lateral retroperitoneal space.

Surgical Experience and Precautions When opening the lateral peritoneum sharply and pulling the ovary suspensory ligament, the author's team believes that better traction can be achieved by pulling 1–2 cm at the head side of the ovary, which can fully expose the pelvic segment of the ovary suspensory ligament.

Sharp separation of the white loose connective tissue within this space can be achieved using an ultrasonic scalpel, entering into the plane of the adipose tissue, thereby revealing the important anatomical structures of the lateral parametrium and the iliac vessels. In cases of obese patients, our team's experience is to first deal with the adnexa. Sufficient tension can be provided for handling the space by pulling the posterior leaf of the broad ligament.

For obese patients, the difficulty of the surgery is increased. Figure 10.2a–j shows the experience and key points of handling the gap in a patient with a body mass index of 38 kg/m^2 and a weight

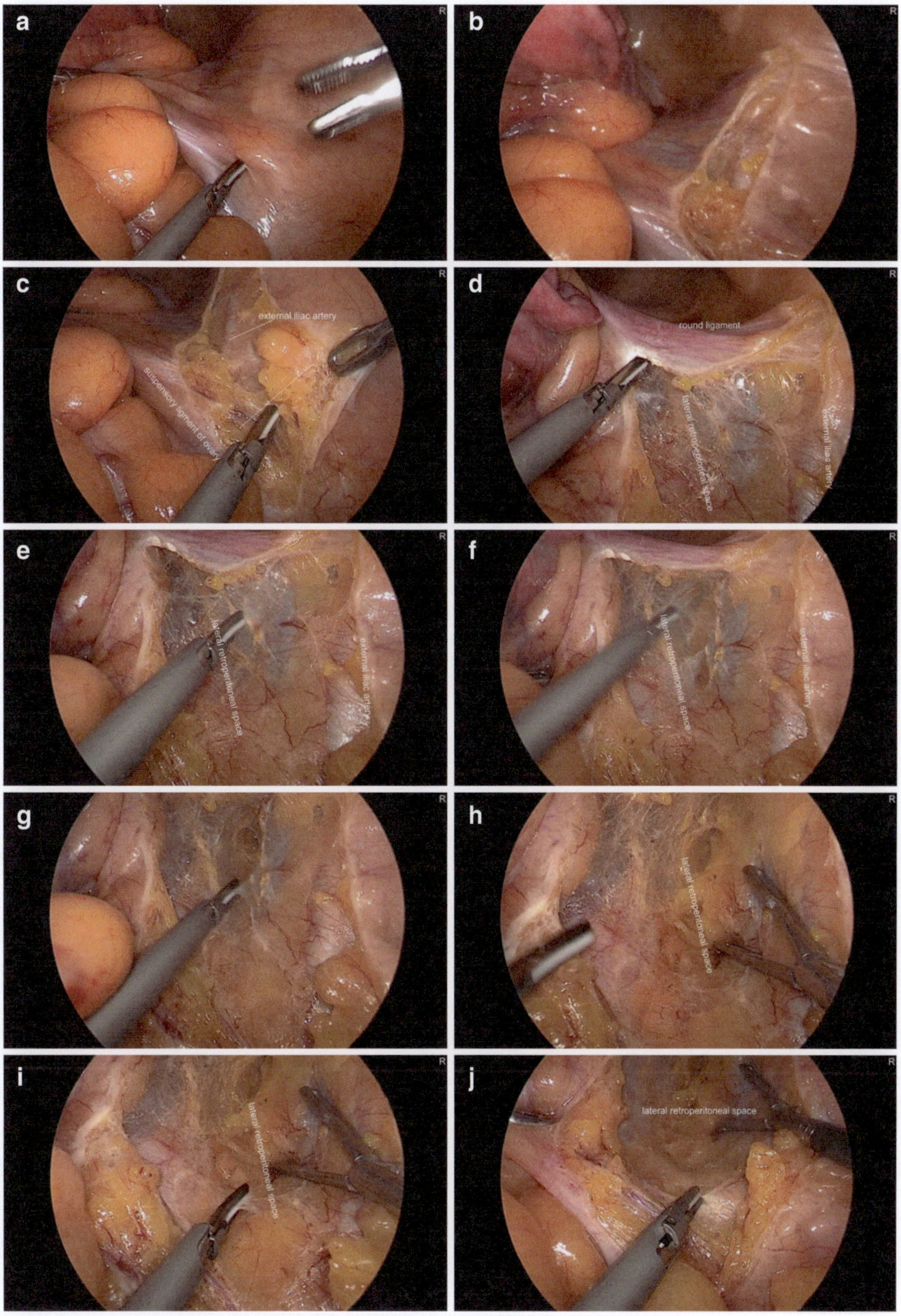

Fig. 10.2 (**a–j**) Expose the lateral retroperitoneal space

of 113 kg. At this time, the ovary suspensory ligament can be pulled inward and the iliac vessels can be gently pressed outward by the assistant. The ultrasonic scalpel is used to sharply separate the gap between the adipose tissue, but it is found that in this obese patient, the tension from pulling is not enough to safely and non-hemostatically separate the gap, so the surgical team carried out the accessory processing first.

10.3 Ovarian/Fallopian Tube Handling

The removal of the adnexa is relatively simple and will not be elaborated further (Figs. 10.3, 10.4, and 10.5).

The ovary suspensory ligament is pulled toward the ventral side. At the intersection of the ovary suspensory ligament and the iliac vessels, the peritoneum on the surface of the ovary suspensory ligament is incised sharply. Under direct vision of the contralateral side or thinning of the lateral peritoneum to allow transillumination, the lateral peritoneum is cut parallel to the ovary suspensory ligament toward the uterine corner, then the fallopian tube is cut tightly from the fimbria to the uterine angle, and finally the ovarian ligament is cut tightly from the uterine angle to remove the ovary and place it in the iliac fossa.

Surgical Experience and Precautions Do not leave a portion of the fimbriae on the surface of the ovary, and make sure to closely seal the blood vessels of the suspensory ligament of the fallopian tube to minimize the impact on ovarian blood supply.

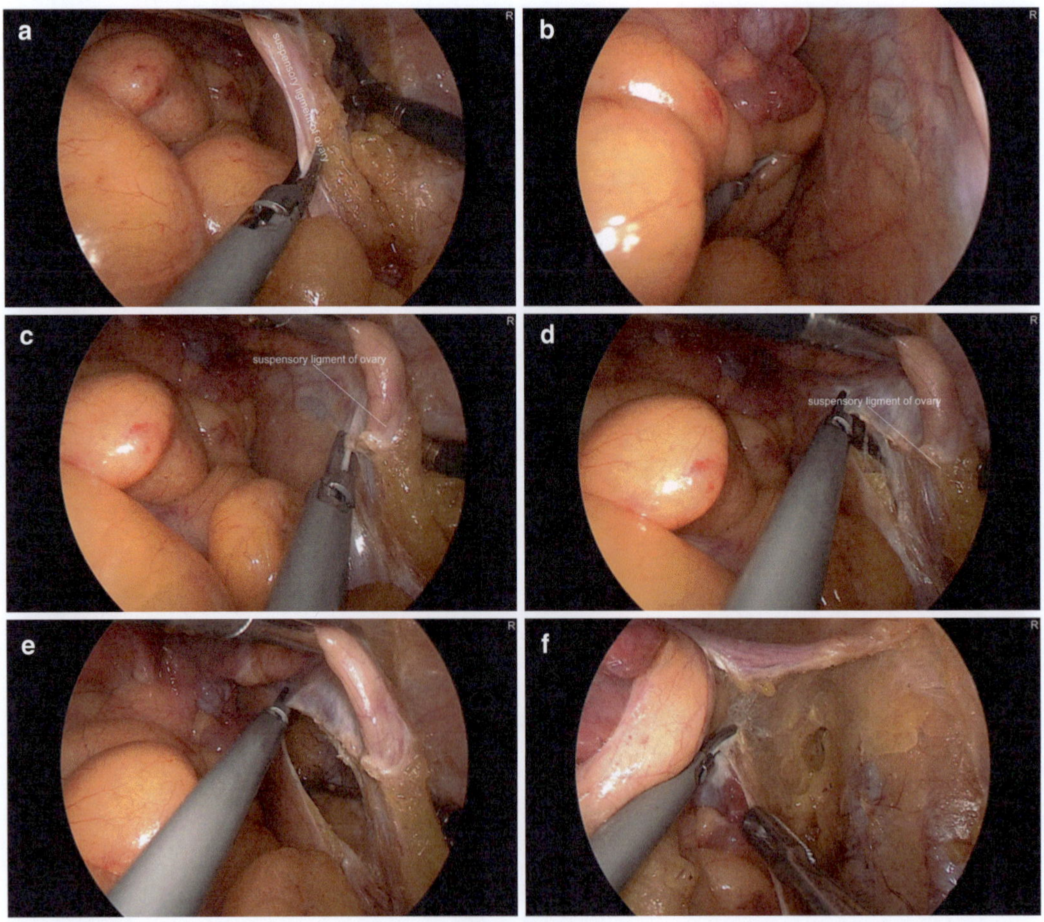

Fig. 10.3 (a–f) Open the lateral retroperitoneal space

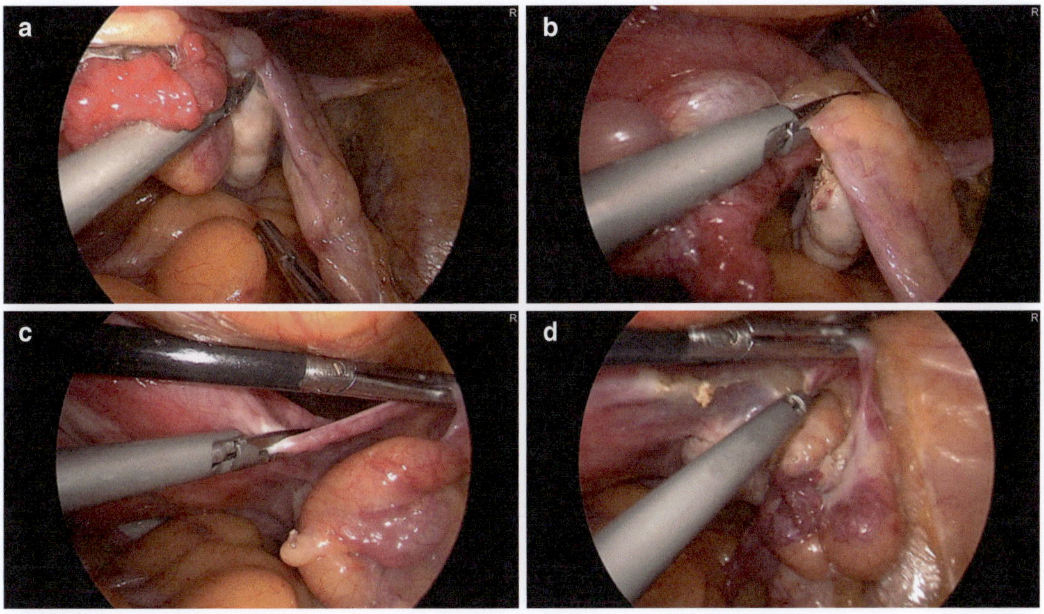

Fig. 10.4 (**a**–**d**) Salpingectomy

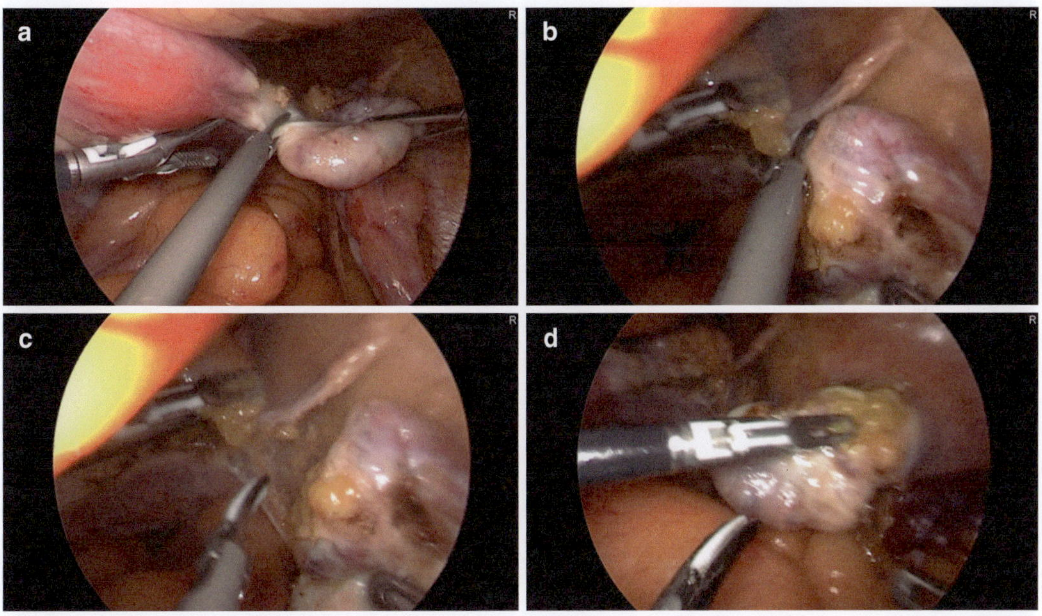

Fig. 10.5 (**a**–**d**) Cut the ovarian ligament

10.4 Exposure of Obturator Space

Continued enlargement of the lateral retroperitoneal space lays the foundation for lateral parametrial dissection. The lateral peritoneum is pulled inward, and sharp dissection is performed within the space using an ultrasonic scalpel. Careful identification all the important anatomical structures is necessary to avoid injury to blood vessels and the ureter (Fig. 10.6a–j).

Surgical Experience and Precautions In obese patients, direct exposure of the internal iliac artery, ureter, and uterine artery planes can

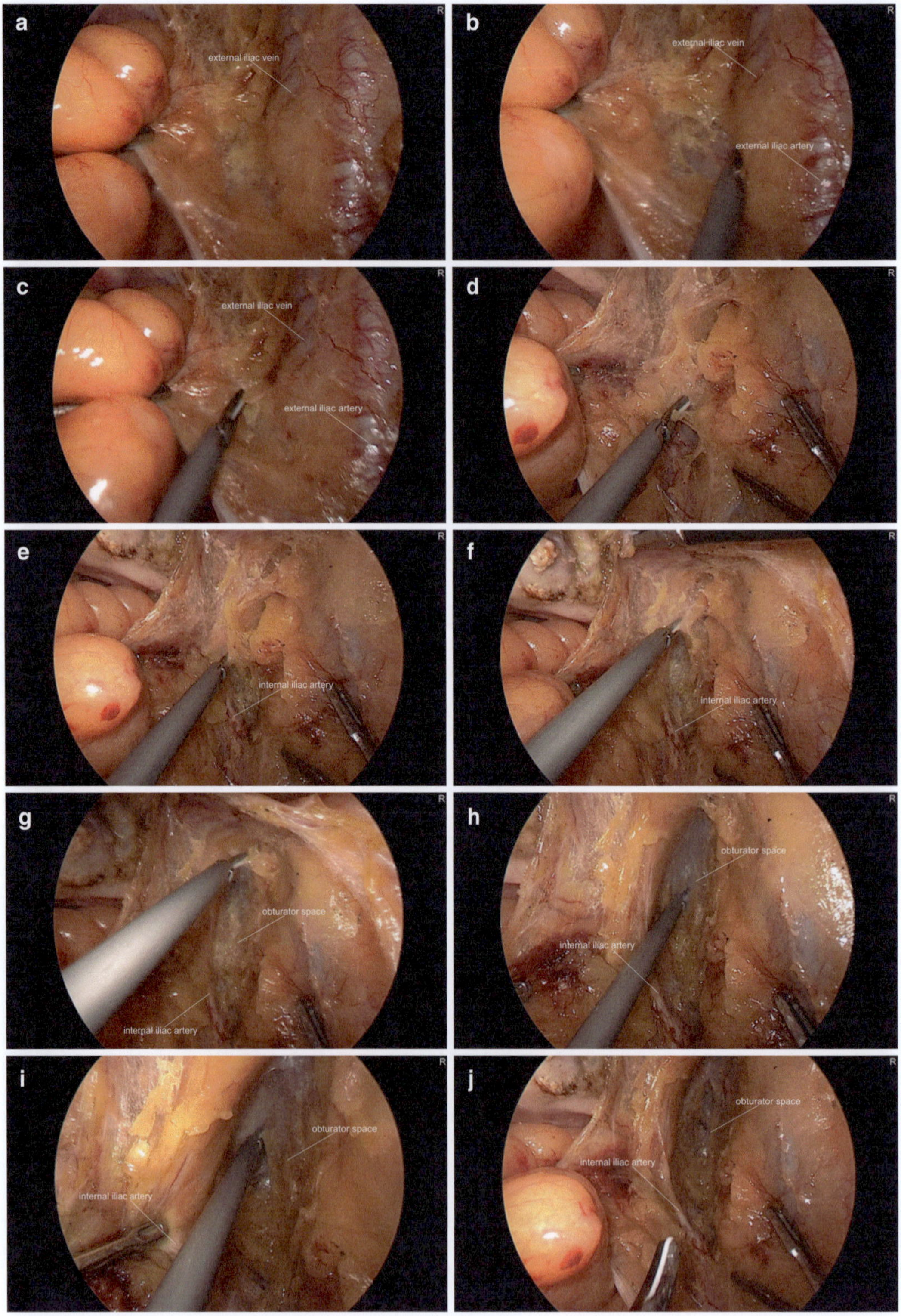

Fig. 10.6 (**a**–**j**) Expose the obturator space

be challenging due to the covering adipose tissue. The adipose tissue covering these structures does not appear to have a "natural" space, but can be differentiated based on subtle morphological differences. Experienced surgeons analyze these adipose tissues from an embryonic perspective and recognize that they may have two different origins: one is the continuation of lymphatic adipose tissue in the iliac vessel region, and the other is the adipose tissue attached to the ureter. By applying countertraction, a gap between these two adipose tissues can be identified, and sharp dissection with an ultrasonic scalpel can be performed within this gap (during dissection, the region is separated from the uterine artery to avoid inadvertent injury). This allows for easier exposure of the underlying internal iliac artery. Continuing dissection along the gap, the internal iliac artery and its continuation to the distal lateral ligament are separated. The internal iliac artery is pulled inward, and dissection continues closely along the outer edge of the internal iliac artery toward the dorsal and caudal directions, allowing for exposure of the obturator gap. The author considers that dissection along the outer side of the internal iliac artery is relatively safe. The branches of the internal iliac artery on the outer side are usually minimal, typically only one obturator artery branching toward the pelvic sidewall, while there are multiple branches on the inner side, which are usually in variable positions. Especially, branches of the uterine artery often lie on the surface of the internal iliac artery, making the surgical field unclear. After dissecting this gap, pulling the lateral ligament outward provides sufficient tension for subsequent lateral parametrial dissection.

10.5 Lateral Parametrial Dissection

Exposing the uterine artery: the lateral peritoneum and ureter are pulled inward. The lateral ligament is pulled outward, and sharp dissection is performed in the space between the ureter and the lateral ligament. Gradually, the uterine artery is exposed (Fig. 10.7a–d).

Expose the paravesical space: By dissecting the space between the ureter and the lateral umbilical ligament at the posterior end of the uterine artery, gradually dissecting the paravesical space (Fig. 10.8a–f).

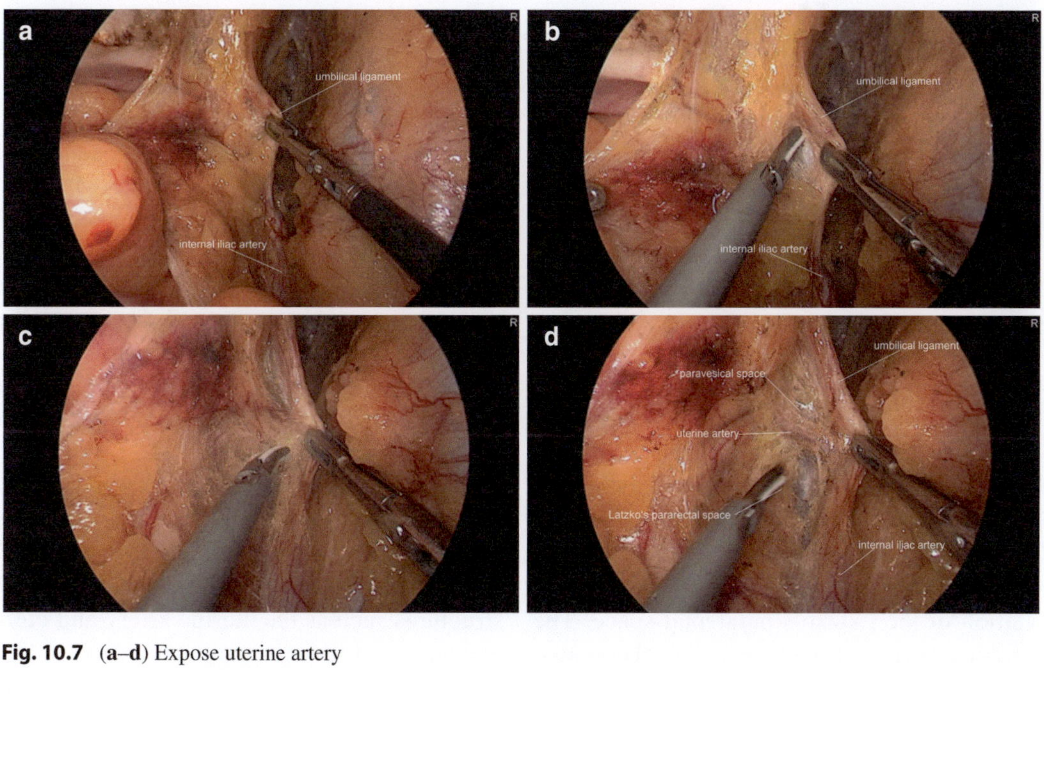

Fig. 10.7 (**a–d**) Expose uterine artery

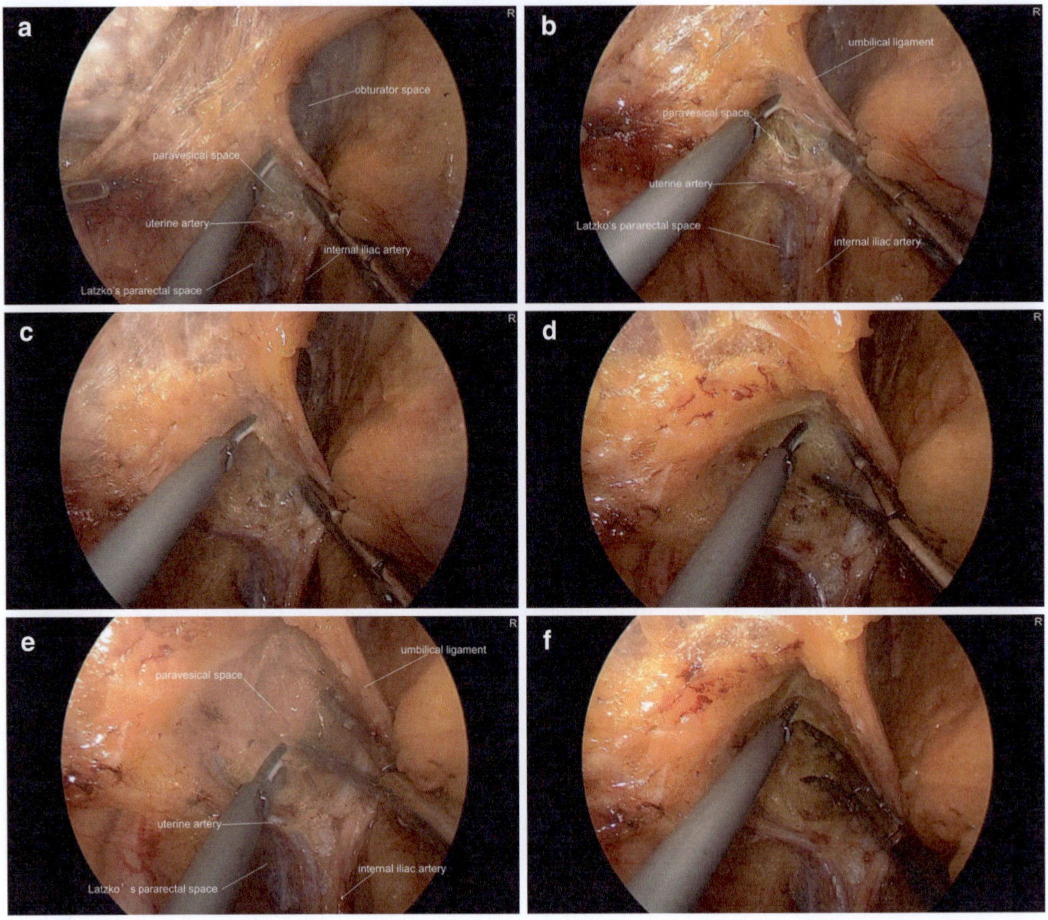

Fig. 10.8 (**a–f**) Separate the paravesical space

Expose the Latzko's pararectal space: By separating the internal iliac artery and the ureter at the anterior end of the uterine artery, revealing the Latzko's pararectal space (Fig. 10.9a–f).

Surgical Experience and Precautions Our team has the habit of first dissecting the paravesical space, as the distance between the ureter and the internal iliac artery in this space is wider compared to the Latzko's pararectal space. It is less likely to cause ureteral injury during the dissection process, and with the countertraction between the internal iliac artery and the ureter, sufficient tension can be achieved, facilitating the separation.

There is a relatively higher risk in the separation of the Latzko's pararectal space. The external side of this space is closely related to the internal iliac artery, internal iliac vein, ureter, and the sidewall of the rectum. Improper manipulation can easily lead to ureteral and internal iliac vessels injury. The key points of the procedure involve adequately pulling the lateral peritoneum inward and pulling the internal iliac artery outward while maintaining sufficient tension. The goal is to widen and deepen this space. During the dissection process, there is no need to rush to identify important anatomical structures such as the superficial uterine veins and deep veins. Especially in obese patients, it is important to patiently and carefully open the paravesical space and the Latzko's pararectal space to expose the important anatomical structures such as the uterine artery and uterine veins that lie between them.

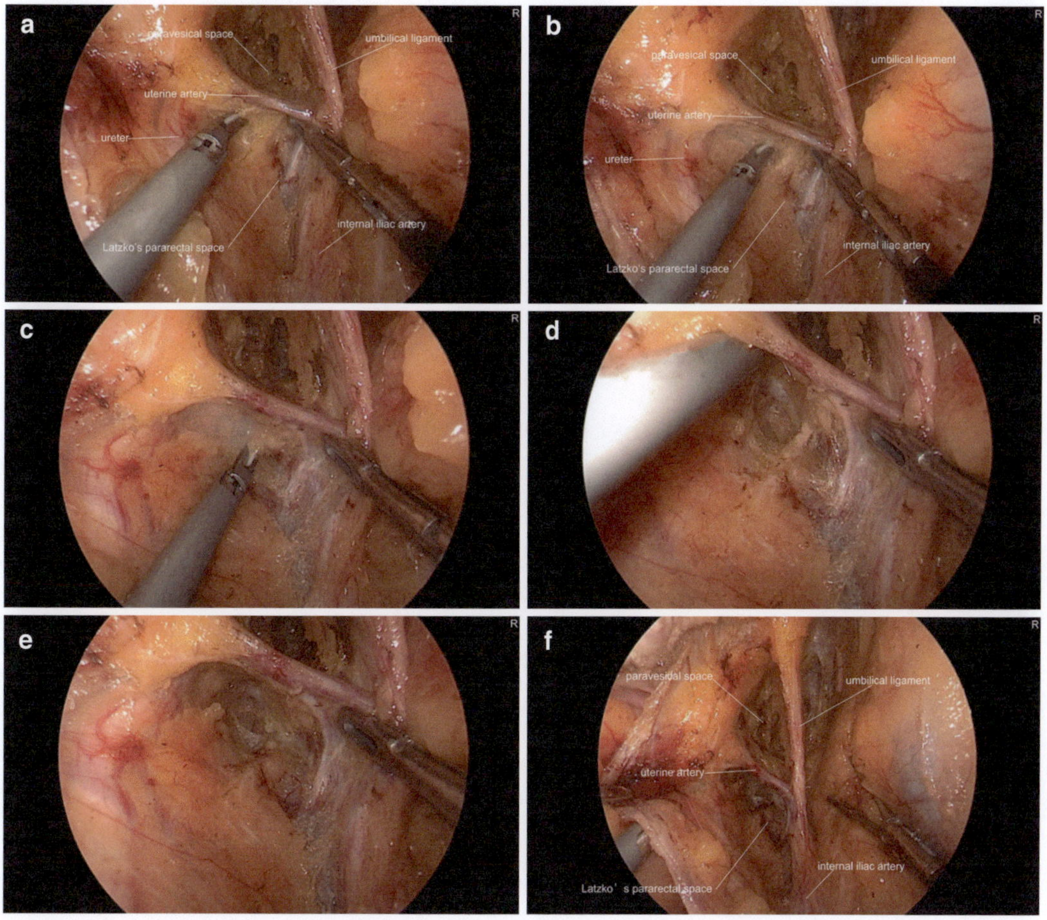

Fig. 10.9 (**a**–**f**) Separate the Latzko's pararectal space

10.6 Expose the Okabayashi's Pararectal Space

By pulling the lateral peritoneum inward and pulling the ureter outward, sharply separating the space between them.

In C2-type surgeries without nerve preservation, only ureteral mobilization is performed. Pull the lateral peritoneum inward and the ureter outward, sharply separate the space between them. Separate to expose the ureteral dorsal mesentery for a distance of more than 2 cm. This allows transection of the ureteral mesentery without affecting the blood supply to the ureter (Fig. 10.10a–j).

Surgical Experience and Precautions In Q-M C1-type surgeries with nerve preservation, it is necessary to fully dissect the Okabayashi's space. Our team has found that it is best to widen the upper part of the Okabayashi's space, ideally until the level of the bifurcation of the internal iliac artery. This provides strong evidence for accurate identification of the nerves. The lower part should be as close as possible to the junction of the sacrospinous ligament, the uterosacral ligament, and the connective tissue near the vagina. The posterior part should reach the level of the rectal sidewall. The lateral aspect should preserve the integrity of the ureter and its posterior layer. The dissection of this space is relatively uncomplicated because there are no major blood vessels

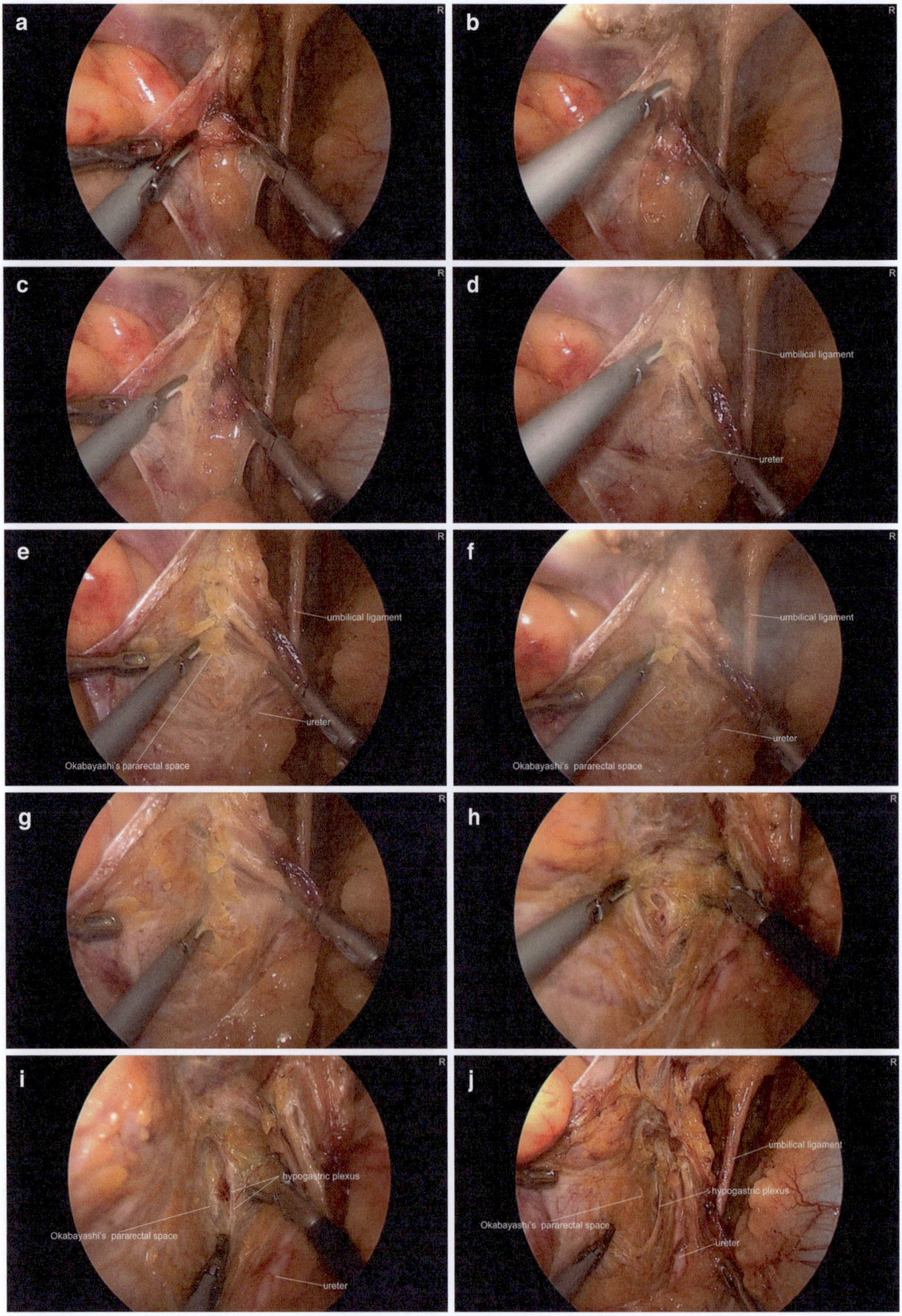

Fig. 10.10 (**a**–**j**) Separate the Okabayashi's pararectal space

within this area. By sharply separating the loose white connective tissue structures in the space using an ultrasonic scalpel, the hypogastric plexus can gradually be exposed.

10.7 Dissection of the Lateral Parametrial Tissue

Pull and expose the paravesical space and the Latzko's pararectal space. Between these two spaces, closely adhere to the medial aspect of the internal iliac vessels and use vascular clamps to sequentially clamp and cut the vessels of the lateral parametrial tissue (Figs. 10.11, 10.12, and 10.13).

Surgical Experience and Precautions In Type C1 surgery, it is necessary to meticulously dissect and ligate the uterine artery, superficial uterine veins, deep uterine veins, as well as the variations such as the middle rectal artery and several branches of the deep uterine veins that drain into the internal iliac vein from different directions.

After ligating the deep uterine veins in Type C1 surgery, it is preferable not to continue the dissection posteriorly because the pelvic splanchnic nerve plexus are located posterior to the deep uterine veins, especially at the point where the deep uterine veins merge into the internal iliac vein. Further sharp dissection with energy devices at this point can lead to nerve injury. The exposure of the nerve-containing portion is reserved for later during nerve preservation.

The use of vascular clamps to manage the blood vessels in the lateral parametrial tissue is relatively safe and reliable. Firstly, clamping and ligating the vessels with vascular clamps reduce the risk of injury to surrounding nerves compared to energy devices, especially during the handling of the deep uterine veins, as the pelvic splanchnic nerve plexus behind them plays a crucial role in preserving pelvic autonomic nerve function. Secondly, after clamping with vascular clamps, the tissue can be cut with scissors. Particularly in the case of the deep uterine veins, even low-energy devices like ultrasonic scalpels can cause vessel contraction upon cutting, which may result in inadequate distance between the vascular clamp and potential melting of the clamp due to heat, leading to detachment and bleeding of the clamped vessel and failure of the Type C1 surgery.

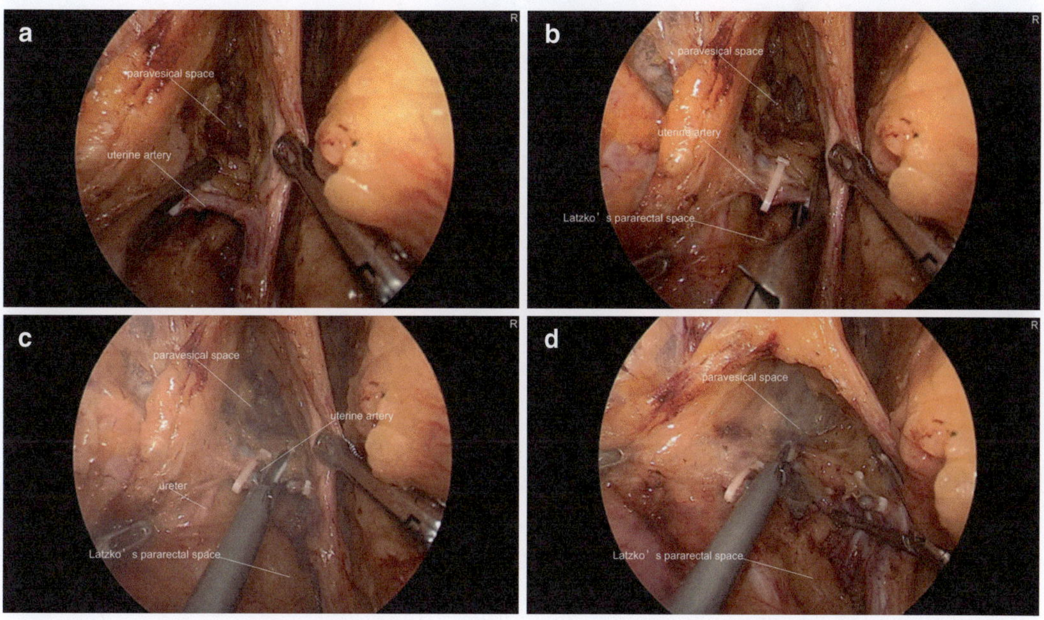

Fig. 10.11 (**a–d**) Transect uterine artery

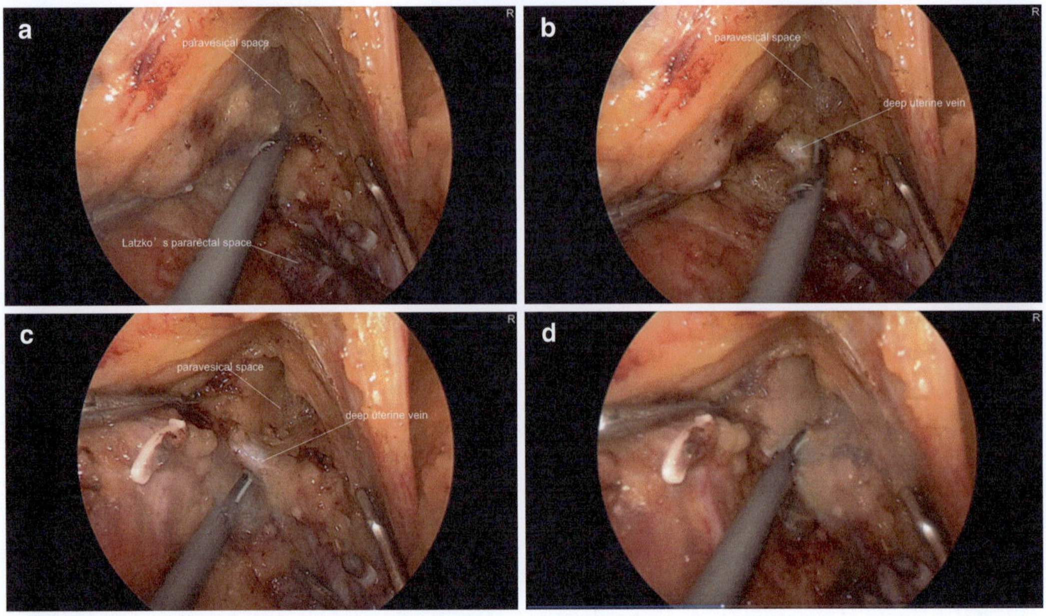

Fig. 10.12 (**a**–**d**) Separate the deep uterine vein

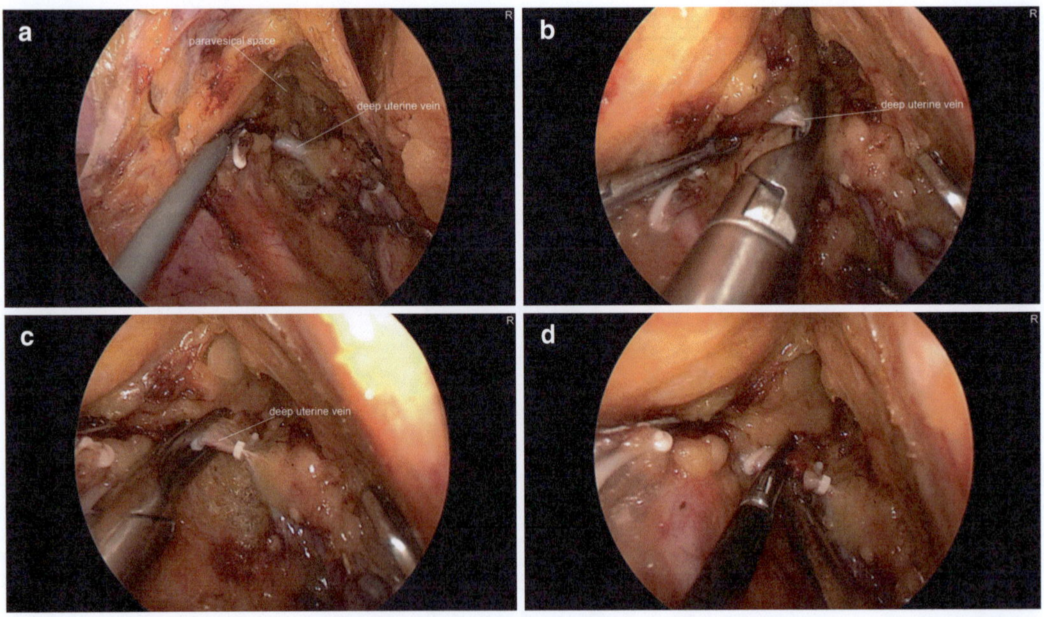

Fig. 10.13 (**a**–**d**) Transect the deep uterine vein

10.8 Exposure of the Dorsal Parametrium

Pull the lateral peritoneum outward and the rectal sidewall inward, and use a ultrasonic scalpel to sharply dissect until the level of the rectal sidewall (Fig. 10.14a–f). Pull the rectum upward, and pull the uterus downward and backward. Open the rectovaginal peritoneum sharply and separate the rectovaginal space (Fig. 10.15a–h).

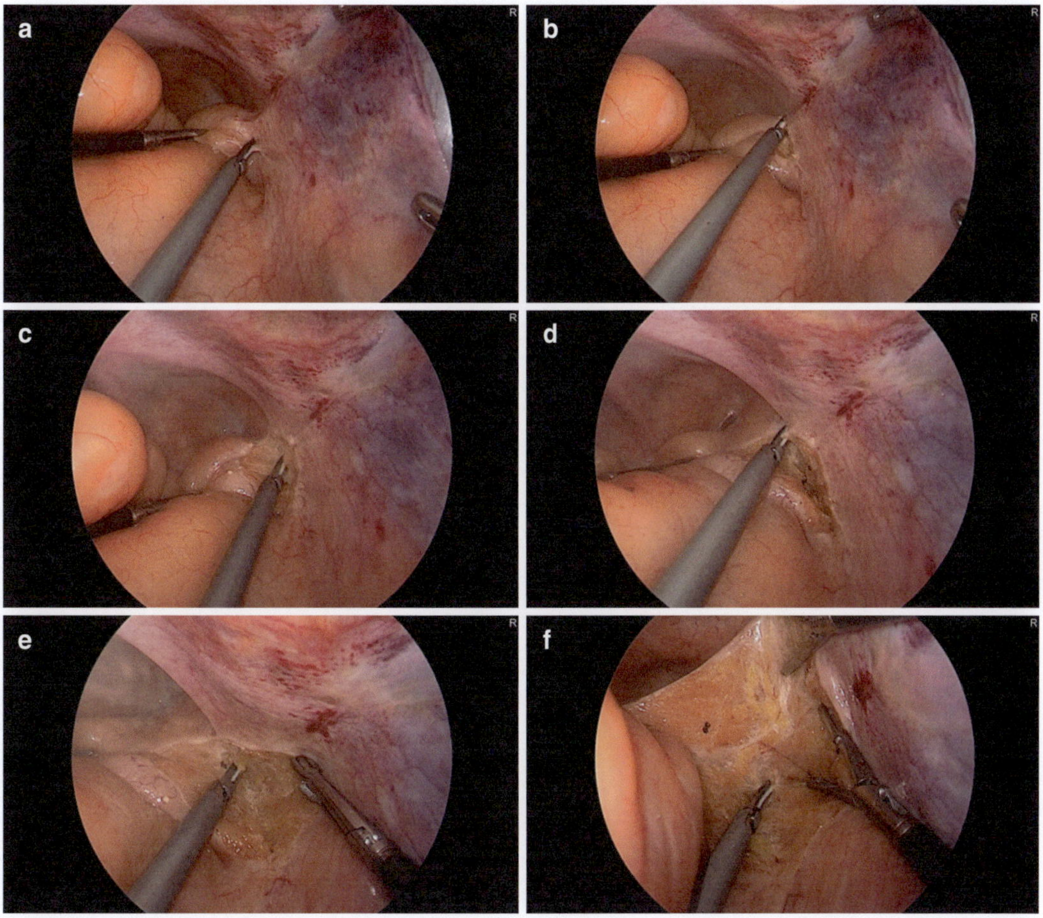

Fig. 10.14 (**a**–**f**) Separate the lateral rectal space

Surgical Experience and Precautions Our team prefers to open the rectovaginal space from the lateral approach. In C1-type surgeries, the range of sacrocervical ligament excision should be at the level of the rectum. The rectal sidewall is usually attached to the medial segment of the sacrocervical ligament, and there is often a distinct "yellow-white" demarcation line in the peritoneal portion. Separate the space between the two and continue the dissection dorsally until the level of the rectal sidewall. Then, open the rectovaginal peritoneum in the midline of the rectovaginal space, deepen the rectovaginal space, widen it bilaterally, and merge it with the lateral approach space. This will safely separate the rectal sidewall from the midsegment of the sacrocervical ligament, avoiding injury to the rectal sidewall, achieving a "horizontal state" of the rectum, and ensuring an adequate and safe excision range during sacrocervical ligament management.

During the opening and separation of the space, it can be helpful to consider the concept of membrane dissection. The advantages are as follows: (1) when opening the space, the position of the peritoneum can be identified at the "membrane bridge," which is the junction of the peritoneum's "yellow-white" border at the fusion point of the two embryonic compartments. (2) During space separation, sharply dissect the white loose connective tissue within the space (located between two different embryonic compartments).

By following these operative procedures and considerations, the surgeon can effectively expose and navigate the rectovaginal space, ensuring optimal surgical outcomes and minimizing the risk of complications.

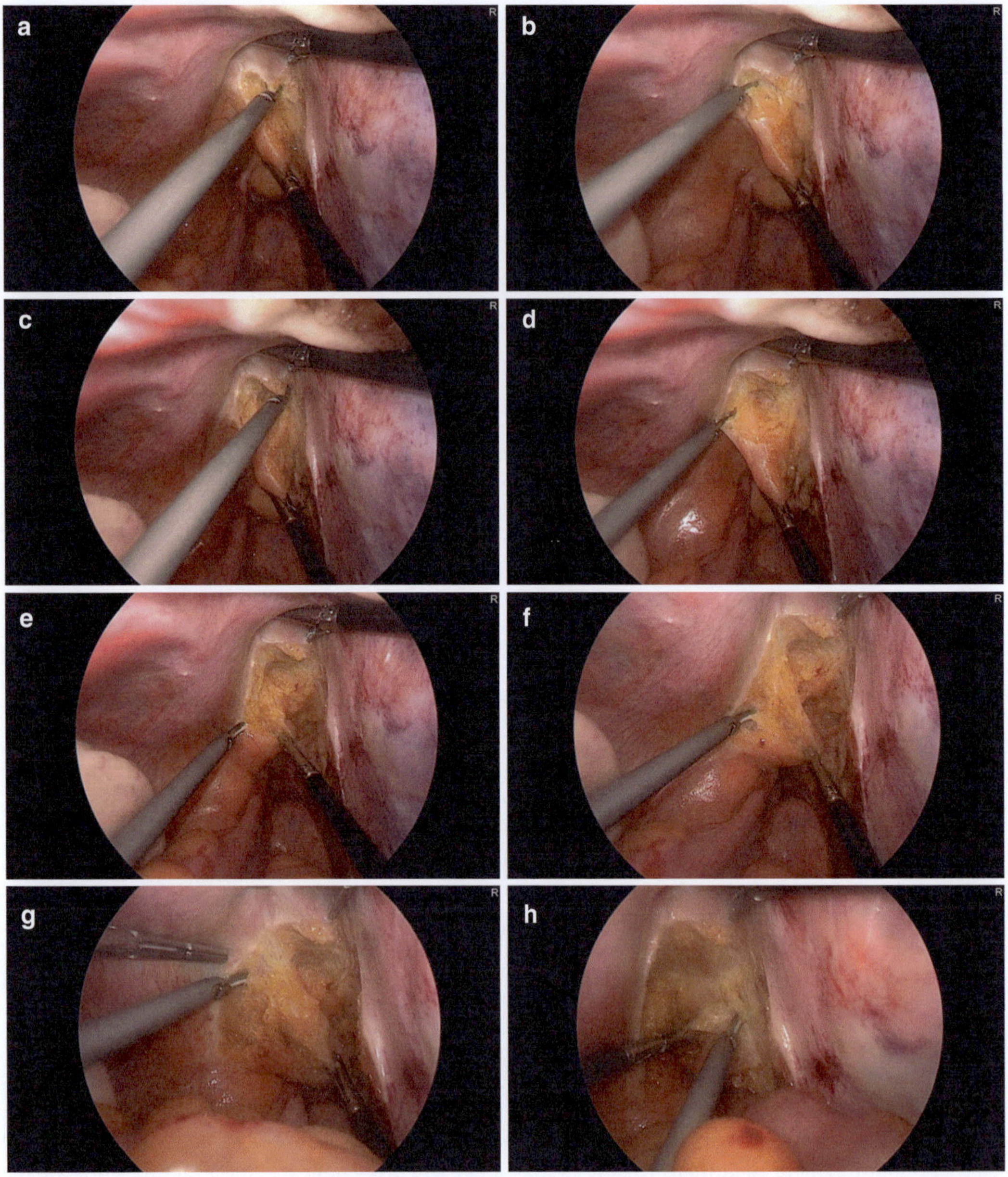

Fig. 10.15 (**a**–**h**) Open the rectovaginal peritoneum sharply and separate the rectovaginal space

10.9 Manipulation of the Ventral Parametrium

Expose the vesicocervical space and vesicovaginal space by pulling the bladder laterally and caudally. Use an ultrasonic scalpel to make a sharp incision at the "yellow-white" junction, followed by sharp dissection of the white loose connective tissue to expose the vesicocervical space and vesicovaginal space (Fig. 10.16a–j).

Surgical Experience and Precautions The vesicovaginal space does not necessarily need to be directly opened to a sufficient depth and width because the uterosacral ligaments have not been completely detached at this stage. This may make

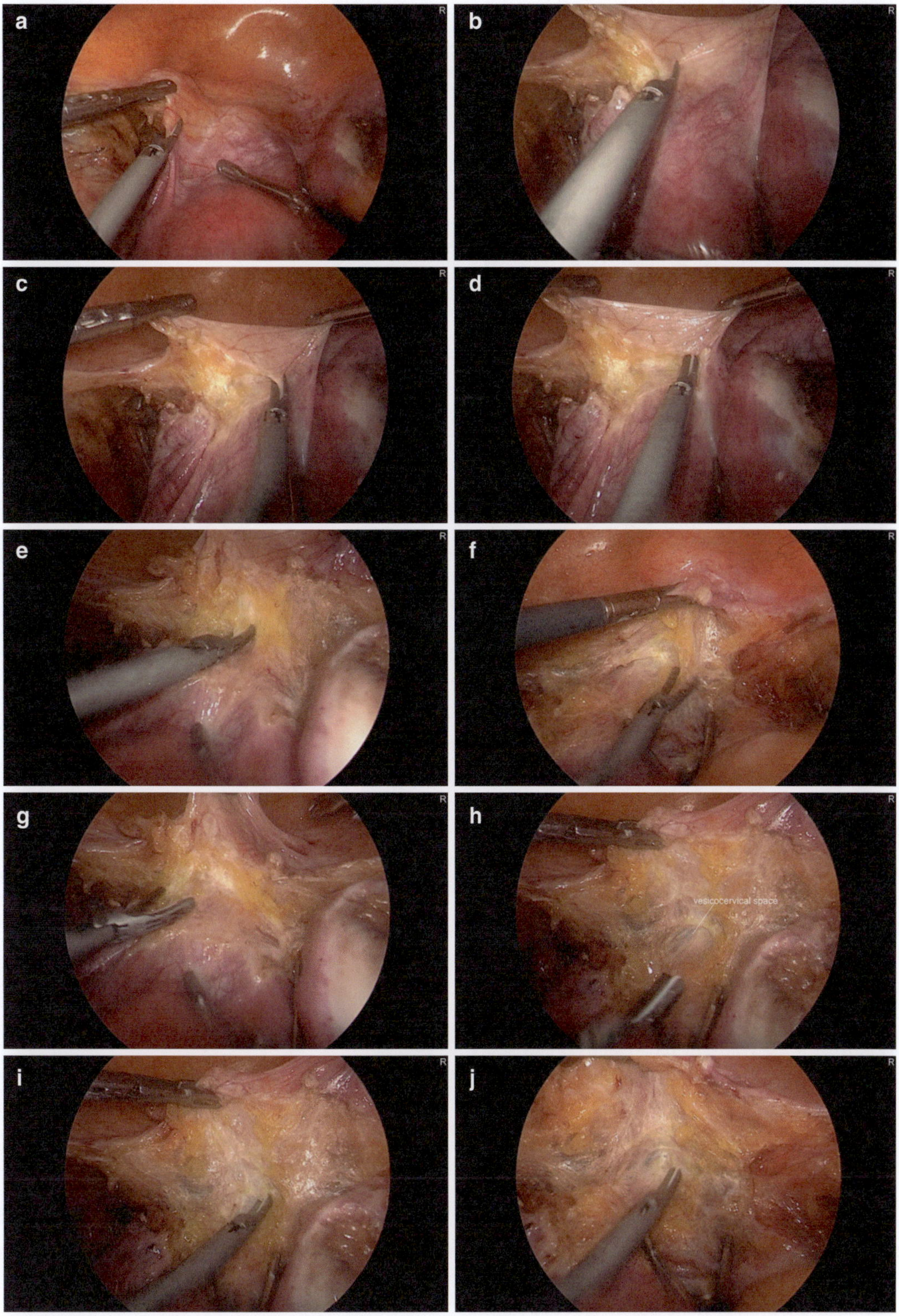

Fig. 10.16 (**a**–**j**) Expose the vesicocervical space and vesicovaginal space

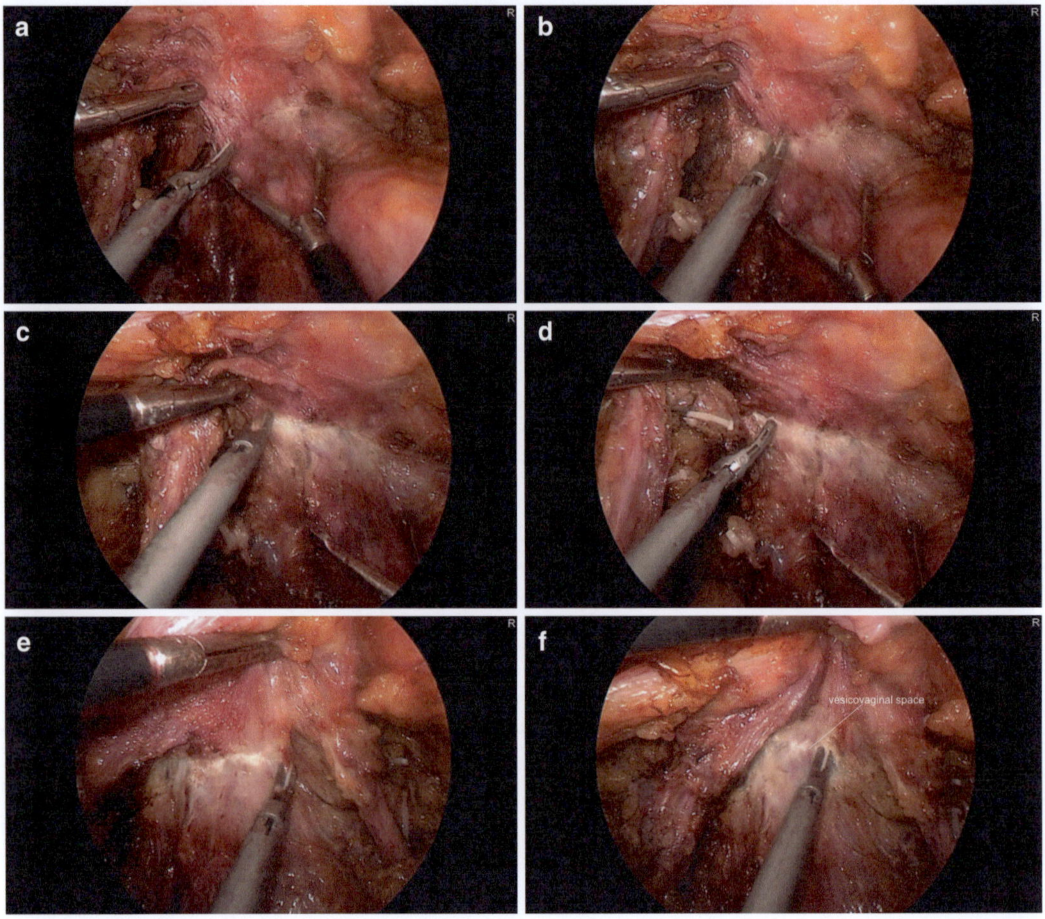

Fig. 10.17 (**a**–**f**) Widen the vesicovaginal space

the exposure difficult due to inadequate tension from uterine traction, especially in obese patients and those with a sacrospinous ligament variant. After the detachment of the uterosacral ligaments and the lateral parametrial vessels, the uterus can be adequately elevated, providing sufficient tension for the exposure of the vesicovaginal space. At this point, continue pulling the bladder laterally and caudally, and use the ultrasonic scalpel to sharply dissect the space toward the caudal direction (Fig. 10.17a–f), preparing for the removal of an adequate length of vaginal wall (C-type surgery requires a 2 cm margin from the lower edge of the lesion for vaginal wall resection). Our team understands this 2 cm as the natural length of the vaginal wall, not the elongated length due to traction. Since there is no specific projection on the vaginal surface, our team uses anatomical landmarks for localization. After the dissection of the vesicovaginal ligaments, the connective tissue adjacent to the vaginal wall that needs to be detached is exposed. It should be vertically dissected in the direction of the vagina to mark the length of vaginal wall resection. Postoperatively, the measurement of the "natural length of the vaginal wall" in the three dimensional specimen is 2–2.5 cm).

10.10 Dissection of the Uterine Artery

10.10.1 Management of the Bladder Branch of the Uterine Artery

Continuing the approach of the lateral space, pull the uterine artery laterally, sharply separate the bladder by pulling it toward the ventral and caudal directions, and further dissect the tissue on the ventral aspect of the bladder angles and the bladder branch of the uterine artery (Figs. 10.18, 10.19, 10.20, and 10.21).

Surgical Experience and Precautions This area requires attention to two anatomical structures: the ureter at the entrance of the "tunnel" and the branch vessel (commonly known as the bladder branch of the uterine artery) originating from the uterine artery toward the bladder. The outer tissues of the bladder branch of the uterine artery are relatively dense, while the inner tissues are relatively loose and can be easily separated. Typically, the ureter is located on the medial aspect of the bladder branch of the uterine artery at the inner side of the tunnel entrance. Therefore,

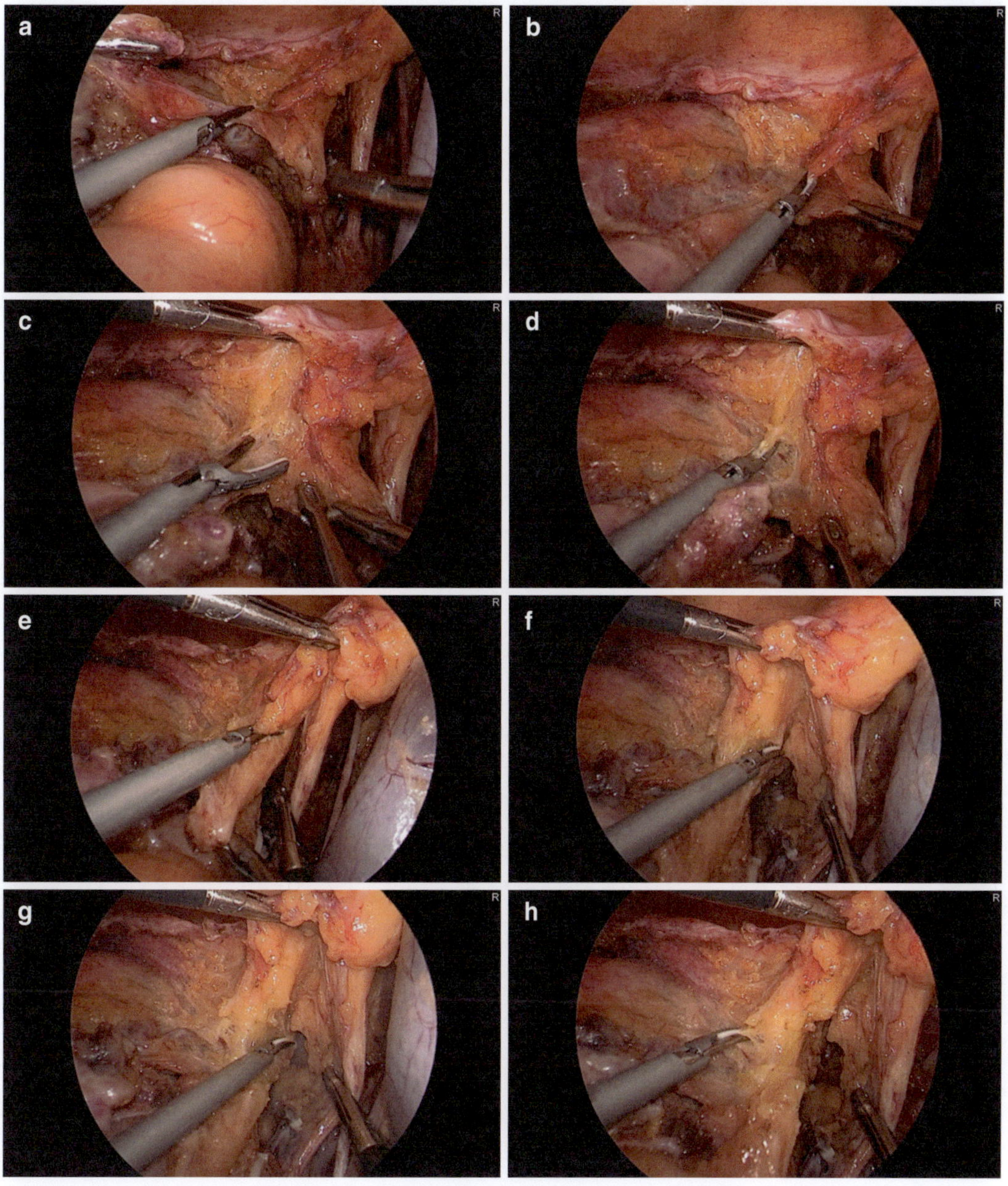

Fig. 10.18 (**a–h**) Separate the ventral tissue of the uterine artery

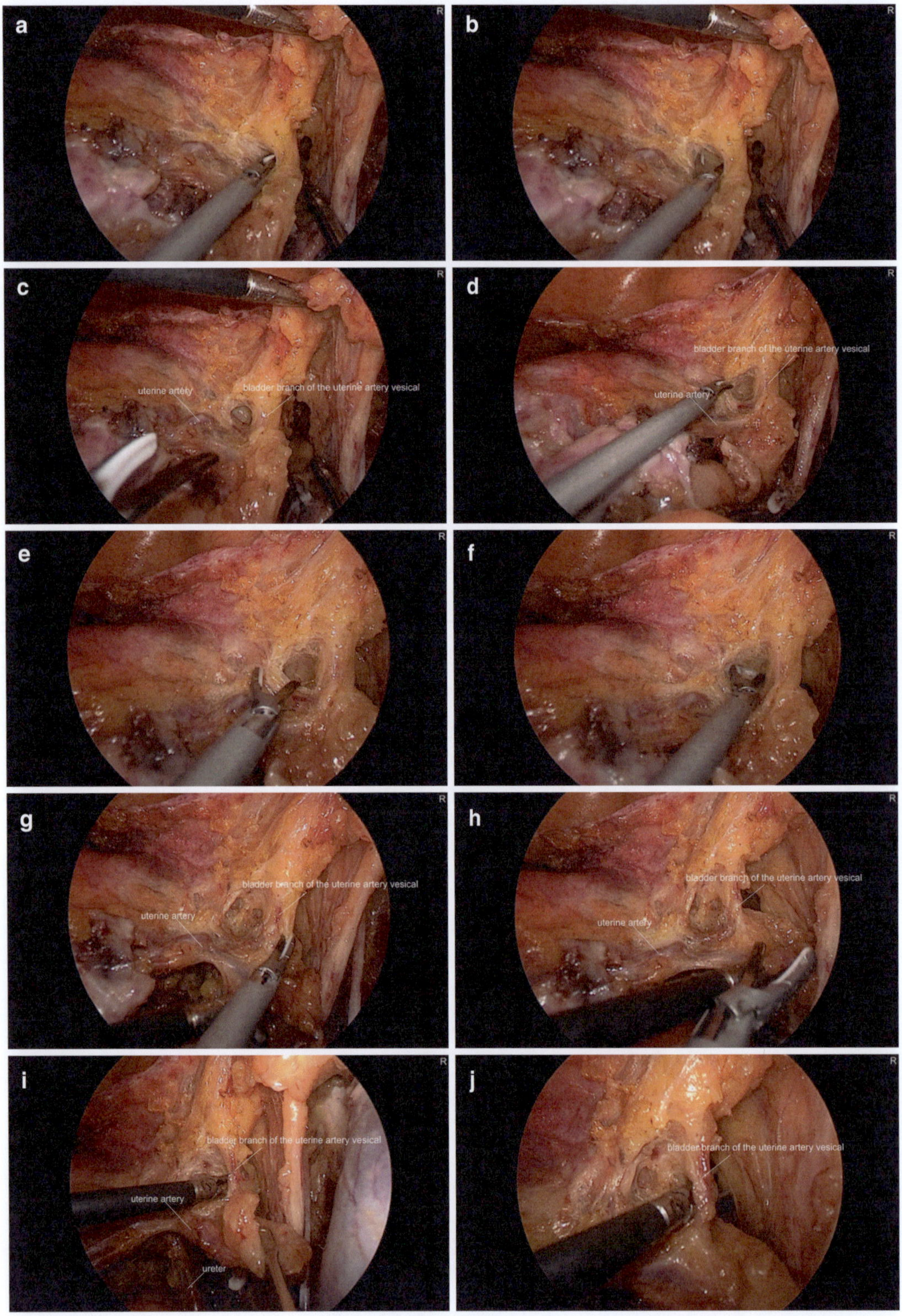

Fig. 10.19 (**a**–**j**) Separate uterine artery bladder branch

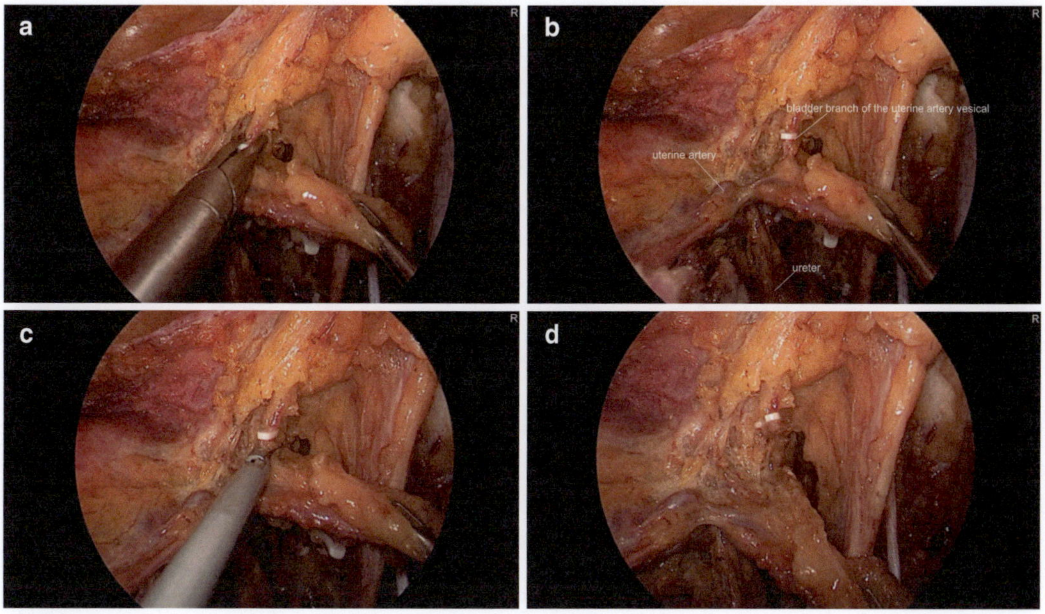

Fig. 10.20 (**a–d**) Transect uterine artery bladder branch

when separating and dissecting the bladder branch of the uterine artery, a blunt dissection technique is mainly used to dissect and anatomize the vessel from the inside to the outside. After separation, the vessel is clamped and ligated, and then dissected with an ultrasonic scalpel.

The bladder branch of the uterine artery is rarely mentioned in existing anatomy textbooks and literature both domestically and internationally. However, our team believes that this vessel is crucial for the safe and bloodless handling of the ureteral "tunnel" based on repeated clinical practice of bloodless surgery. In extensive reference to various textbooks and literature, we found that this vessel was mentioned in the book "New Techniques of Extensive Radical Hysterectomy: Anatomical and Surgical Techniques for Preservation of Nerves in Extensive Radical Hysterectomy." The diameter of the bladder branch of the uterine artery is usually similar to that of the main uterine artery. Therefore, if this vessel is not individually addressed during the exposure of the ureteral "tunnel" entrance, it may result in bleeding and lead to a blurry space and difficulty in handling the "tunnel." In some cases, the diameter of this vessel is relatively thin, and surgeons may overlook it while handling the separation of the uterine artery and the ureteral "tunnel" entrance.

10.10.2 Dissection of the Ureter and Uterine Artery

Reverse traction is applied to the ureter and uterine artery, using a combination of blunt and sharp dissection until the ureter is freed to the entrance of the tunnel (Fig. 10.22a–h).

Surgical Experience and Precautions During the dissection, multiple uterine artery ureteral branches may be seen. It is important to sharply divide them close to the uterine artery to avoid thermal radiation damage caused by energy devices. Additionally, it is necessary to avoid immediate blunt dissection of the ureter after sharp dissection using an ultrasonic scalpel. Our team adopts the following methods to prevent thermal injury during this step: (1) allowing 3–5 seconds of natural cooling after sharp dissection; (2) placing the functional blade of the ultrasonic scalpel on the uterine serosa for 2–3 seconds to assist in heat dissipation, which is commonly used in robot-assisted surgery;

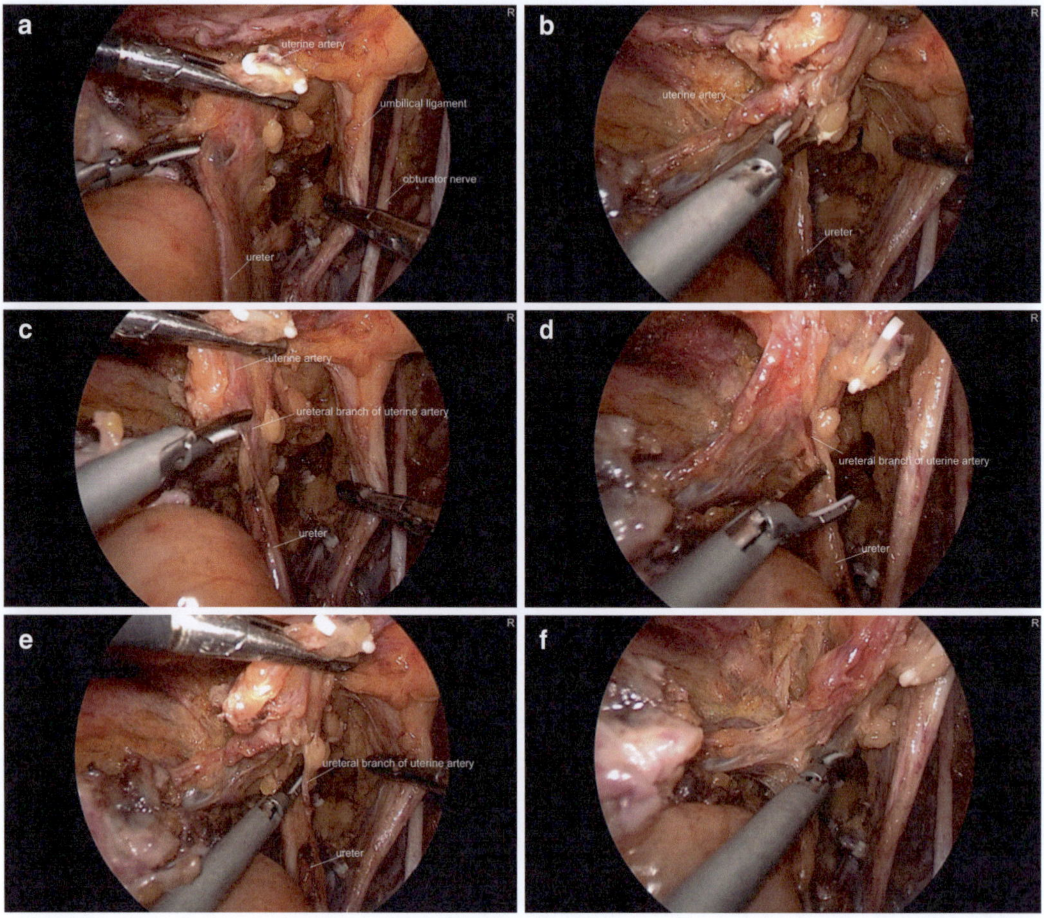

Fig. 10.21 (**a**–**f**) Transect uterine artery ureteral branch

(3) using room temperature physiological saline for irrigation to cool the scalpel, which is more commonly used in open and laparoscopic surgery.

Regarding the understanding of the ureteral "tunnel," our team believes that during the ureteral dissection process, it is necessary to perform three-dimensional dissection circumferentially (medial, lateral, ventral, and dorsal) to fully free the ureter from the "tunnel." In QM-C1-type surgery, preserving the pelvic autonomic nerves is required, and the hypogastric nerves are located within the mesentery on the dorsal aspect of the ureter. Therefore, the dorsal aspect of the ureter is temporarily not dissected.

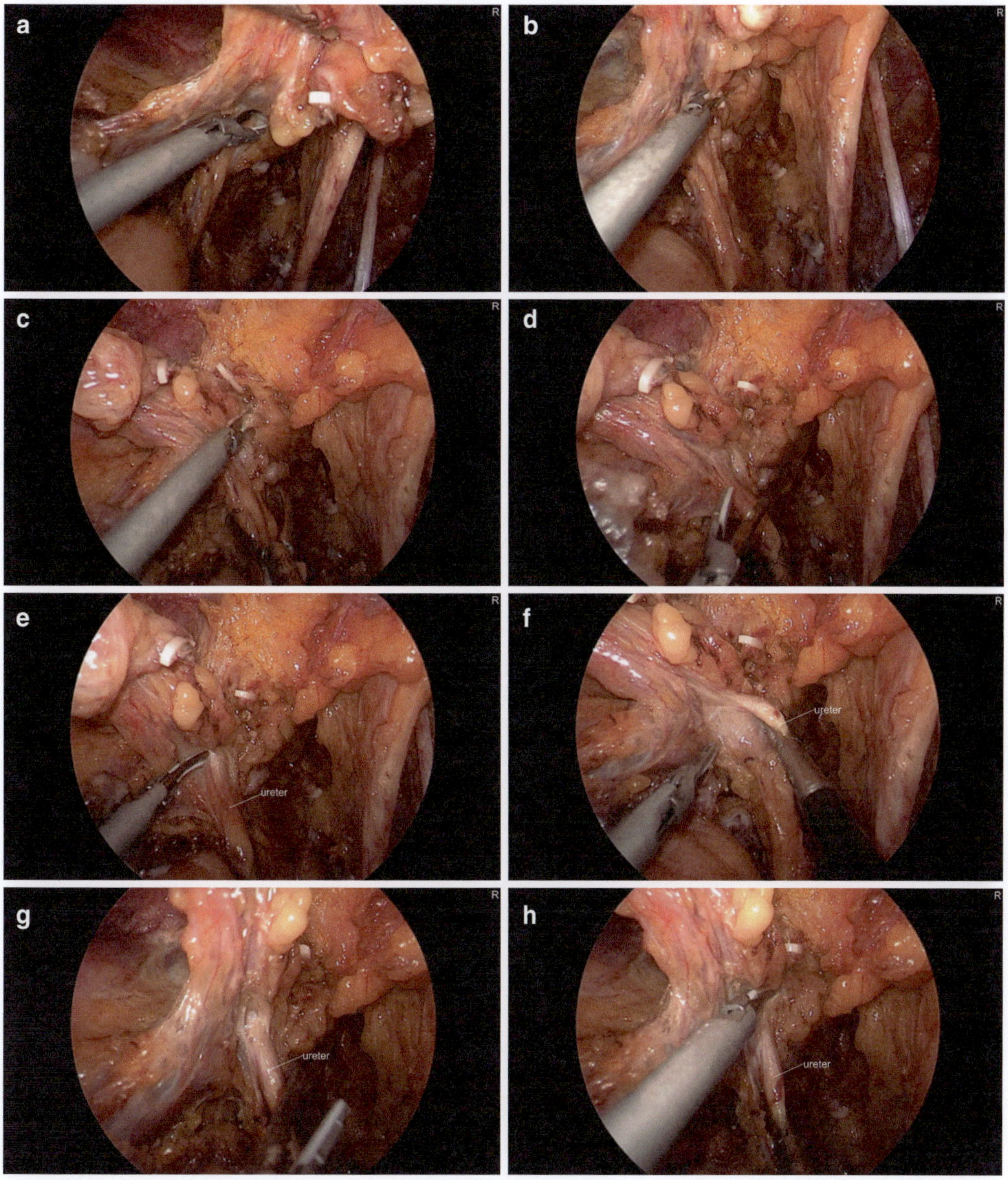

Fig. 10.22 (**a**–**h**) Separate ureter to "tunnel" entrance

10.11 Expose the Fourth Space (to Locate the Exit of the Ureteral "Tunnel")

Exposing the fourth space *by pulling the ureter outward, and pulling the bladder upward and caudally, and the uterus cranially and dorsally to create tension. Use an ultrasonic scalpel to sharply enlarge the already separated vesicovaginal space laterally. During the gradual separation process, the ureter may become visible. Continue pulling the bladder towards the ventral side and perform a combined blunt and sharp dissection to separate the bladder from the parametirum, then exposing the fourth space (Fig. 10.23a–l).*

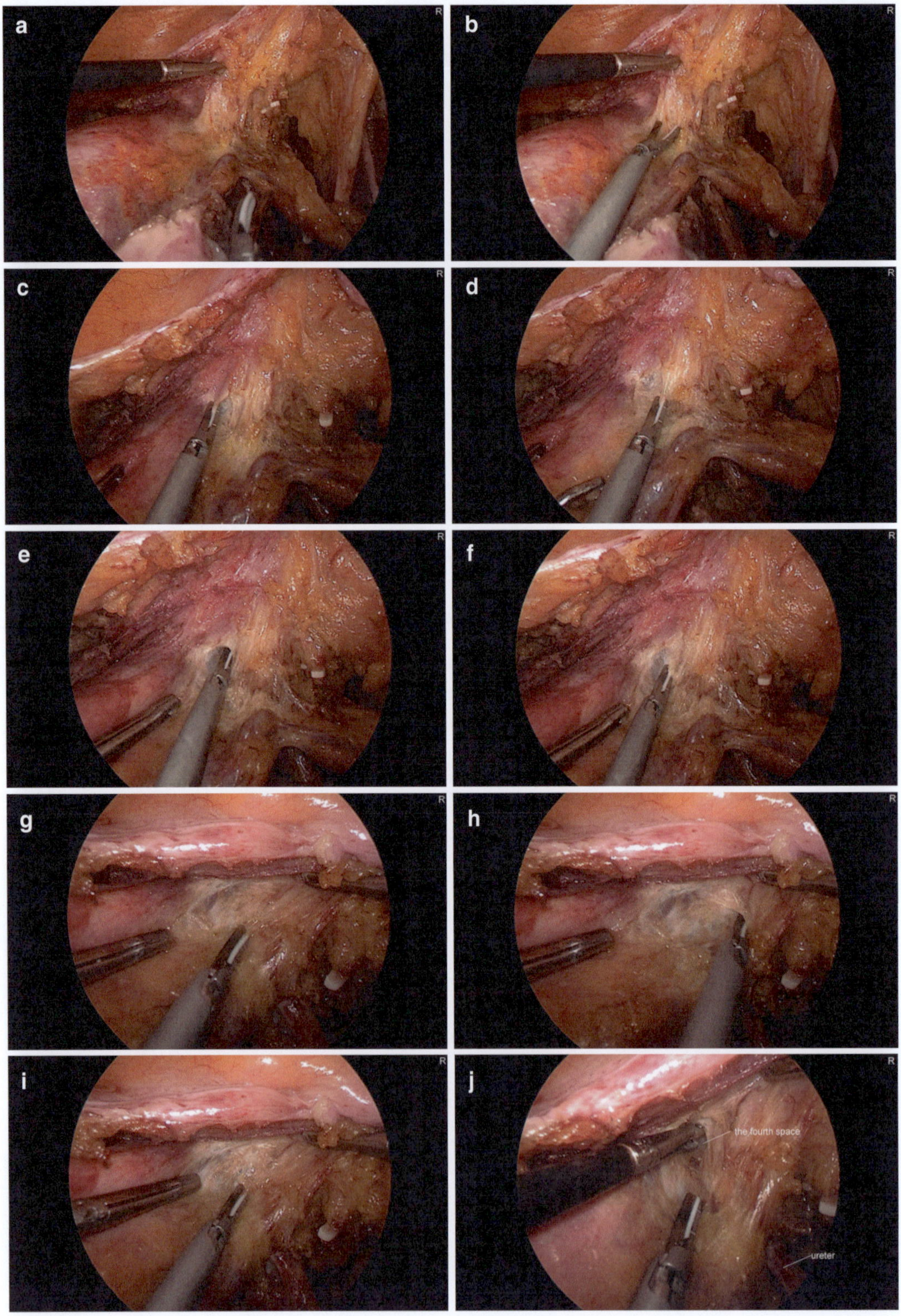

Fig. 10.23 (**a**–**l**) Expose the fourth space

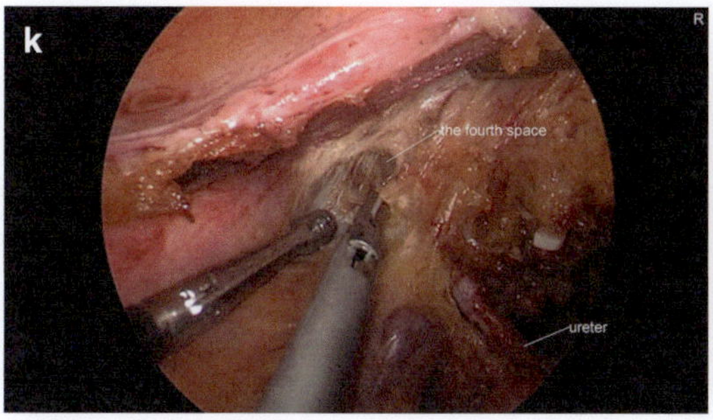

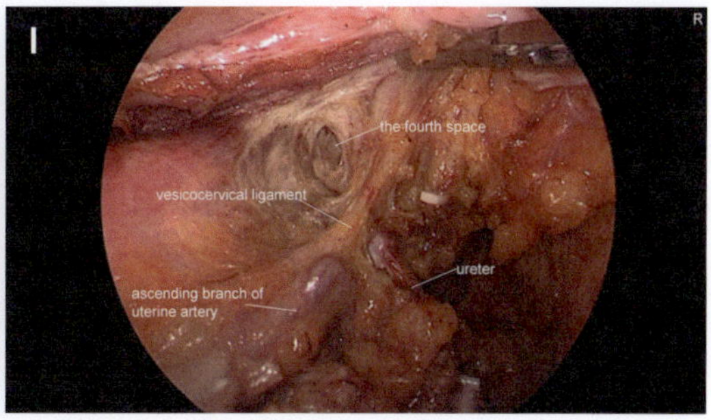

Fig. 10.23 (continued)

Surgical Experience and Precautions This step is particularly important and depends on the safe handling of the vesicocervical ligaments. Our team is accustomed to utilizing this space for the safe shallow dissection of the vesicocervical ligaments while directly visualizing the entrance and exit of the ureteral "tunnel." Even if bleeding occurs during the dissection, it can be calmly sutured and electrocoagulated without concern for ureteral injury.

In type C1 surgery, it is important to avoid reaching the deepest part of the paravaginal space (where it communicates with the paravesical space) to prevent damage to the preserved nerves.

Management of the Vesicocervical Ligament Management of the vesicocervical ligament involves pulling the bladder toward the ventral side. Using a ureteral clamp, the ureter at the entrance of the tunnel is pulled laterally and abdominally. The ultrasonic knife is then used to approach the cervix and coagulate the vesicocervical ligament (Fig. 10.24a–i).

Surgical Experience and Precautions During the management of the vesicocervical ligament, it is crucial to fully push and pull the ureter laterally to prevent ureteral injury during the energy instrument coagulation.

In case of bleeding during the coagulation of the vesicocervical ligament, electrocoagulation can be used on the uterine side, and absorbable suture can be applied on the ureteral side to achieve hemostasis.

Management of vesicovaginal ligament, with attention to the vesical venous plexus, using ureteral forceps to pull the ureter toward the ventral and lateral sides, exposing the suburethral fascia, hypogastric plexus, and vesicovaginal ligament. Between the hypogastric plexus and ureter or at the ventral side of the uterine side of the deep uterine vein, the ureteral mesentery is opened horizontally (Fig. 10.25a–f), and continued separation is performed toward the caudal side. The vesicovaginal ligament is sharply dissected using an ultrasonic scalpel, exposing the vesical venous plexus that drains into the deep uterine vein, and the individual branches of the vesical venous plexus are sequentially ligated, usually 2–3 branches (Fig. 10.26a–h).

Surgical Experience and Precautions

1. For ligation of branches of the vesical venous plexus, it is necessary to first open the ureteral mesentery up to the vesicovaginal ligament. For cases with a clearly visible hypogastric plexus, the ureteral mesentery can be opened between the hypogastric plexus and the ureter. For cases with an indistinct hypogastric plexus, to avoid accidental injury to the hypogastric plexus (located within the ureteral fascia on the dorsal side of the ureter, approximately 1.5–2 cm), the uterine side of the deep uterine vein can be identified to open the ureteral mesentery on its ventral side.
2. The branches of the vesical venous plexus should be adequately exposed, and after clamping the blood vessels, they should be

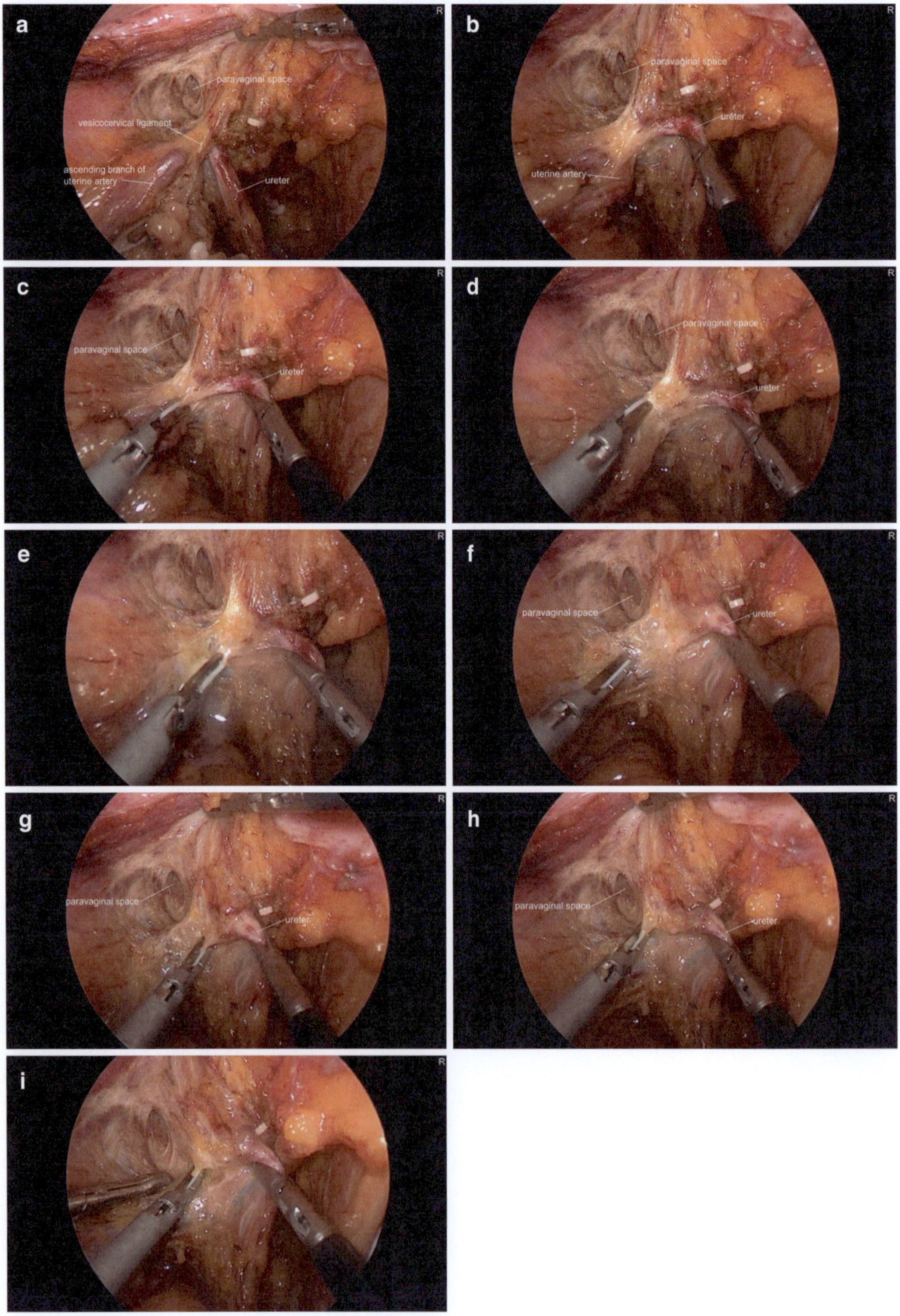

Fig. 10.24 (**a**–**i**) Transect the vesicocervical ligament

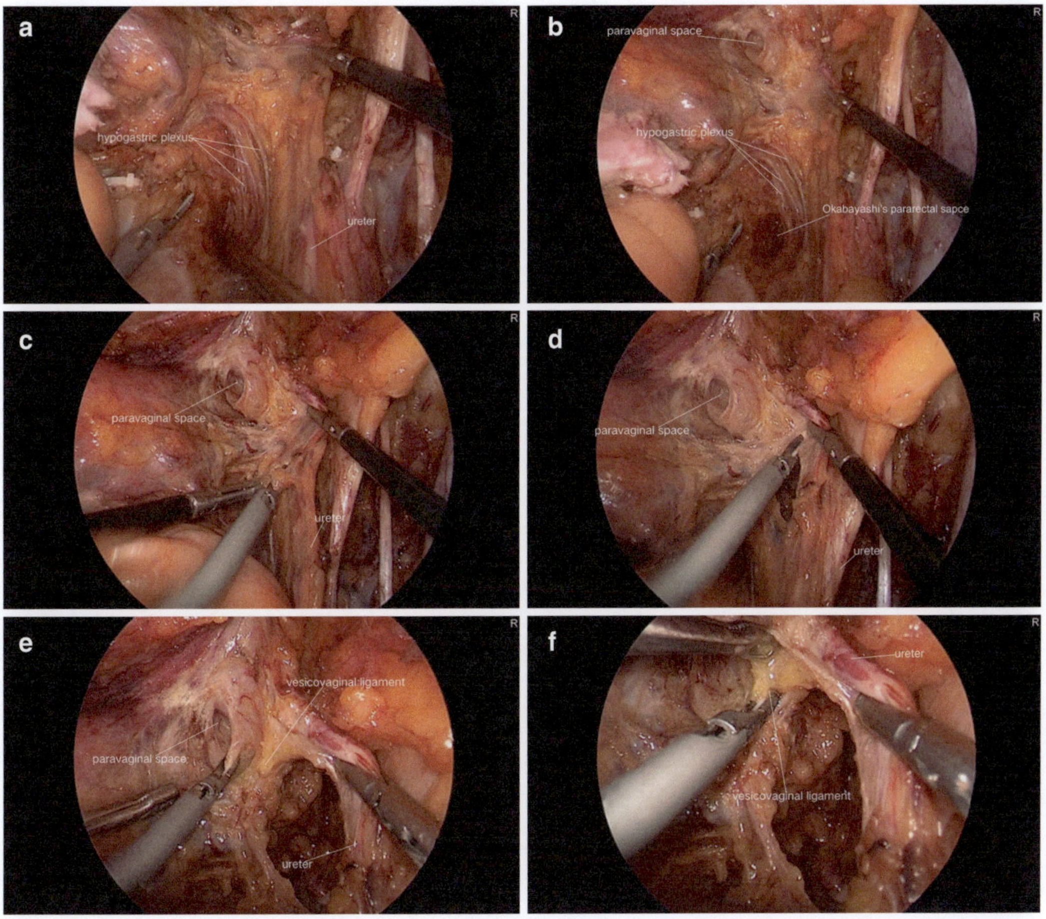

Fig. 10.25 (**a–f**) Open the ureteral mesentery

ligated to prevent bleeding and avoid the use of energy devices to prevent nerve damage.

The management of the vesicovaginal ligament and the vesical venous plexus within it is particularly important in nerve-sparing surgeries. The procedure should be performed with minimal bleeding to ensure safe preservation of the nerves under direct visualization. If there are multiple branches of the vesical venous plexus, it is necessary to ligate them all individually. The advantage is that they can be ligated one by one after pushing the nerves aside, maximizing the bloodless preservation of the autonomous pelvic nerves.

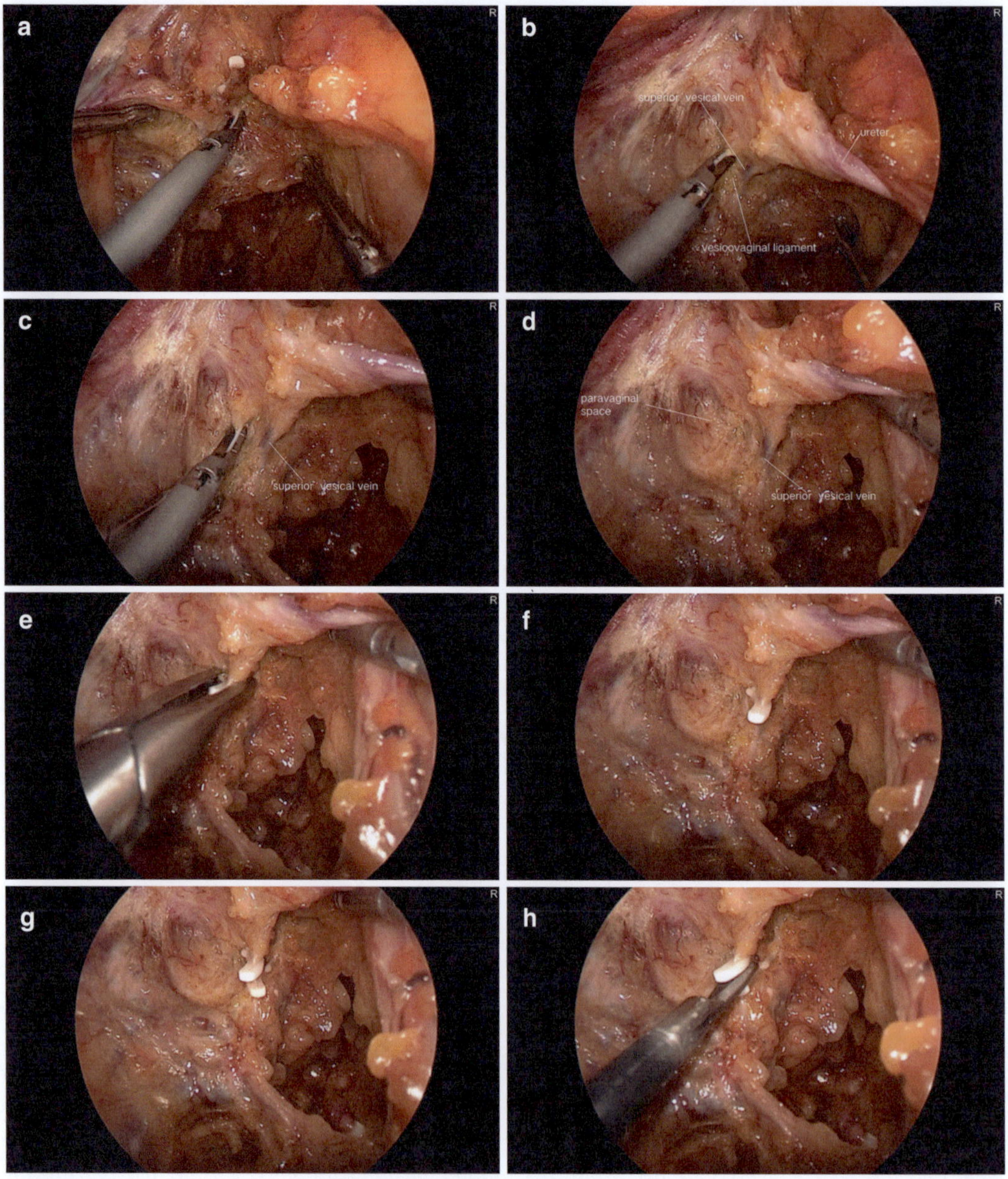

Fig. 10.26 (**a**–**h**) Management of the vesicovaginal ligament

10.12 Separation and Preservation of Nerves

Simple preservation of the autonomous pelvic nerves: The uterine side of the deep uterine vein is pulled toward the ventral and medial sides, and the relationship between it and the nerves below is separated along the caudal direction, closely following the lower edge of the deep uterine vein. The connective tissue adjacent to the dorsal side of the deep uterine vein is dissected, while gradually ligating the remaining vesicovaginal ligament. The uterine branches, rectal branches, and cervical branches of the pelvic plexus are sequentially ligated and separated, while preserving the bladder branches by pushing them aside. The connective tissue adjacent to the vaginal side and the dorsal sacroiliac ligament are dissected in the vertical direction of the vagina (Figs. 10.27, 10.28, and 10.29).

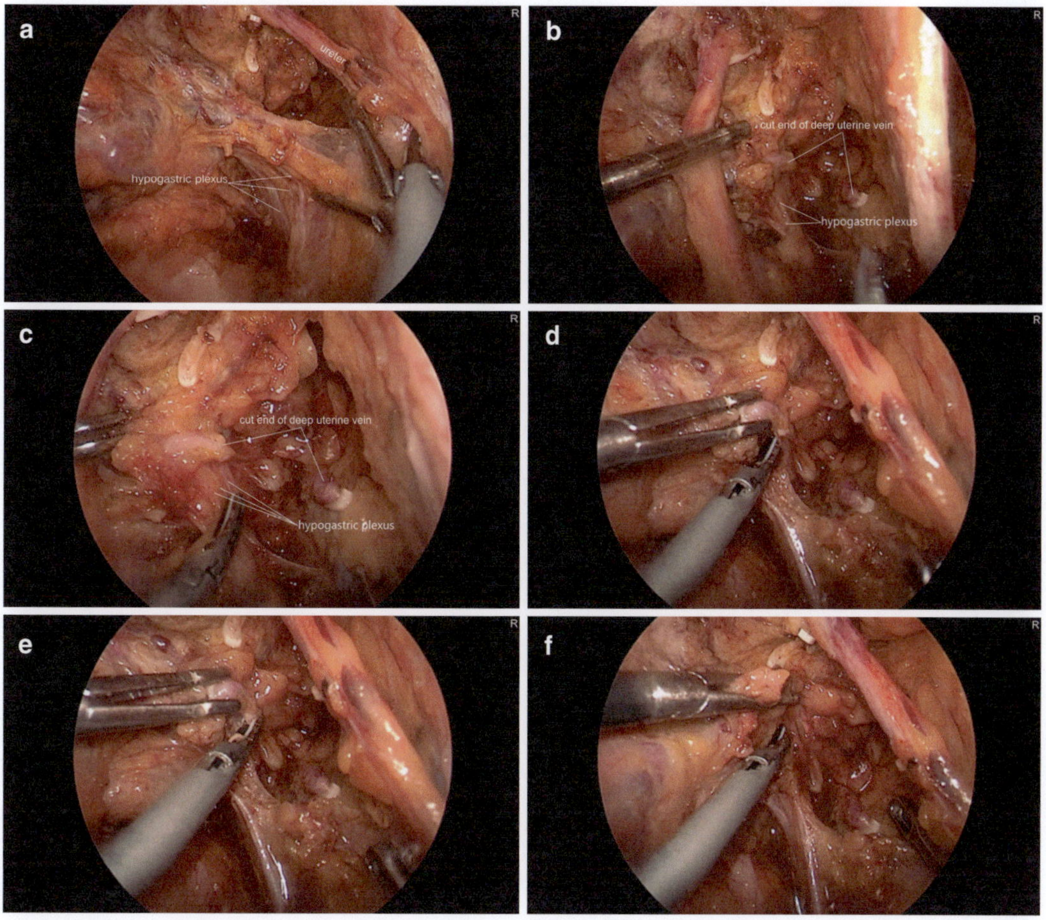

Fig. 10.27 (**a**–**f**) Separate pelvic autonomic nerves

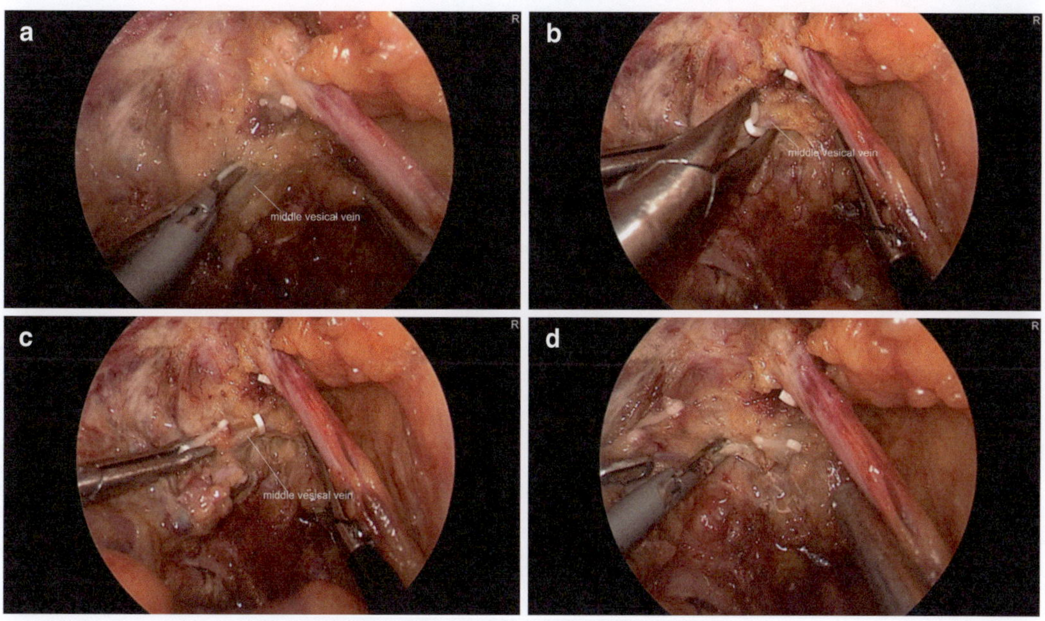

Fig. 10.28 (**a**–**d**) Vascular clamp occludes the superior vesical vein and dissect it

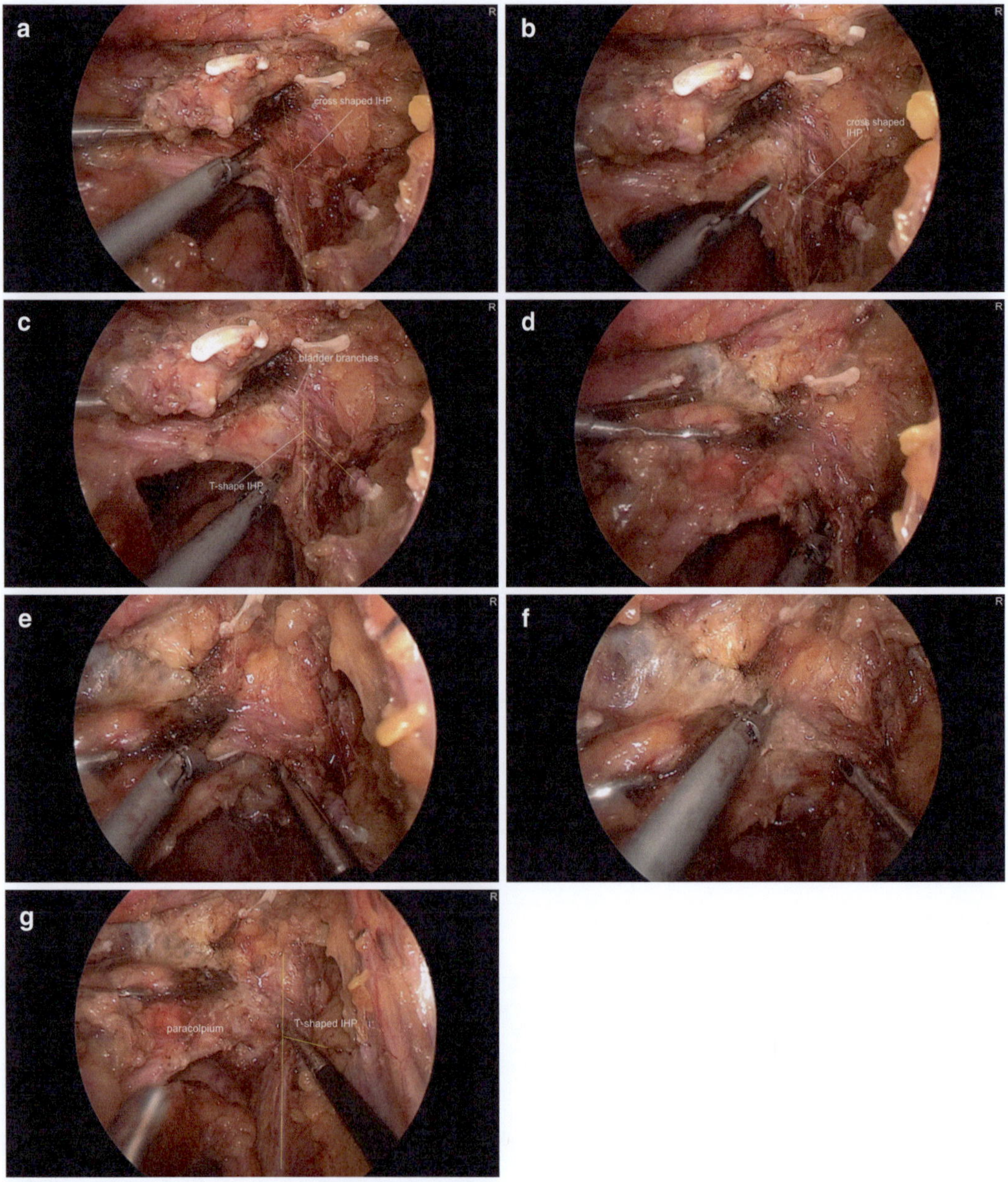

Fig. 10.29 (**a**–**g**) Preserve the pelvic autonomic nerve

10.13 Preservation of the Autonomous Pelvic Nerves

Demonstration of a case involving systematic preservation of the autonomous pelvic nerves on the left side. To maintain continuity, the description begins with the establishment of the paravaginal space.

Exposure of the Paravaginal Space The uterus is pulled horizontally toward the cranial and medial sides, while the bladder and peritoneum at the bladder angle are pulled toward the ventral and caudal sides to create tension. This allows visualization of the loose connective tissue between the posterior wall of the bladder and the vagina, as well as the paracolpium.

Using a combination of blunt and sharp dissection, the already exposed vesicovaginal space is further expanded toward the lateral side (Figs. 10.30 and 10.31).

Surgical Experience and Precautions In our team's experience, the ultrasonic scalpel is used with a sharpness of only 1/5 or even smaller, and the tension between the posterior wall of

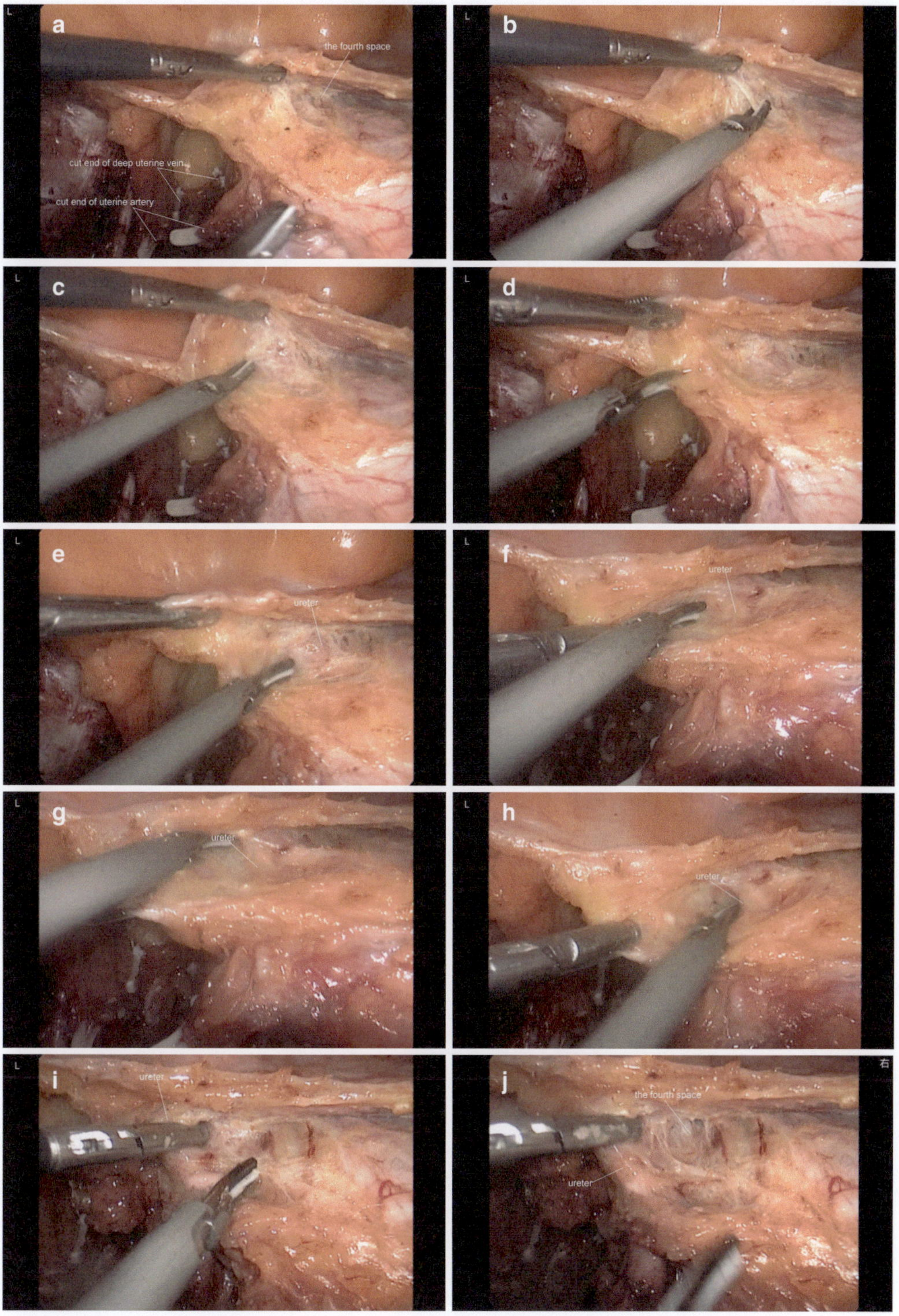

Fig. 10.30 (**a**–**j**) Expose the fourth space

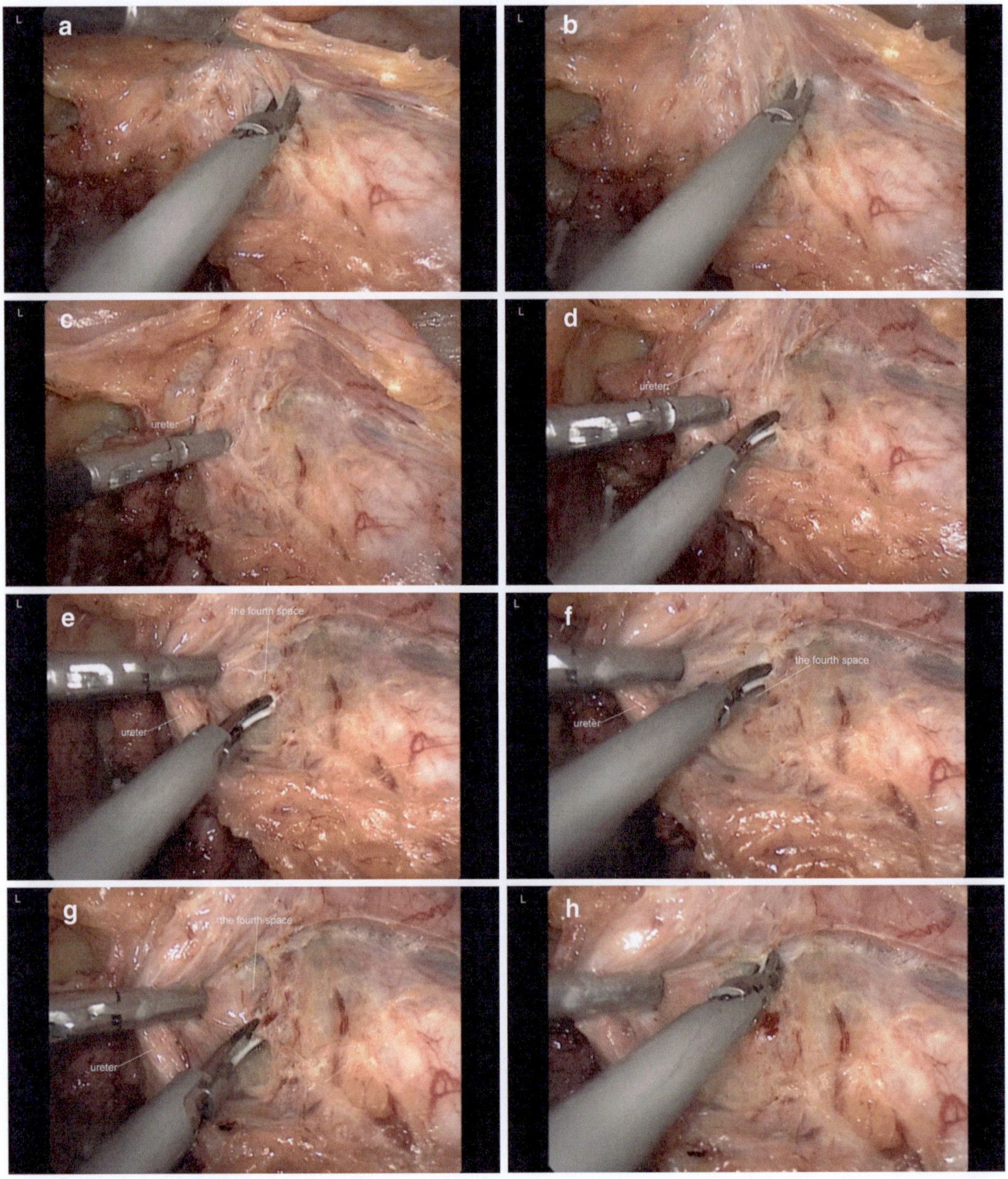

Fig. 10.31 (**a**–**h**) Separate the fourth space

the bladder and the vagina, as well as the paracolpium, is continuously adjusted. This ensures safe dissection within the correct space.

When approaching the vicinity of the ureter, it is prone to unintentionally deviate toward the ventral side of the ureter, leading to ureteral injury. Our team is accustomed to deepening and widening the fourth space during the dissection process. By utilizing the space between the caudal end of the posterior bladder wall and the paracolpium it can be expanded in the opposite direction toward the cranial side. This readily exposes the space between the ureter and the paracolpium.

Once the ureter is progressively exposed, it is pulled together with the posterior bladder wall toward the ventral and lateral sides, and sharp dissection is performed in the fourth space using

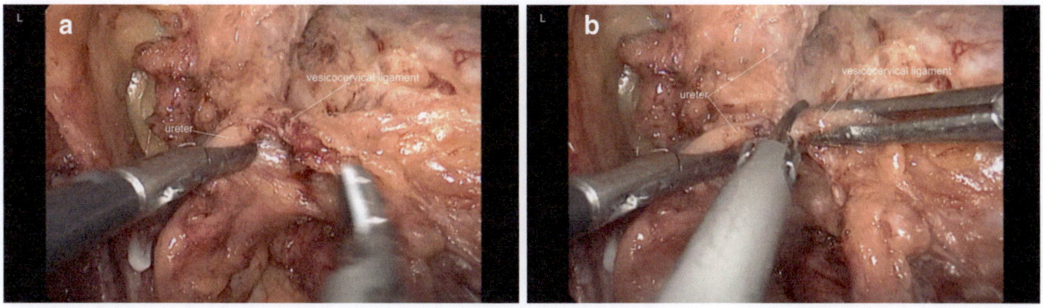

Fig. 10.32 (**a**, **b**) Management of the vesicocervical ligament

the ultrasonic scalpel. Directly connecting the fourth space to the pelvic floor and the paravesical space should be avoided. If such connection occurs, it is highly likely to disrupt the bladder branches of the preserved autonomous pelvic nerves.

10.14 Management of the Vesicocervical Ligament

Clamp the ureter with ureteral forceps, pull it outward and toward the ventral, and sharply divide it using an ultrasonic scalpel (Fig. 10.32a, b). During the handling of the vesicocervical ligament, it is crucial to fully push and pull the ureter, avoiding ureteral injury during the process of energy instrument coagulation. If bleeding occurs during the coagulation of the vesicocervical ligament, electrocoagulation can be applied on the uterine side, and absorbable suture can be used for hemostasis on the ureteral side.

10.15 Management of the Vesicovaginal Ligament

Use a ureteral clamp to pull the ureter toward the ventral and outward, exposing the fascia below the ureter, the pelvic plexus, and the vesicovaginal ligament (Fig. 10.33a–h). Open the ureteral mesentery between the pelvic plexus and the ureter or on the uterine side of the uterine vein's uterine end horizontally toward the ventral. Continue separating it toward the caudal direction, and sharply divide the vesicovaginal ligament using an ultrasonic scalpel, exposing the vesical veins that drain into the uterine vein (Fig. 10.34a–h). Sequentially divide the branches of the vesical veins, usually 2–3 branches (Fig. 10.35a–c).

Surgical Experience and Precautions The division of the branches of the vesical veins should be performed after opening the ureteral mesentery at the vesicovaginal ligament. In cases where the pelvic plexus is clearly visible, the ureteral mesentery can be opened between the pelvic plexus and the ureter. For cases where the pelvic plexus is not clearly visible, to avoid inadvertent injury to the pelvic plexus (located approximately 1.5–2 cm inside the ureteral mesentery on the dorsal side of the ureter), the uterine side of the uterine vein's uterine end can be identified, and the ureteral mesentery can be opened on its ventral side. The branches of the vesical veins should be adequately exposed, clamped, and divided after vascular clamping to avoid bleeding and the use of energy instruments, thus preventing nerve damage.

The handling of the vesicovaginal ligament and the vesical veins within it is particularly important in nerve-sparing surgery. It is crucial to ensure a bloodless procedure throughout to achieve safe preservation of the nerves under direct vision. If there are multiple branches of the vesical veins, it is not necessary to directly and individually divide all of them. Instead, after exposing the nerves outward, they can be sequentially divided, maximizing the bloodless preservation of the pelvic autonomous nerves.

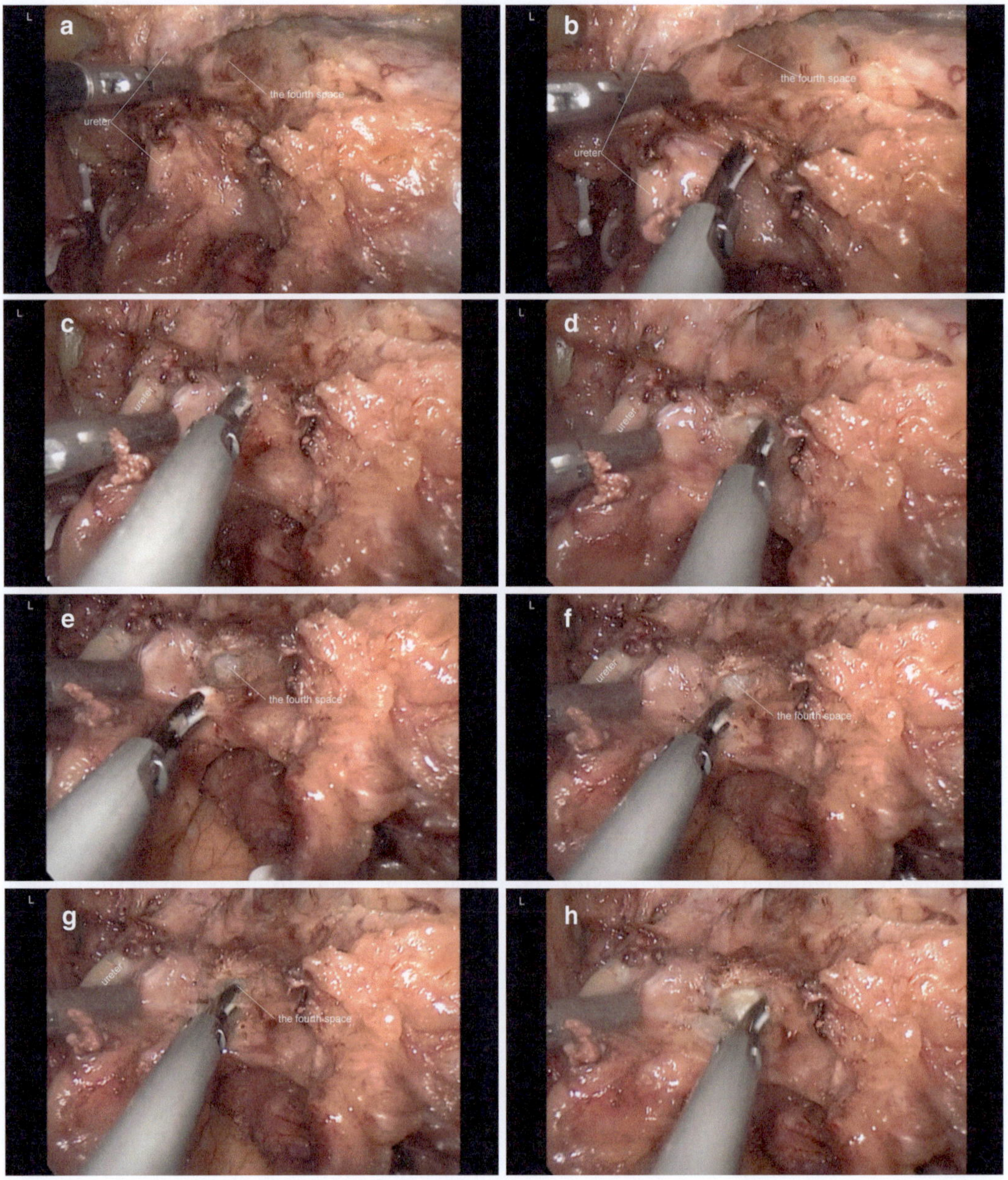

Fig. 10.33 (**a**–**h**) Treat the vesicovaginal ligament

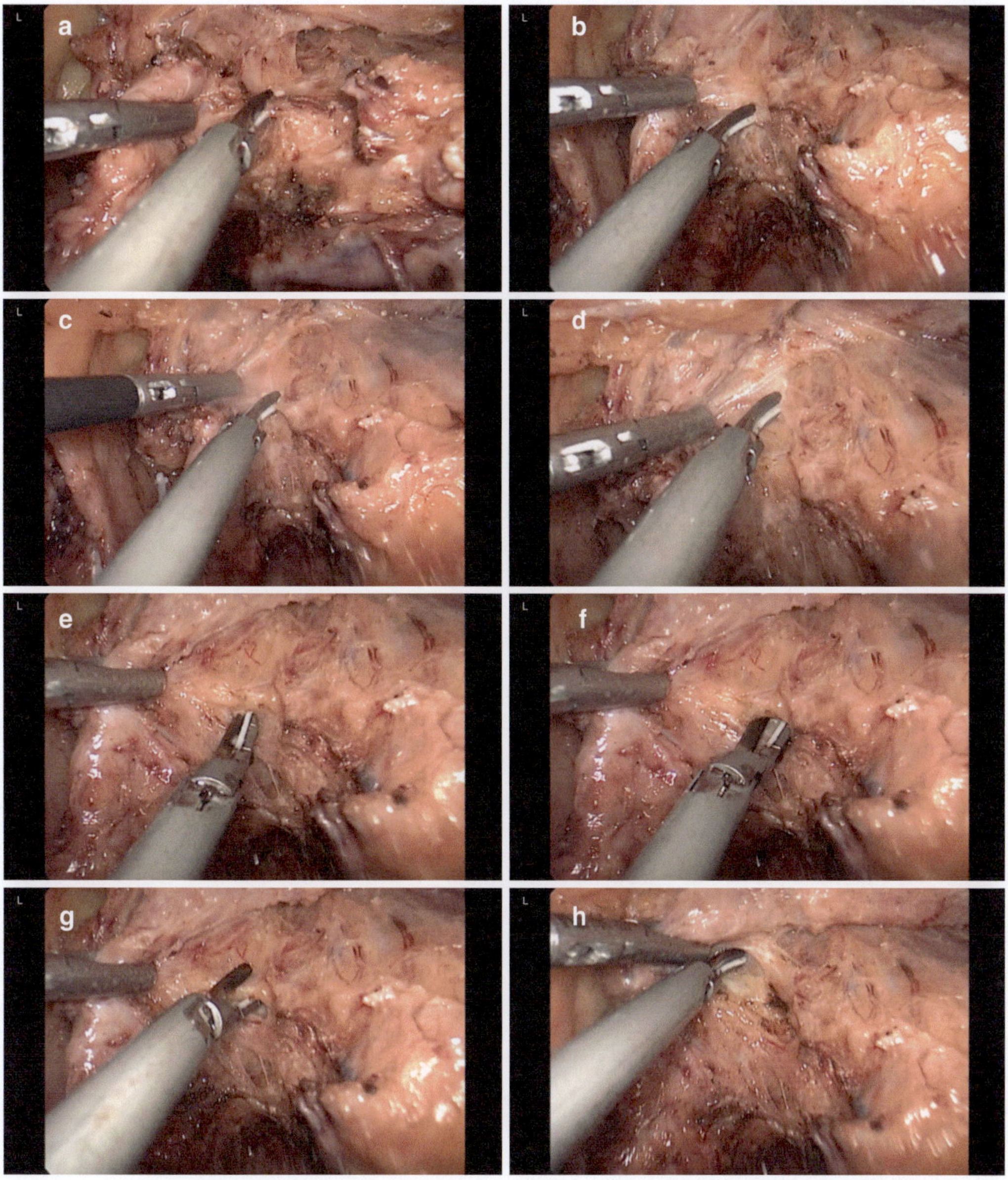

Fig. 10.34 (**a**–**h**) Dissect the superior vesical vein

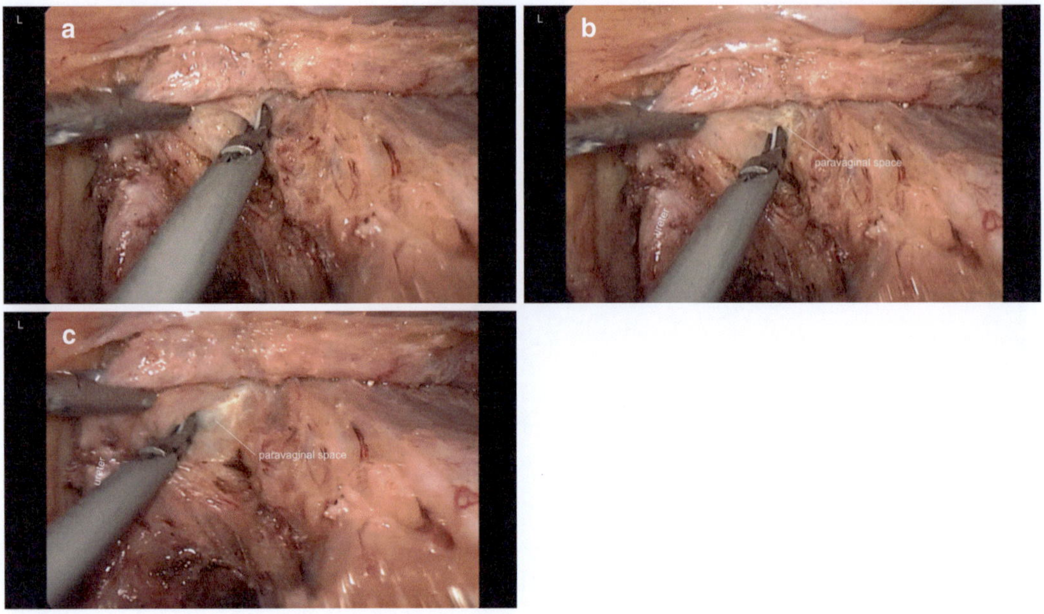

Fig. 10.35 (**a–c**) Sequentially divide the branches of the vesical veins

10.16 Exposure of the Pelvic Plexus Nerves

Pull the ureter and its mesentery medially to expose the Latzko's pararectal space and the paravesical space. The structures that need to be visualized at this point include the hypogastric plexus, the pelvic splanchnic nerve plexus, and the uterine side of the deep uterine veins. The nerves usually run along the posterior surface of the deep uterine veins. Therefore, it is necessary to open the ureteric mesentery on the ventral surface of the deep uterine veins and expand it ventrally and caudally, approaching the vesicovaginal ligament. Use an ultrasonic scalpel to continue the sharp dissection of the remaining portion of the vesicovaginal ligament and divide the remaining branches of the vesical venous plexus. At this point, the uterine side of the deep uterine veins can be pulled medially, and the ureter can be pulled laterally and ventrally. Bluntly and sharply separate the posterior wall fat tissue of the bladder from the paracolpium, continuing the dissection to the pelvic floor. This will expose the pelvic floor fascia, and the nerves are located within the paracolpium between the pelvic floor fascia and the deep uterine veins. Continue to pull the uterine side of the deep uterine veins medially and the ureter laterally to fully expose the nerve junction area and its superficial fat tissue. At this point, use the irrigation suction device (hospitals with appropriate conditions may choose "water knife") and use a push, peel, and suction technique to remove the superficial fat tissue from the nerve surface, revealing the classic "cross" structure (Figs. 10.36, 10.37, 10.38, 10.39, and 10.40).

Surgical Experience and Precautions To divide the branches of the vesical venous plexus, it is necessary to first open the ureteric mesentery at the vesicovaginal ligament. For cases with a clearly visible hypogastric plexus, the ureteric mesentery can be opened between the hypogastric plexus and the ureter. For cases with an unclear hypogastric plexus, to avoid accidental injury to the hypogastric plexus (located within the ureter's posterior fascia approximately 1.5–2 cm from the ureter), the ventral surface of the uterine side of the deep uterine veins can be explored to open the ureteric mesentery. Regarding the exposure of the "cross" of

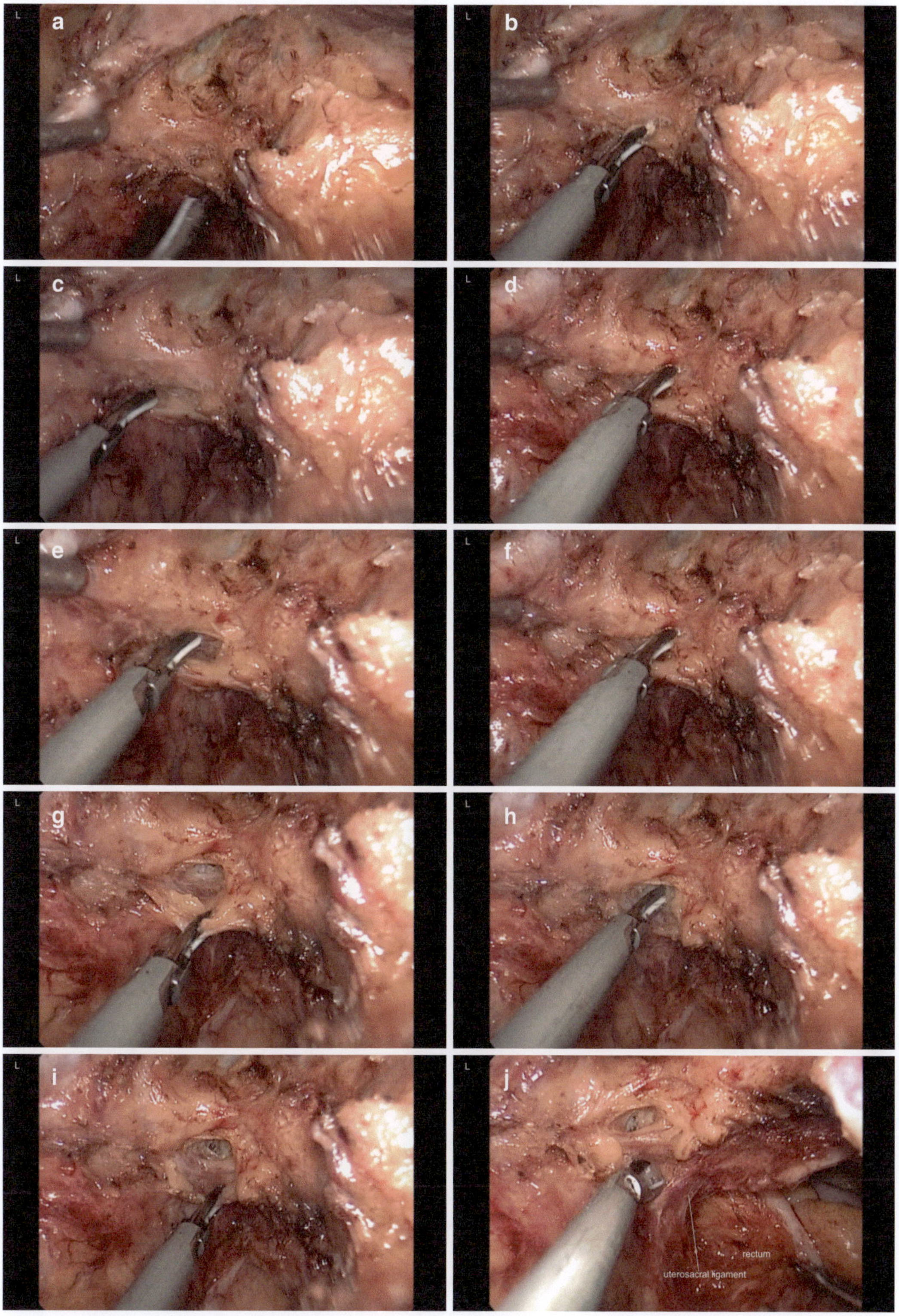

Fig. 10.36 (**a–j**) Management of the vesicovaginal ligament

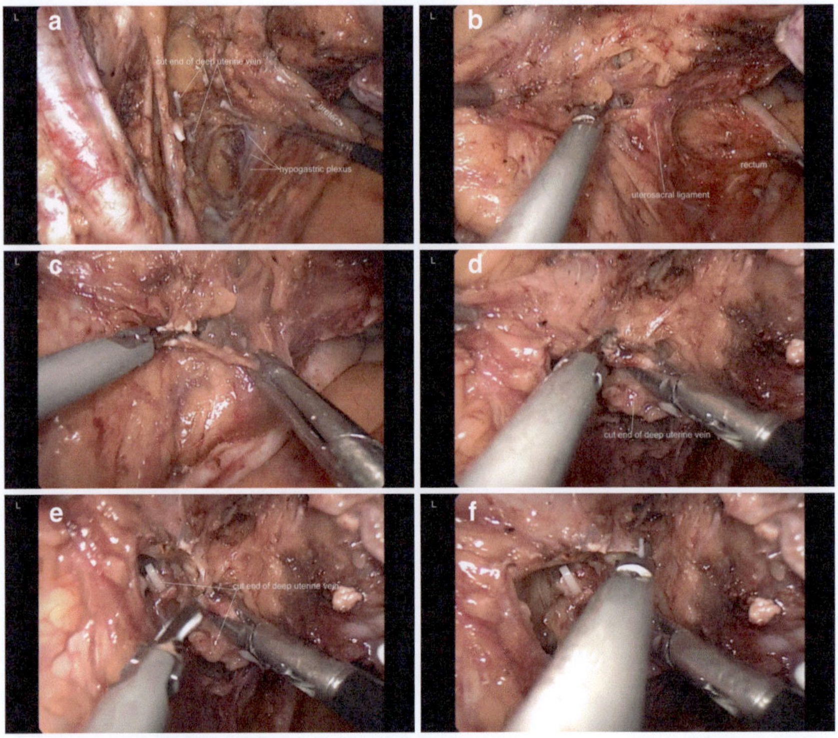

Fig. 10.37 (**a**–**f**) Open the ureteric mesentery on the ventral surface of the deep uterine veins

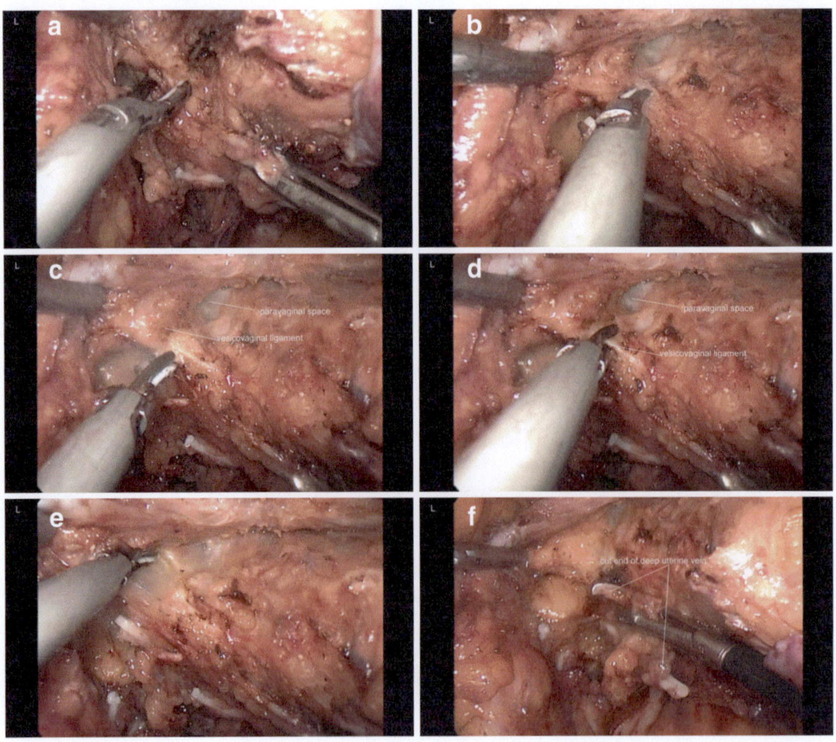

Fig. 10.38 (**a**–**f**) Sharply dissect of the remaining portion of the vesicovaginal ligament

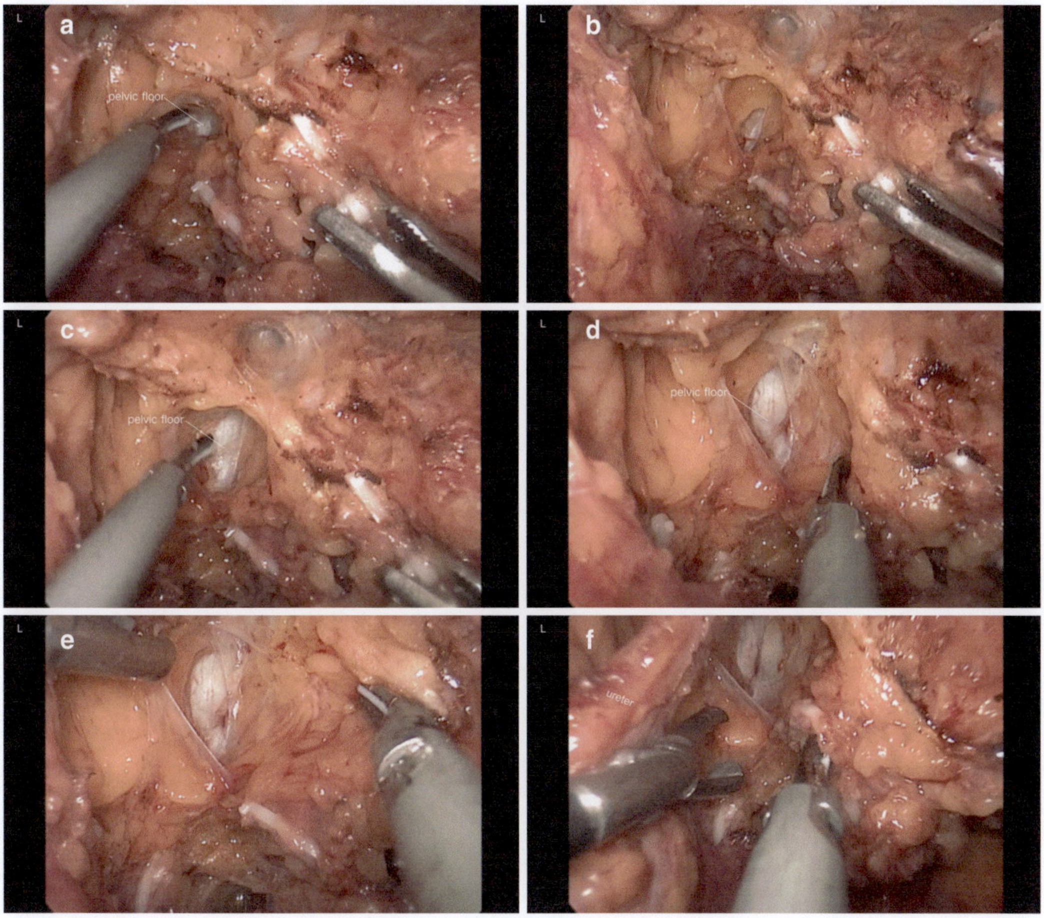

Fig. 10.39 (**a**–**f**) Expose the pelvic floor fascia

the nerves: The pelvic plexus formed by the intersection of the pelvic splanchnic nerve plexus and the hypogastric plexus is located within the paracolpium. Its separation and exposure should be performed using cold instruments. Our team prefers to use a irrigation suction device, which allows repeated flushing of the surgical field to facilitate nerve exposure. If bleeding occurs during nerve exposure, when hemostasis with energy devices is necessary, it is recommended to use spot coagulation or short-duration electrocoagulation. At the same time, use the irrigation suction device to repeatedly flush the surgical field to maintain a clear view and achieve cooling and temperature reduction, with the aim of reducing nerve damage.

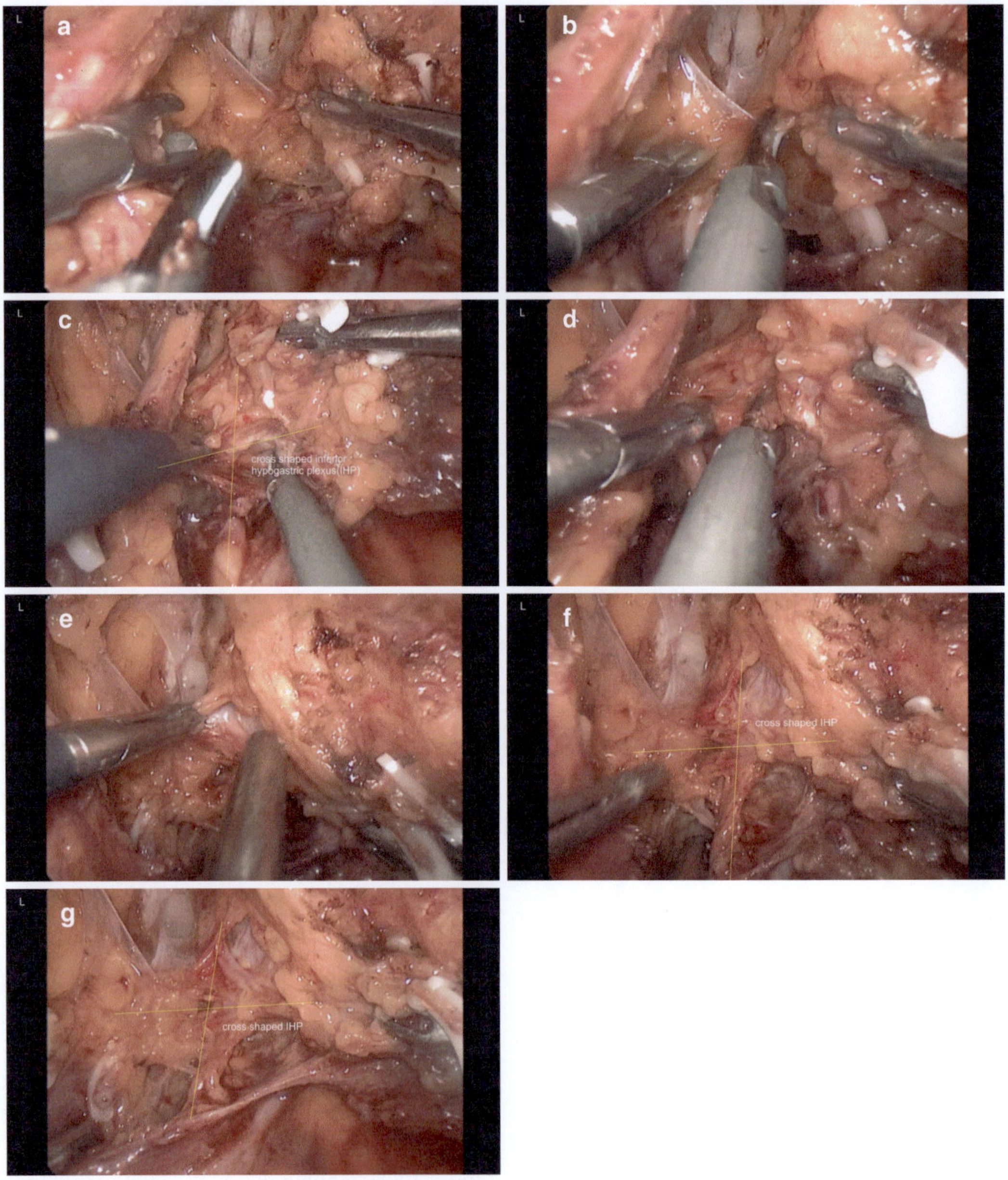

Fig. 10.40 (**a**–**g**) Expose pelvic plexus

10.17 Preservation of the Bladder Branches of the Pelvic Plexus

After exposing the "cross," the nerve branches that innervate the cervix and uterus can be clearly seen at the nerve junction. They should be sequentially divided (Figs. 10.41, 10.42, 10.43, 10.44, and 10.45).

Surgical Experience and Precautions It is often thought that once the "cross" is exposed, the preservation of the nerves is accomplished. However, this is actually the true beginning of nerve preservation. The division of the nerve branches that supply the cervix and uterus should be performed before horizontally dividing the sacrocardinal ligament and some para-

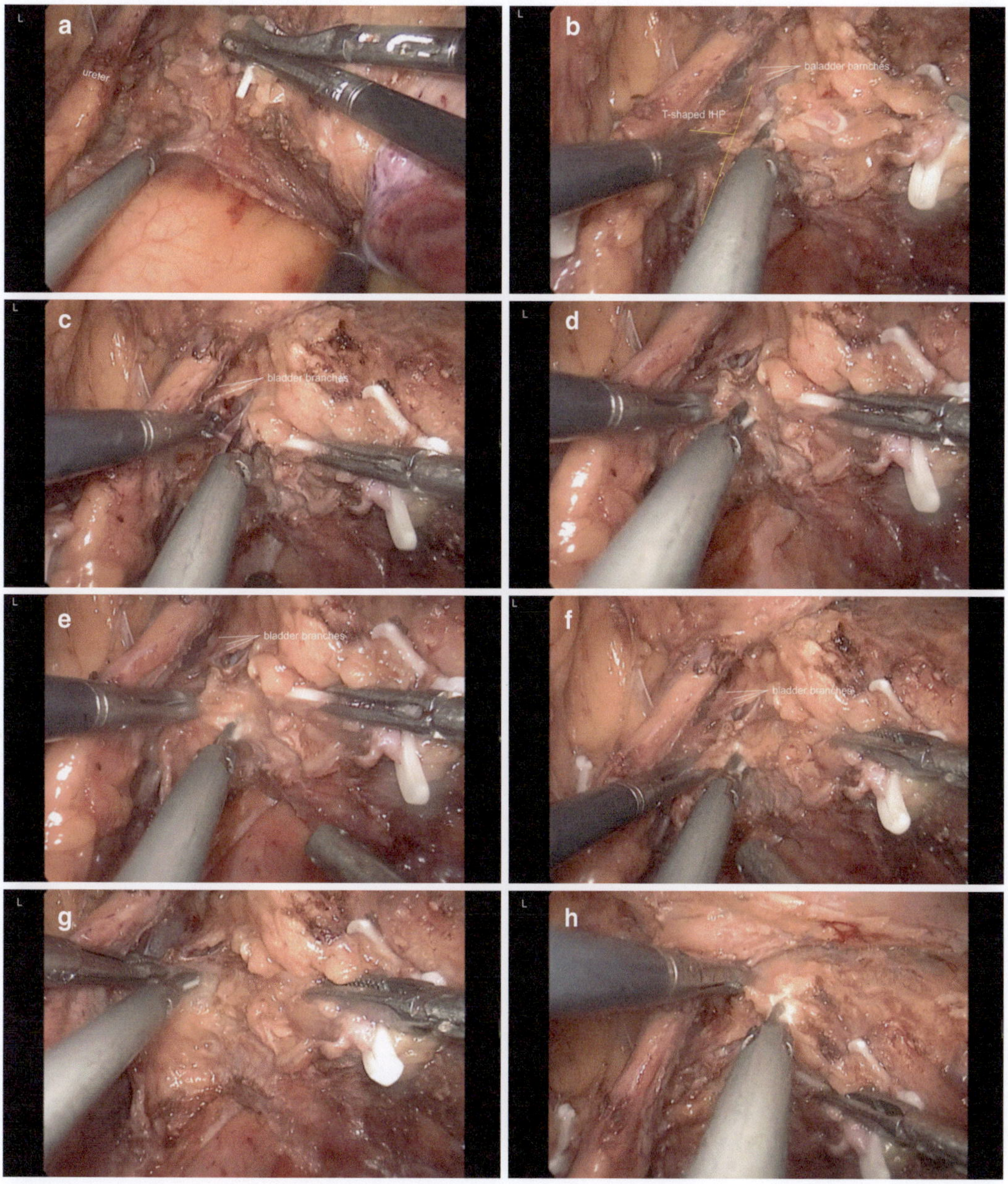

Fig. 10.41 (**a–h**) Cut pelvic plexus uterine branch

colpium. This increases the tension at the nerve junction when pulling it laterally, facilitating sharp dissection with the ultrasonic scalpel.

Separating the pelvic plexus nerves away from the paracolpium allows the resection range of the paracolpium to remain unaffected.

The pelvic plexus nerves travel within the deep layer of the lateral parametrial tissue and externally to the paracolpium. The paracolpium contains a rich network of veins. Therefore, it is crucial to carefully and sharply dissect each clamped tissue during this process to avoid bleed-

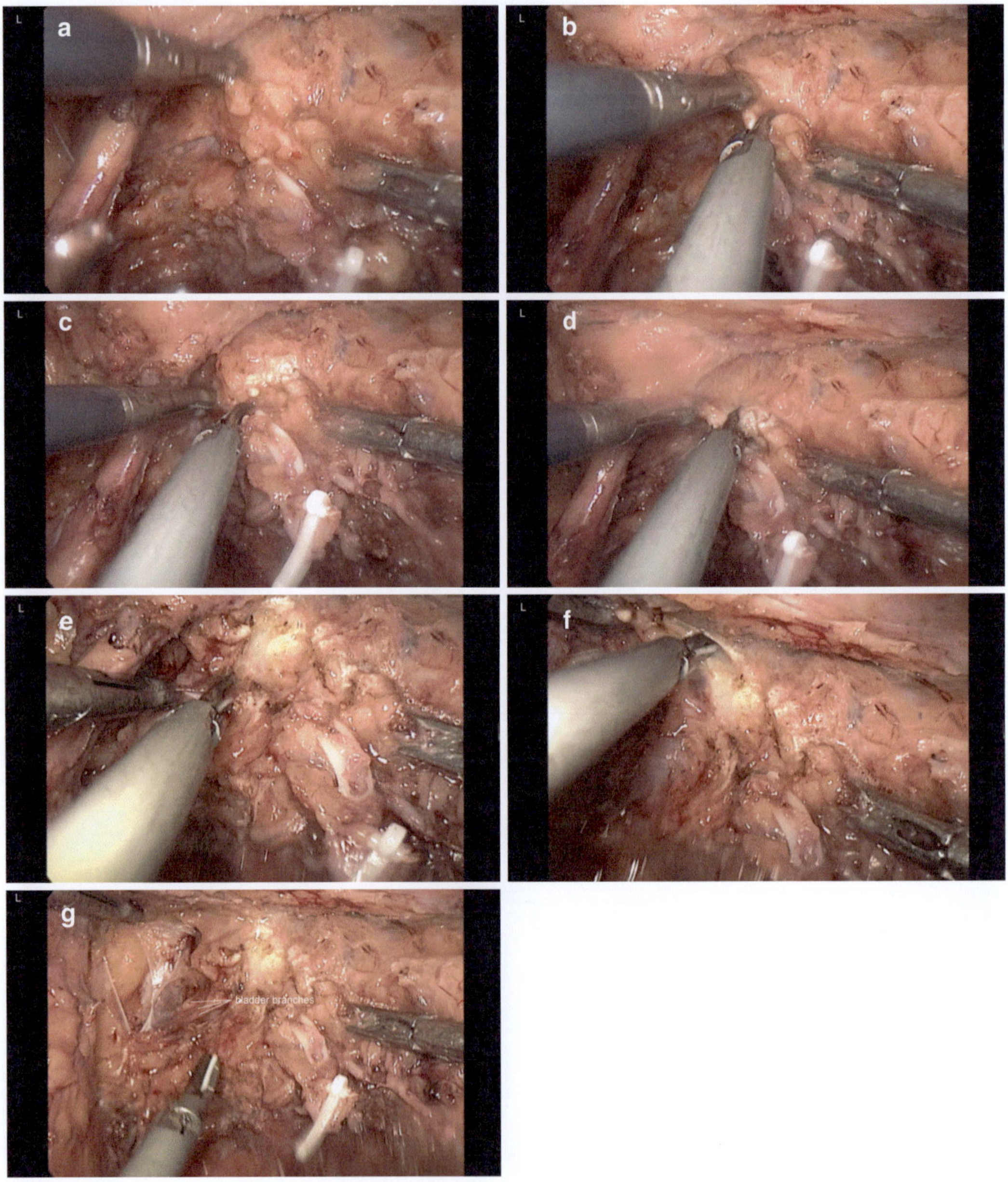

Fig. 10.42 (**a**–**g**) Separate and extrapolate pelvic plexus bladder branch

ing. If bleeding occurs, it is necessary to use a high-energy device such as bipolar electrocoagulation for hemostasis. Bleeding can be catastrophic for nerve preservation surgery. In our team's practice, we prefer to simultaneously separate the nerves laterally while dividing the sacrocardinal ligament and some paracolpium. This provides sufficient tension for subsequent nerve separation.

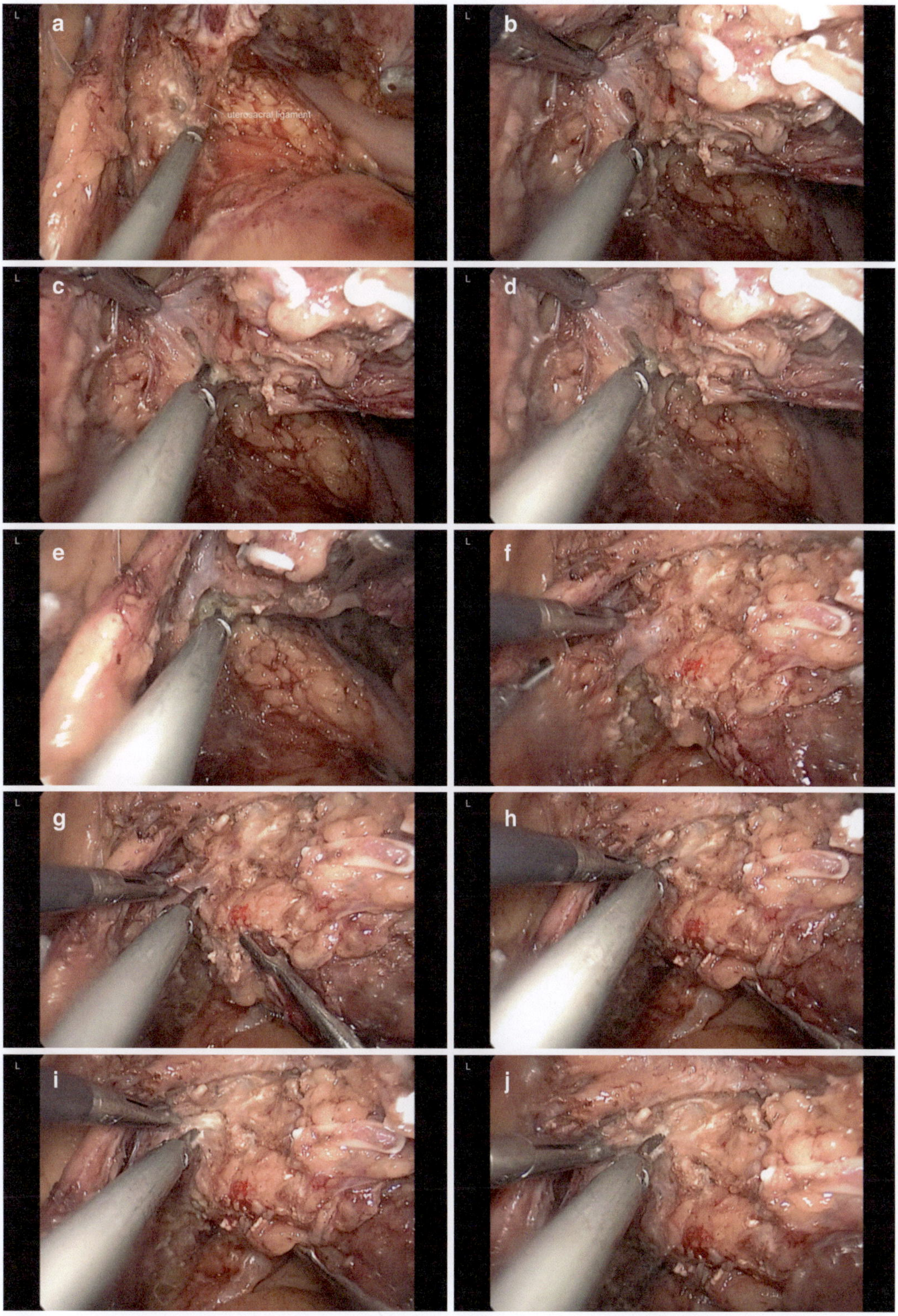

Fig. 10.43 (**a**–**j**) Cut the cervical, vaginal, and rectal branches and the bladder branches of the pelvic plexus

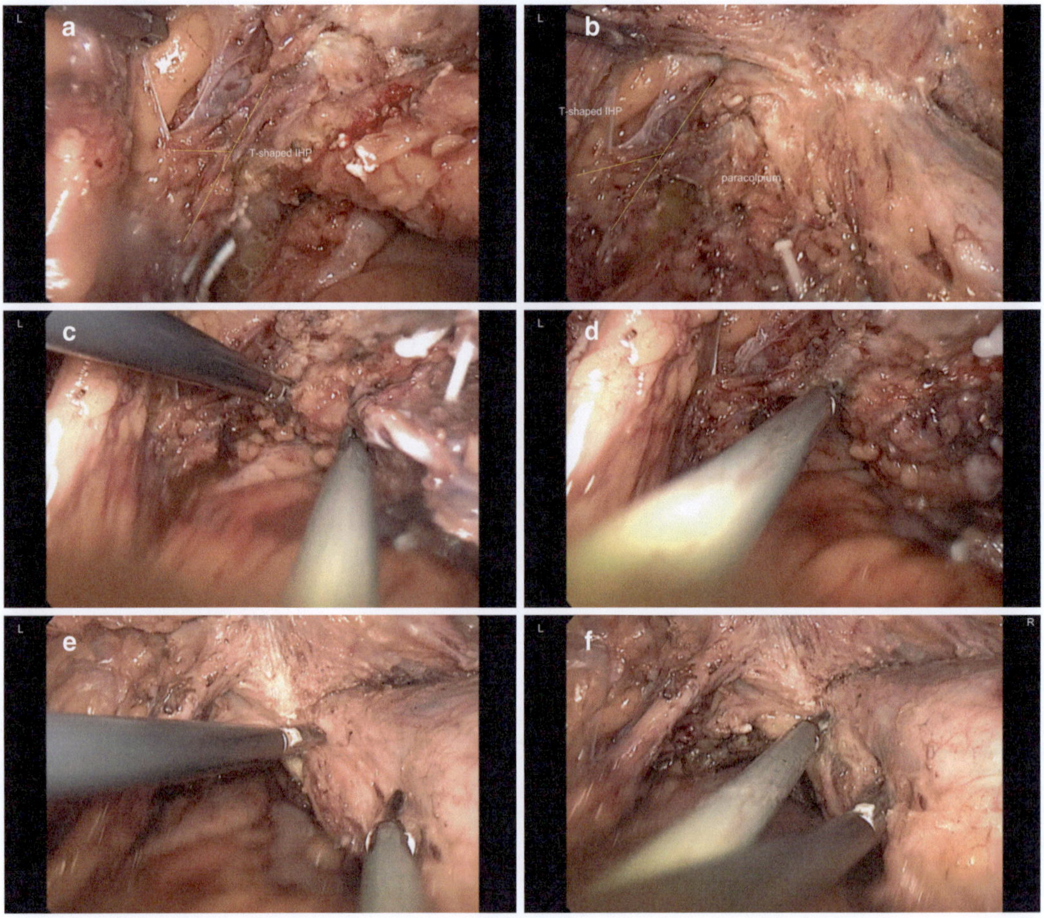

Fig. 10.44 (**a**–**f**) Separate and extrapolate nerves, and transect the remaining paracolpium

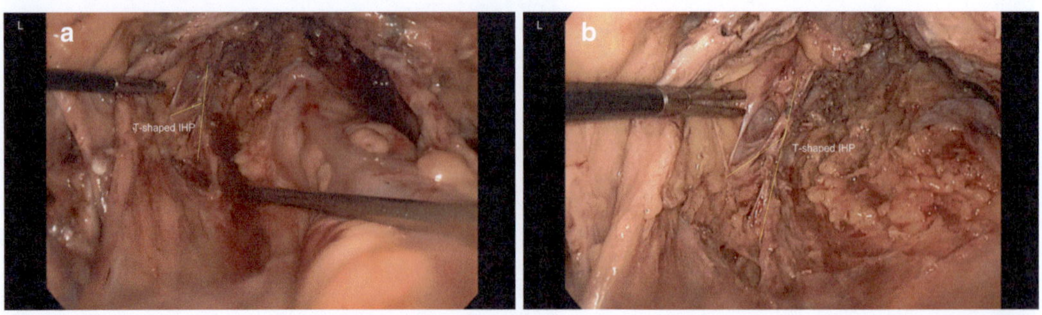

Fig. 10.45 (**a**, **b**) Expose the "T-shaped IHP"

10.18 Closure of the Vagina and Vaginal Cuff Excision for Complete Removal of the Uterus

The vaginal cuff is closed using absorbable suture, and the closed vagina is repeatedly irrigated with sterile distilled water at 42 °C. The vagina is incised 2 cm below the cervix or lesion, and the uterus is completely removed (Figs. 10.46, 10.47, and 10.48).

Surgical Experience and Precautions The closed vagina is repeatedly irrigated with sterile distilled water at 42 °C, and the vagina is sutured after incision to isolate cervical cancer lesions. During the process of removing the uterus through the vagina, care should be taken to maintain the integrity of the uterus and avoid cutting or damaging it. For Type C surgery, the length of vaginal wall excision is 2 cm from the lower edge of the lesion. The 2 cm refers to the natural length of the vagina in its relaxed state, not when it is stretched or extended. Since the vaginal surface does not have specific landmarks, our team uses anatomical landmarks for positioning. Usually, after handling the vesicovaginal ligament, the paracolpium of the vagina that needs to be excised is exposed. The vaginal wall excision is performed in a vertical direc-

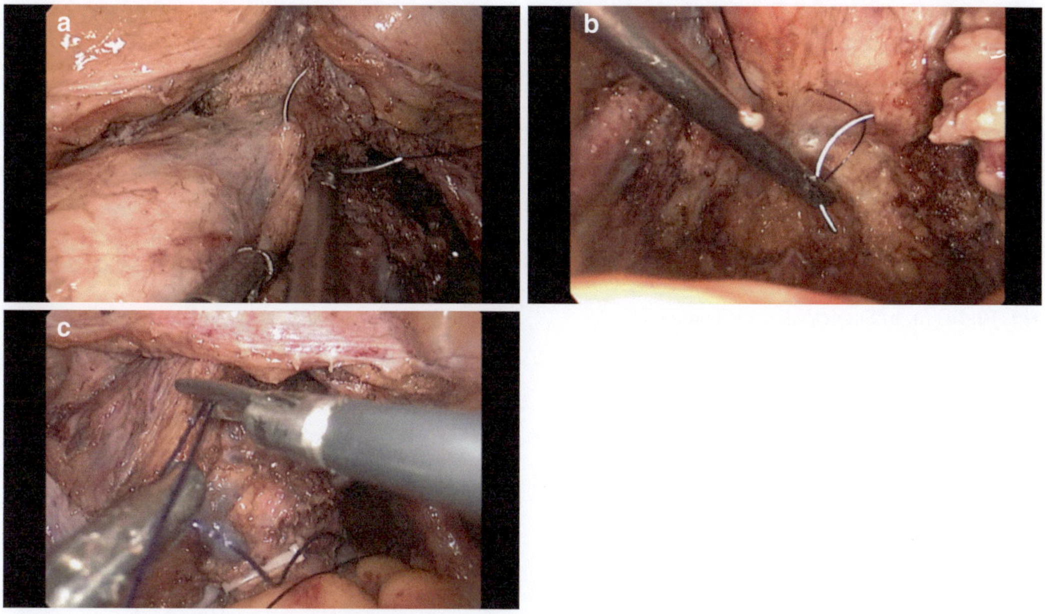

Fig. 10.46 (**a**–**c**) Close the vagina using absorbable suture

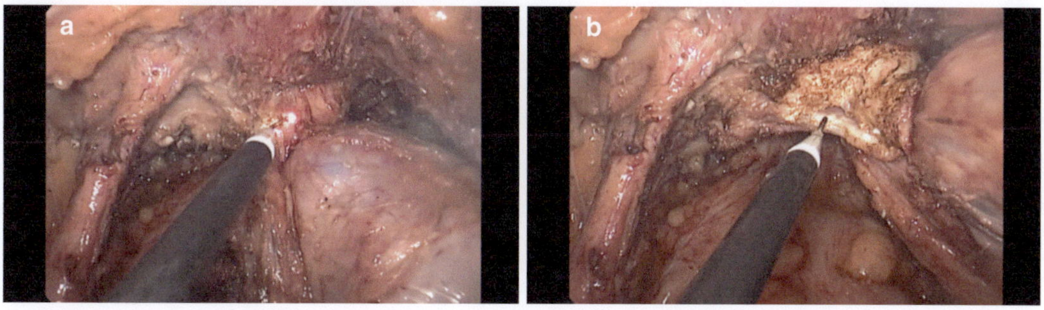

Fig. 10.47 (**a**, **b**) Circumferentially cut vagina

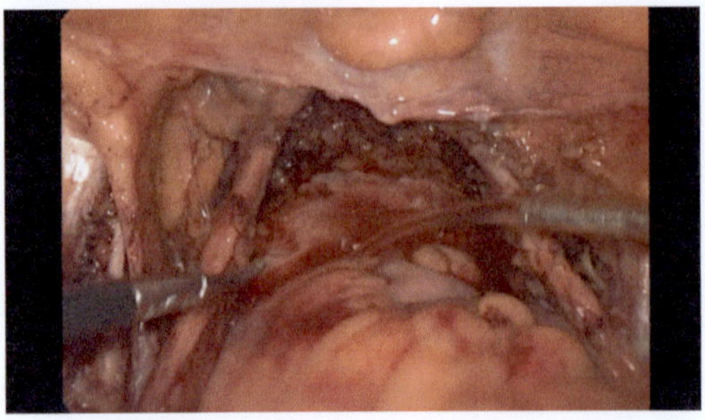

Fig. 10.48 Repeatedly irrigate the pelvic wound with 42 °C sterilized distilled water

tion, and our team marks the length of vaginal wall excision based on this landmark. Postoperatively, the measurement of the "natural length of the vaginal wall" in the three-dimensional specimen is 2–2.5 cm.

Surgical specimen presented in Fig. 10.49.

The QM-C1 type radical hysterectomy (laparoscopic) is shown in Videos 10.1 and 10.2.

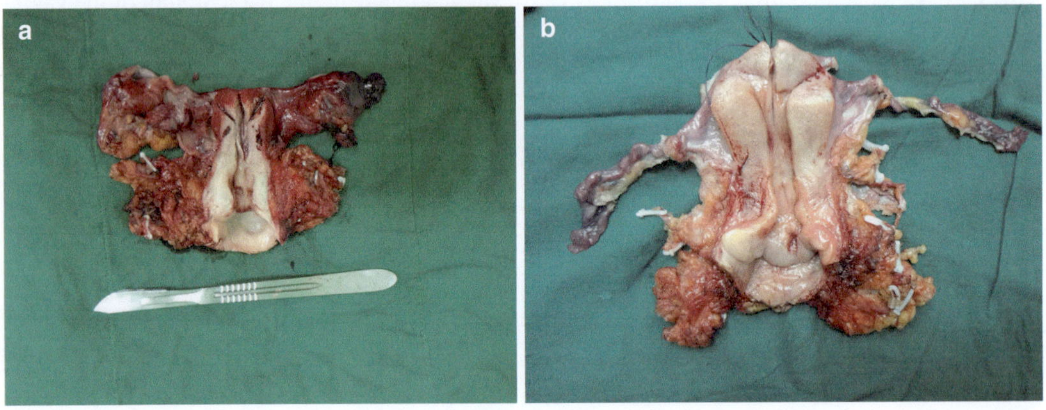

Fig. 10.49 (**a**, **b**) Surgical specimen presentation

Reference

1. Cibula D, Abu-Rustum NR, Benedetti-Panici P, et al. New classification system of radical hysterectomy: emphasis on a three-dimensional anatomic template for parametrial resection. Gynecol Oncol. 2011;122:264–8.

11 Type QM-C2 Radical Hysterectomy

Jun Wang, Shichao Han, Jing Na, and Ya Li

Cervical cancer surgery can be categorized into lymph node dissection and radical hysterectomy [1]. The author's team conducted a comprehensive review of the literature and sought advice from numerous experts in the field regarding the optimal sequence for these procedures, i.e., whether to perform lymph node dissection first or proceed with radical hysterectomy. However, there is no strict consensus on the order of these two procedures. In this description, the author's team will adopt the approach of performing radical hysterectomy first, followed by lymph node dissection.

11.1 Uterine Suspension

See Sect. 10.1 (Fig. 11.1a, b).

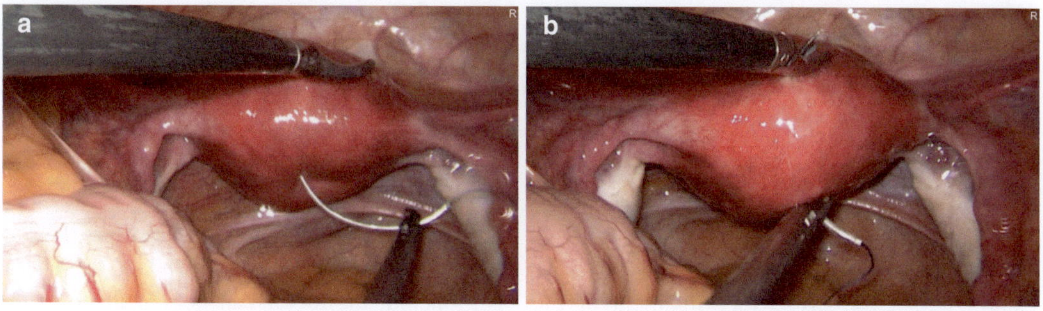

Fig. 11.1 (**a**, **b**) Suspend uterus

Supplementary Information The online version contains supplementary material available at https://doi.org/10.1007/978-981-97-7687-0_11.

J. Wang (✉) · S. Han · J. Na · Y. Li
Department of Gynecology and Obstetrics, Second Affiliated Hospital of Dalian Medical University, Dalian, China

S. Han, J. Wang (eds.), *Open, Laparoscopic, and Robotic Surgery for Cervical Cancer*, https://doi.org/10.1007/978-981-97-7687-0_11

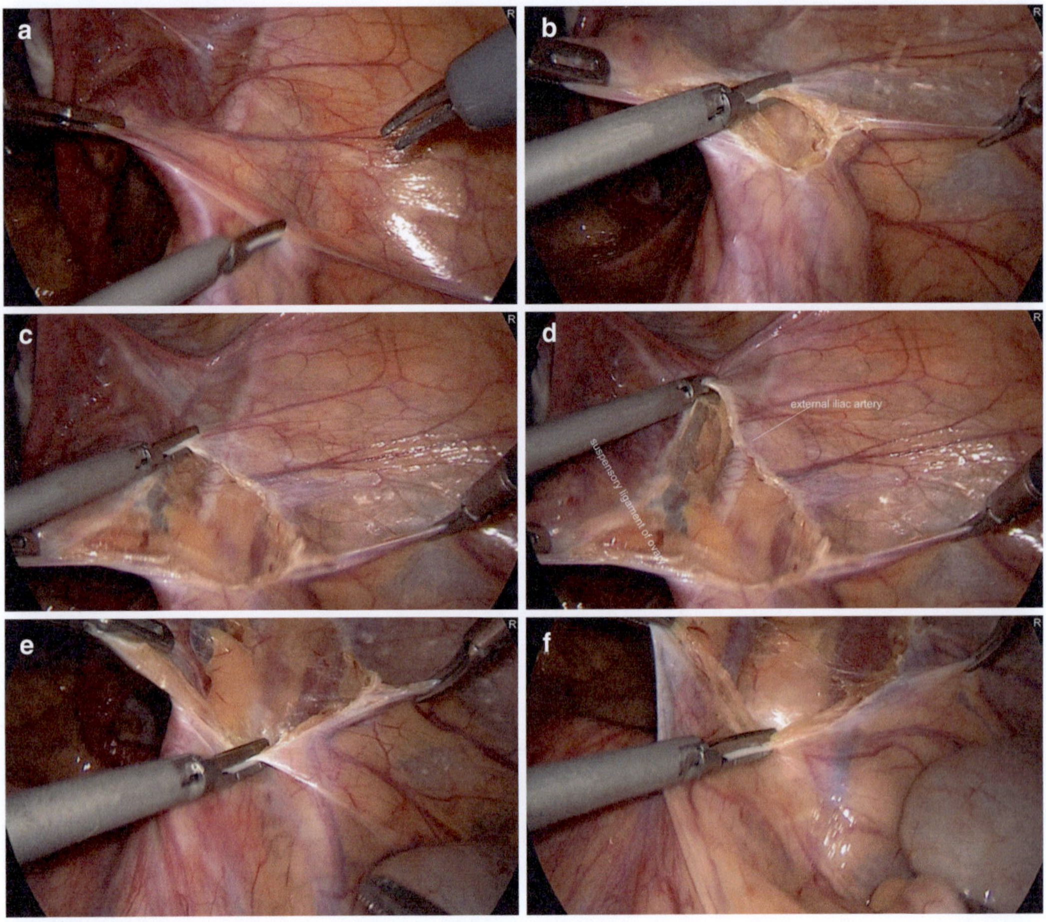

Fig. 11.2 (a–f) Expose the lateral retroperitoneal space

11.2 Adnexal Management

Gently retract the suspensory ligament of the ovary medially and the lateral peritoneum laterally, while maintaining close adherence to the suspensory ligament of the ovary to facilitate the opening of the lateral peritoneum (Fig. 11.2a–f). Employing sharp dissection, proceed in both caudal and cranial directions, with the caudal dissection reaching the round ligament and the cranial dissection reaching the upper margin of the intersection between the suspensory ligament of the ovary and the iliac vessels (Fig. 11.3a–c).

Surgical Experience and Precautions During the dissection of the cranial end of the lateral peritoneum, the ureter can be visualized in the retroperitoneal space, ensuring a safer and more reliable treatment of the adnexa. The course of the ureter can also be observed on the medial side of the lateral peritoneum. Under direct visualization of the ureter, the peritoneum is sharply opened at the site of the suspensory ligament of the ovary (Fig. 11.4a–g).

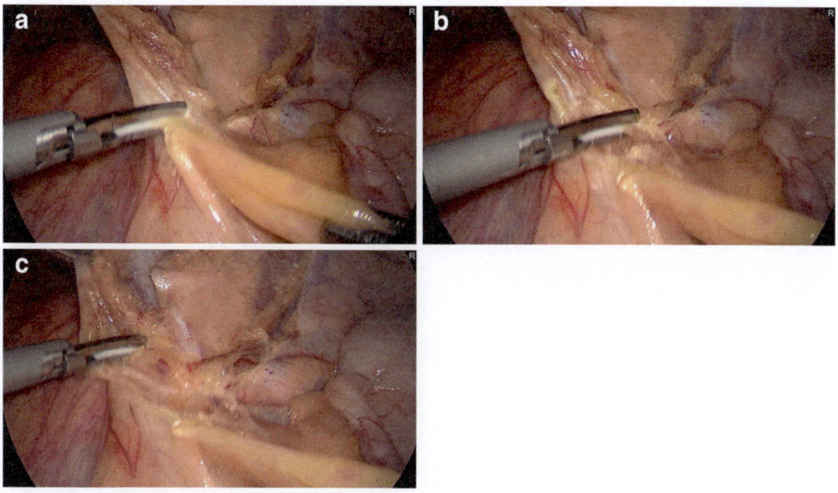

Fig. 11.3 (**a**–**c**) Dissect the lateral retroperitoneal space cranially reaching the upper margin of the intersection between the suspensory ligament of the ovary and the iliac vessels

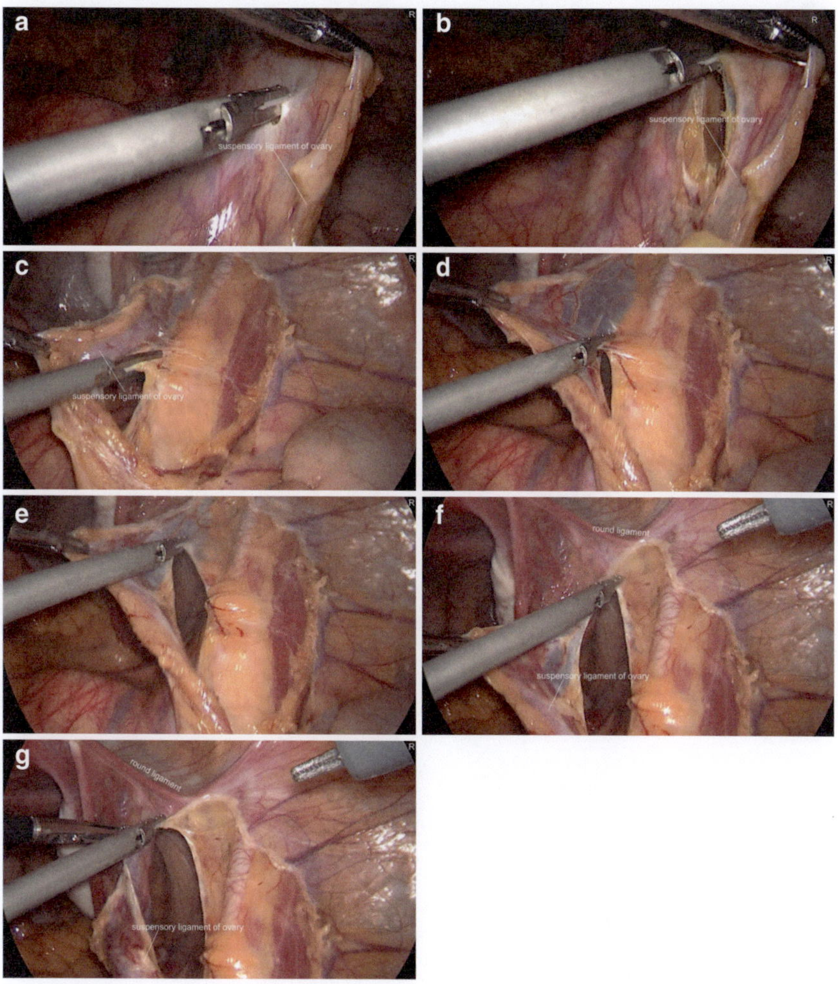

Fig. 11.4 (**a**–**g**) Under direct visualization of the ureter, the peritoneum is sharply opened at the site of the suspensory ligament of the ovary

11.3 Salpingectomy

The lateral peritoneum is sharply dissected along the suspensory ligament of the ovary toward the direction of the uterine angle until reaching near the angle. Sharp excision of the fallopian tubes is performed using a ultrasonic scalpel (Fig. 11.5a–d). Subsequently, the ovarian suspensory ligament is sharply detached near the uterine angle, and the ovaries are placed in the iliac fossa (Fig. 11.6a–g) for subsequent ovarian repositioning.

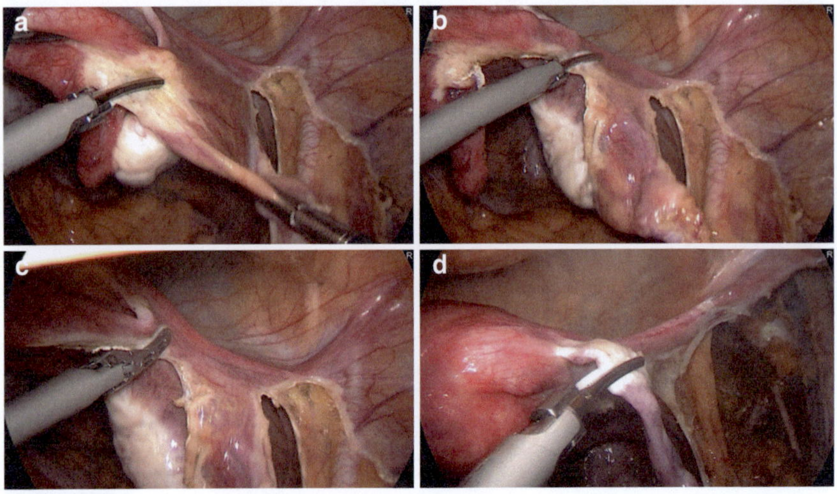

Fig. 11.5 (**a**–**d**) Salpingectomy

Fig. 11.6 (**a**–**g**) Sharply detach he ovarian suspensory ligament near the uterine angle, and the ovaries are placed in the iliac fossa

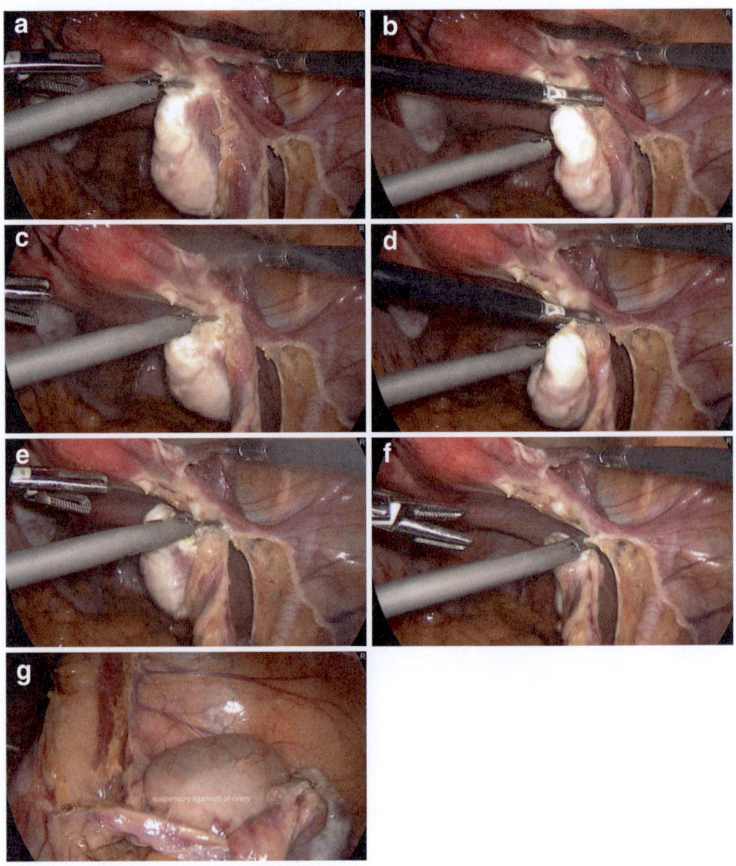

11.4 Removal of the Adnexa

Using a ultrasonic scalpel, sharply dissect the lateral peritoneum adjacent to the suspensory ligament of the ovary in a caudal direction to create space for subsequent clamping of the suspensory ligament of the ovary. Sharp dissection is then performed to expose the surface of the suspensory ligament of the ovary (Fig. 11.7a–f). Only the adipose tissue of the peritoneum covering the suspensory ligament of the ovary needs to be separated and removed, and after vascular clamping, it is dissected (Fig. 11.8a–c). Next, the proximal end of the suspensory ligament of the ovary is pulled inward, and sharp dissection of the lateral peritoneum is performed adjacent to the suspensory ligament of the ovary, reaching near the uterine angle. The ovarian suspensory ligament and the fallopian tube are sharply dissected after bipolar coagulation (Fig. 11.9a–e).

Surgical Experience and Precautions There are multiple techniques available for dissecting the suspensory ligament of the ovary, including bipolar coagulation followed by dissection, dissection after suture ligation, Ligasure dissection, stepwise dissection of blood vessels after individually exposing them using an ultrasonic scalpel, and dissection after vascular clamping. After thorough experimentation with these diverse methods, the author's team has concluded that dissection after vascular clamping is the most dependable and efficacious approach.

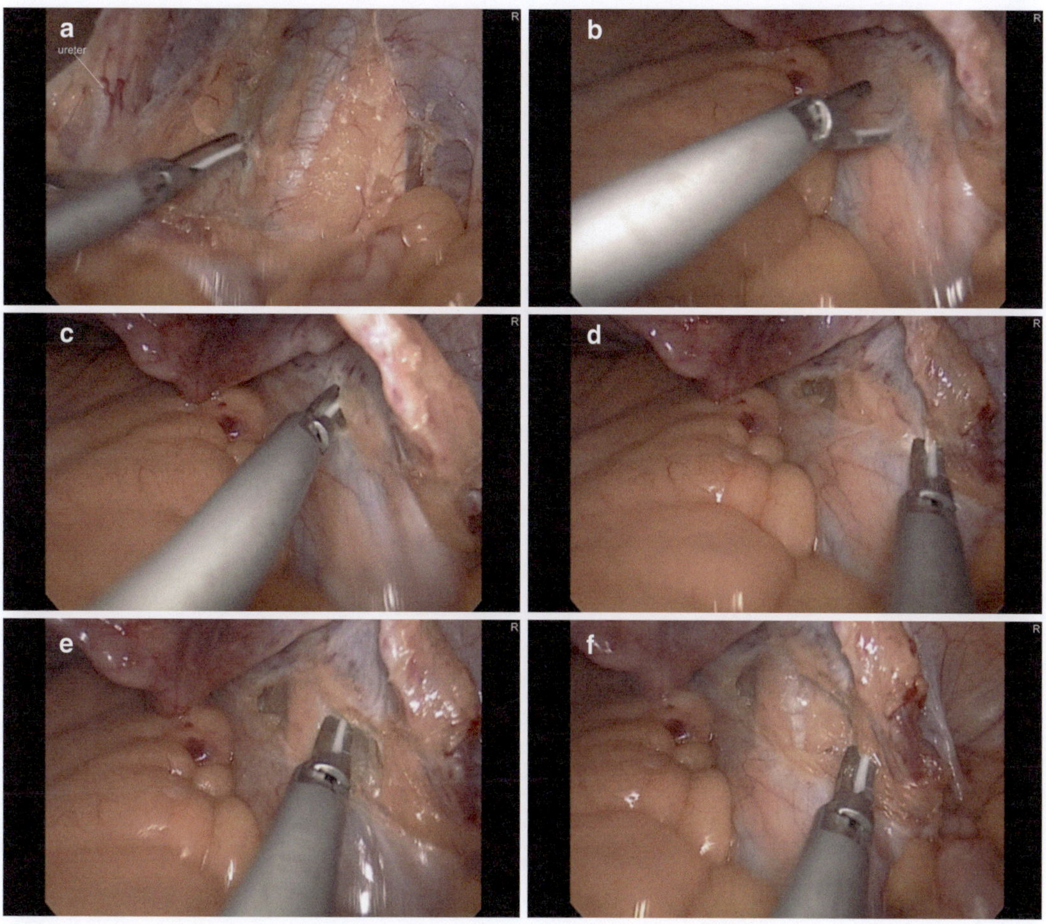

Fig. 11.7 (a–f) Sharply dissect the lateral peritoneum adjacent to the suspensory ligament of the ovary, expose the surface of the suspensory ligament of the ovary

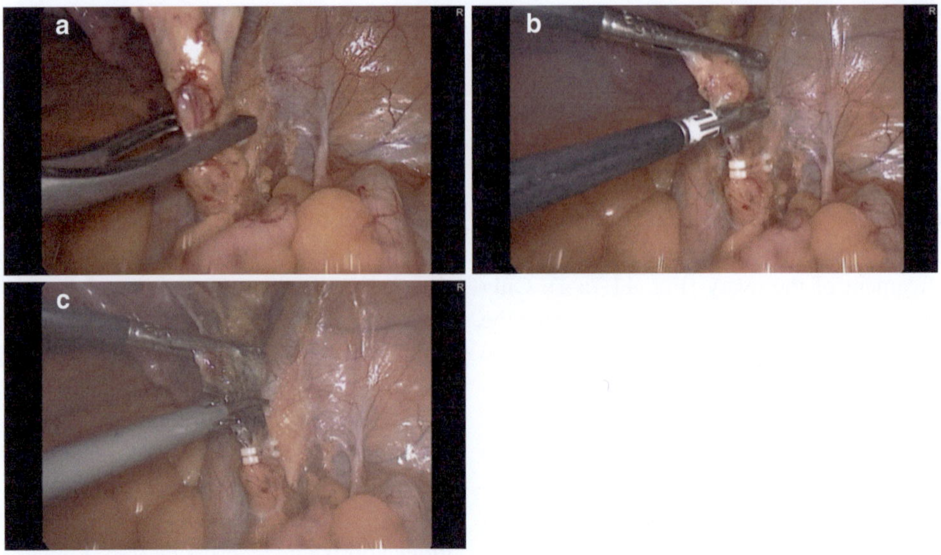

Fig. 11.8 (**a–c**) Vascular clamp and dissect suspensory ligament

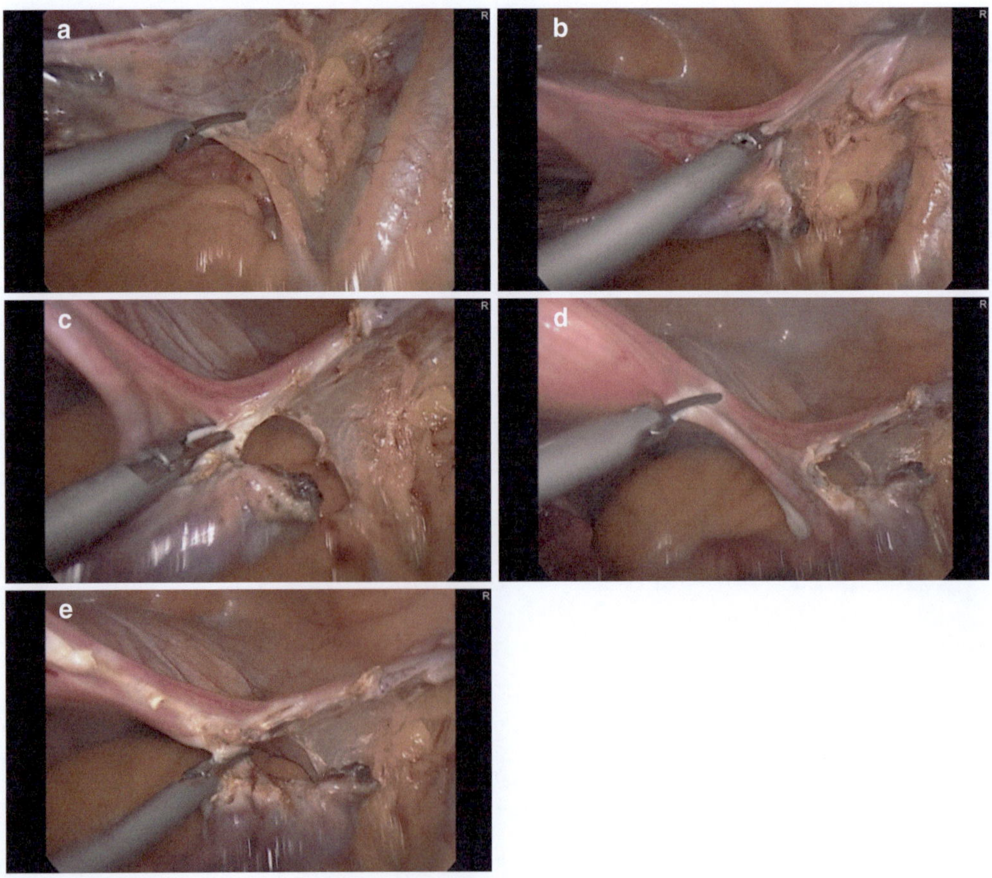

Fig. 11.9 (**a–e**) Sharp dissection of the lateral peritoneum is performed adjacent to the suspensory ligament of the ovary, reaching near the uterine angle. The ovarian suspensory ligament and the fallopian tube are sharply dissected after bipolar coagulation

11.5 Exposure of Key Anatomical Structures in the Lateral Parametrial Region Using the Lateral Retroperitoneal Space Approach

By pulling the lateral peritoneum and ureter medially, and under direct visualization of the ureter, the lateral retroperitoneal space is sharply dissected (Fig. 11.10a–d), gradually revealing the internal iliac artery (Fig. 11.11a–d). Maintaining tension on the lateral peritoneum and ureter, sharp dissection is carried out closely adhering to the extraperitoneal side of the internal iliac artery, proceeding caudally, which exposes the internal iliac artery and the lateral umbilical ligament. Continuing along the external aspect of the internal iliac artery and its distal lateral umbilical ligament, sharp dissection is

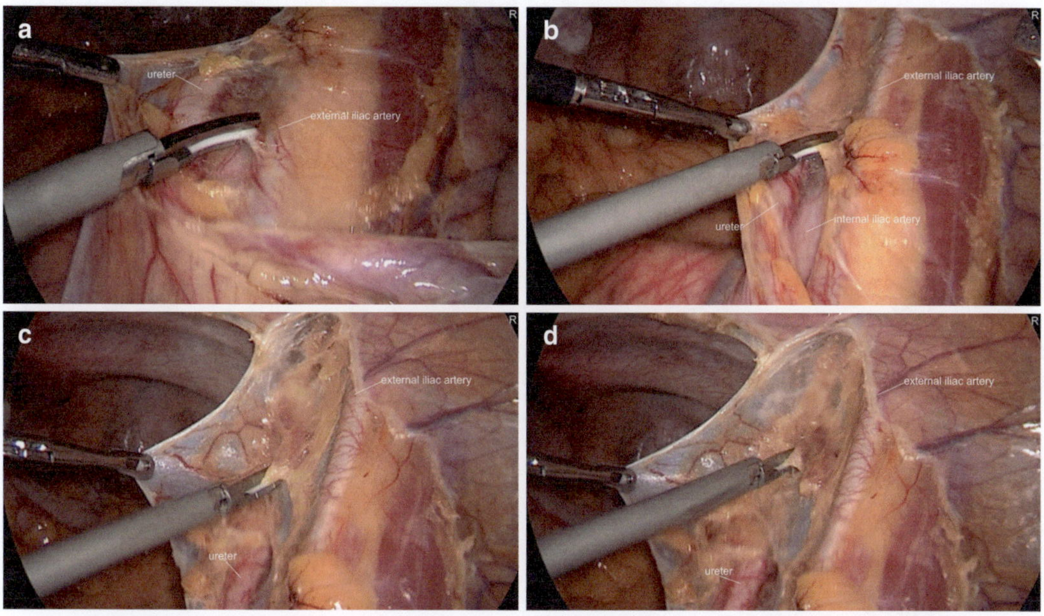

Fig. 11.10 (**a**–**d**) Widen the lateral retroperitoneal space

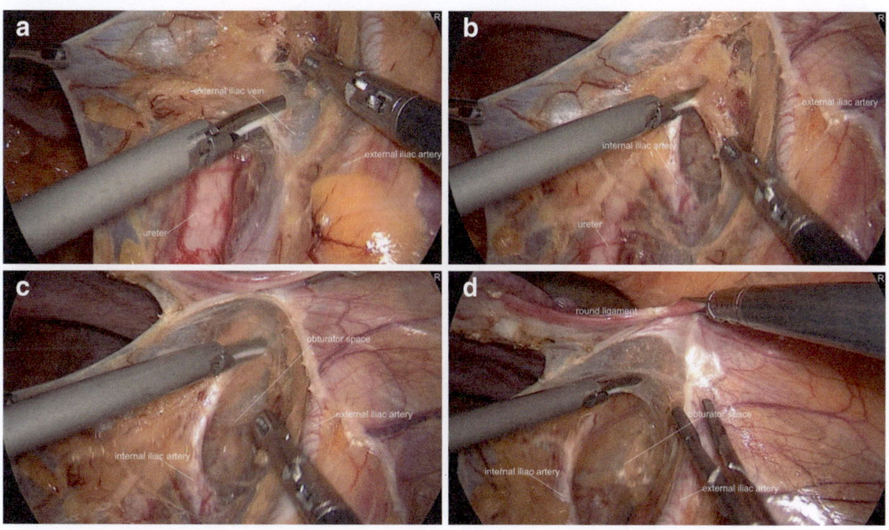

Fig. 11.11 (**a**–**d**) Expose the internal iliac artery

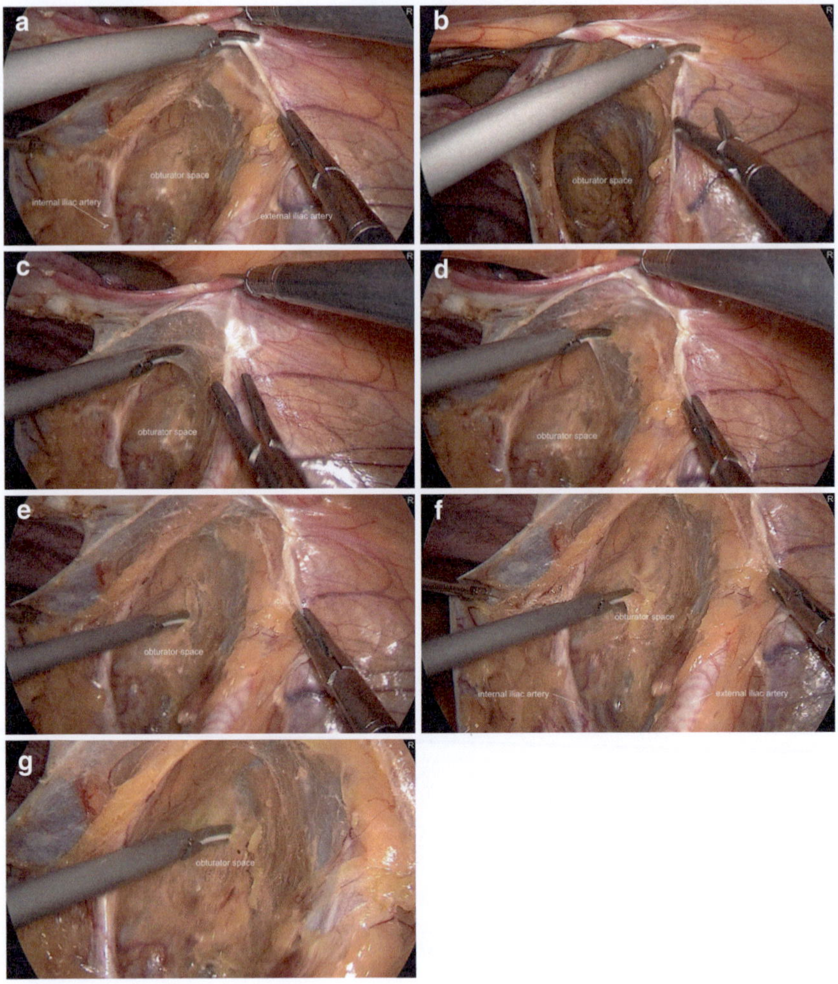

Fig. 11.12 (**a–g**) Expose the obturator space

directed posteriorly and caudally, revealing the obturator space (Fig. 11.12a–h) and its contents, including the obturator nerves and vessels (Figs. 11.13a–c and 11.14a–f).

Surgical Experience and Precautions During this dissection process, enlarged lymph nodes on the surface of the uterine artery may be encountered. In C-type surgery, the author's team prefers to dissect them laterally and ultimately remove them together with the pelvic lymph nodes.

The purpose of freeing the obturator space is to allow ample lateral traction of the internal iliac artery, providing sufficient tension for subsequent lateral parametrial procedures.

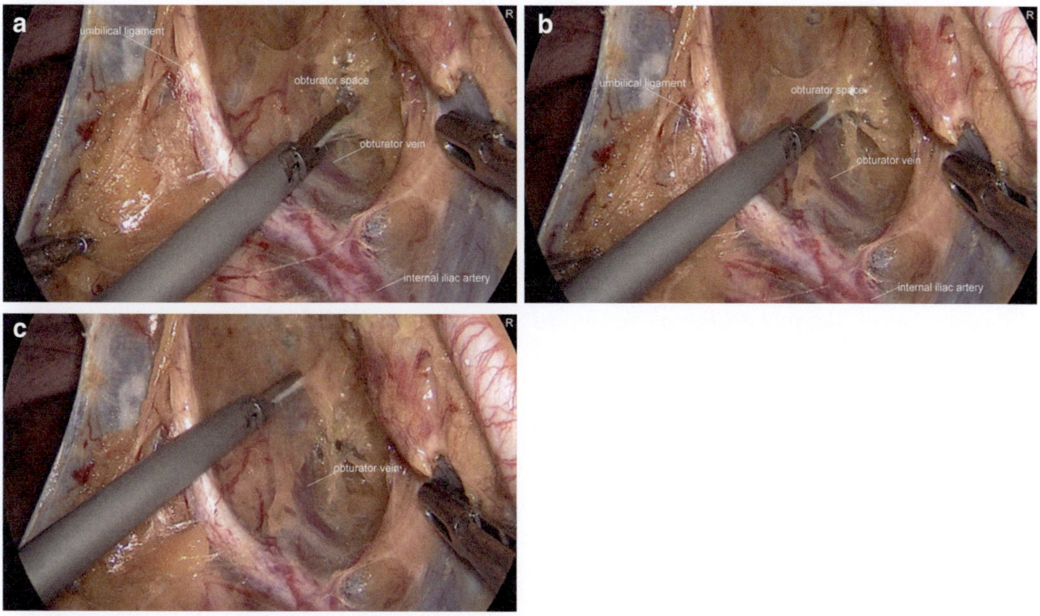

Fig. 11.13 (**a**–**c**) Expose obturator vein in the obturator space

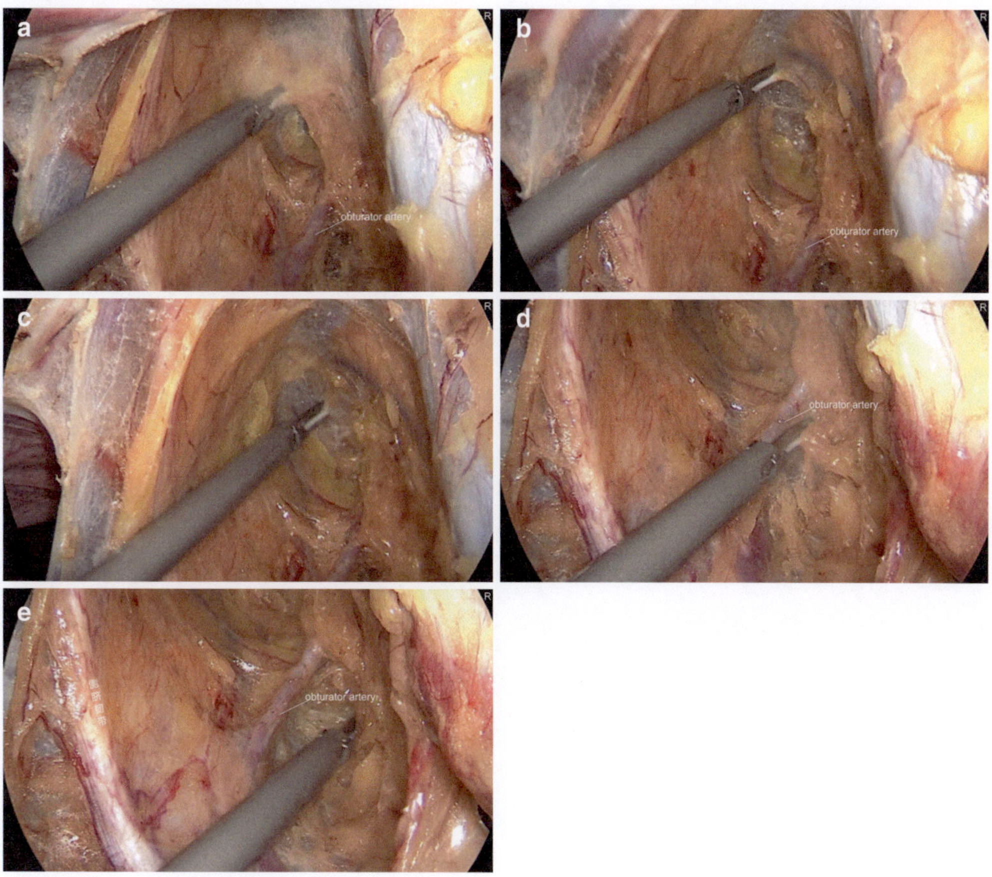

Fig. 11.14 (**a**–**e**) Expose obturator artery in the obturator space

11.6 Management of Vascular Structures in Lateral Parametrial Region

11.6.1 Exposure of the Latzko's Pararectal Space

The lateral peritoneum is pulled medially, and the internal iliac artery is pulled laterally. Using an ultrasonic scalpel, sharp dissection is performed within the white, loose connective tissue between them, allowing for separation of the ureter and the internal iliac artery at a certain distance. Simultaneously, sharp dissection is carried out in a posterior direction within the space to gradually expose the uterine artery. The space between the uterine artery, ureter, and internal iliac artery is further enlarged longitudinally and deepened posteriorly to fully expose the Latzko's pararectal space (Fig. 11.15a–f).

11.6.2 Exposure of the Paravesical Space

The lateral peritoneum is pulled medially, and the distal part of the internal iliac artery along with the lateral umbilical ligament is pulled laterally. Using an ultrasonic scalpel, sharp dissection is performed within the white, loose connective tissue between them, resulting in the separation of the ureter from the lateral umbilical ligament at a certain distance. Continuing the dissection longitudinally and deepening

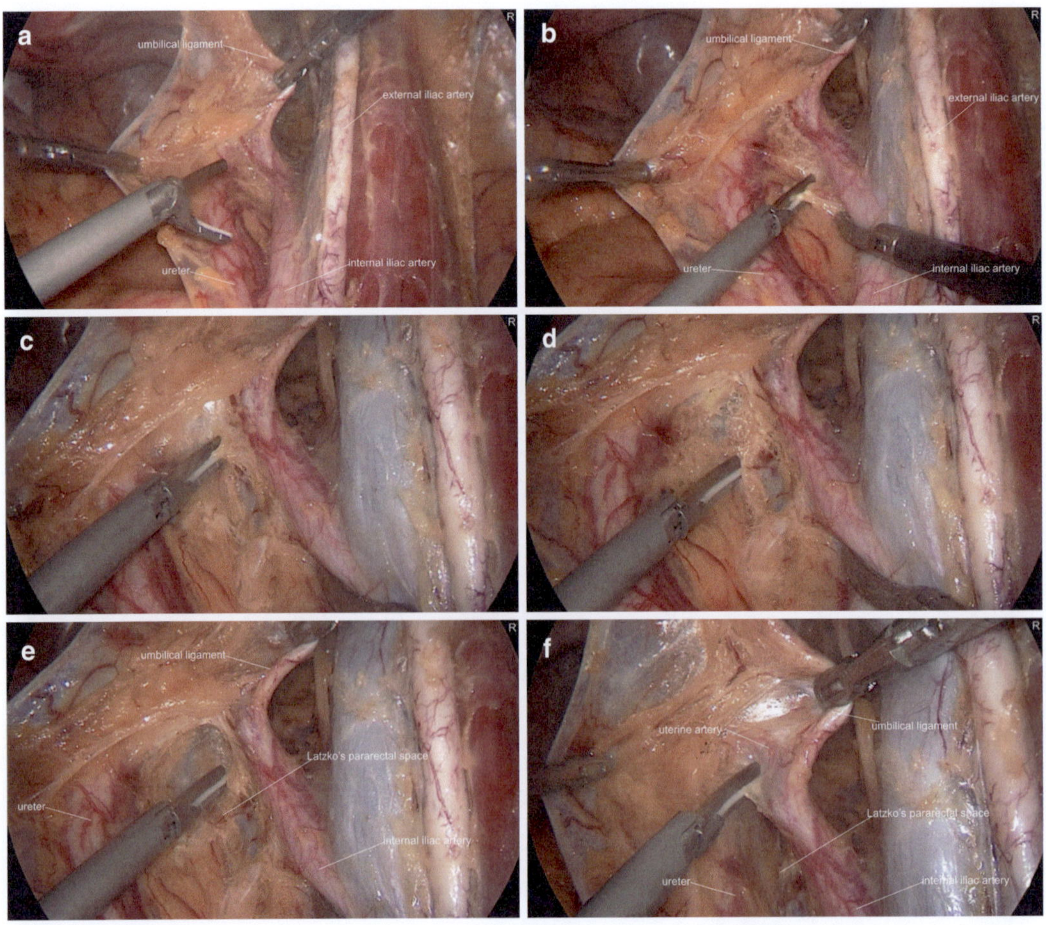

Fig. 11.15 (**a–f**) Separate the Latzko's pararectal space

posteriorly within the space between the uterine artery, ureter, and lateral umbilical ligament, the paravesical space is fully exposed (Fig. 11.16a–f).

11.6.3 Expose the Paravesical Space

Pull the lateral peritoneum inward and the distal side of the internal iliac artery and its lateral umbilical ligament outward. Use a ultrasonic scalpel to sharply dissect the white, loose connective tissue within the space between the two structures, separating the ureter from the lateral umbilical ligament by a certain distance. Continue to vertically expand and deepen the space between the uterine artery, ureter, and lateral umbilical ligament, fully exposing the paravesical space (see Fig. 11.16a–f).

11.6.4 Transection of the Lateral Parametrial Vascular Tissue

At this stage, the pararectal space and the paravesical space have been opened, and the lateral parametrial vascular tissue is fully exposed. The lateral parametrial vascular tissue is carefully dissected adjacent to the internal iliac vessels (Figs. 11.17a–e and 11.18a–i).

Surgical Experience and Precautions For some patients, the course of the lateral parametrial vascular tissue can be complex, and it is not

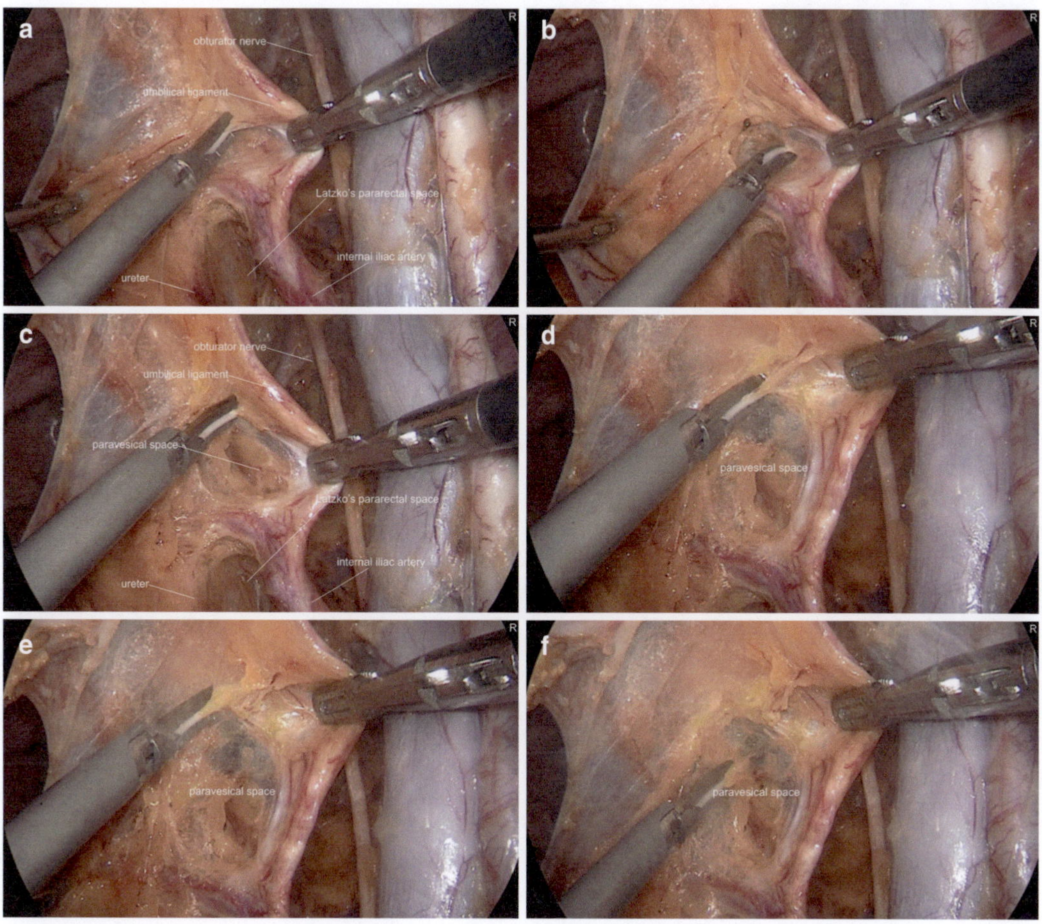

Fig. 11.16 (**a**–**f**) Separate the paravesical space

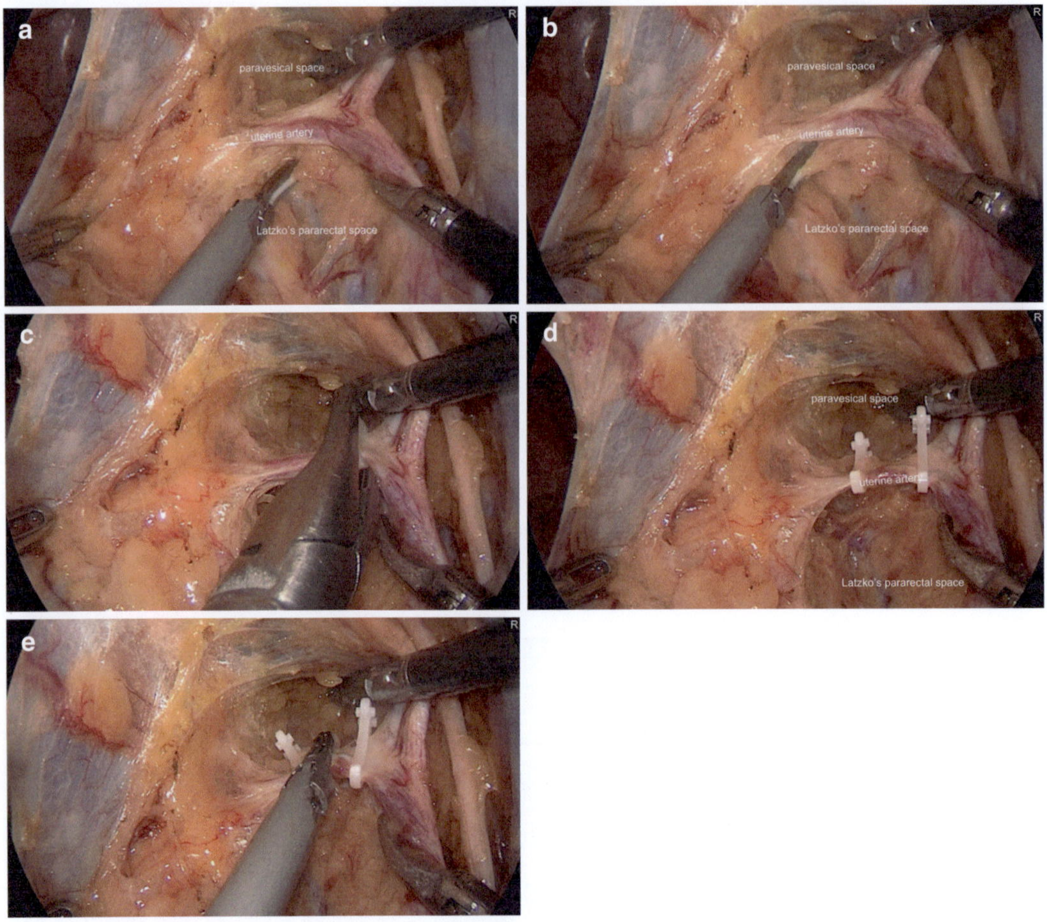

Fig. 11.17 (**a–e**) Dissect uterine artery adjacent to the internal iliac vessels

always necessary to directly separate these two spaces to expose the deep uterine vein. In these cases, after transecting the uterine artery, the dissection process may not directly reveal the deep uterine vein. Instead, multiple lateral parametrial blood vessels may still be visible, and they are carefully transected one by one until the deep uterine vein is exposed. Once the deep uterine vein is identified, it is clamped with vascular clamps and then transected.

After clamping the lateral parametrial blood vessels with vascular clamps, all of them can be sharply dissected using an ultrasonic scalpel, except for the deep uterine vein, which the author's team considers safer to transect using laparoscopic scissors. During the transection of the deep uterine vein with an ultrasonic scalpel as an energy instrument, the two ends of the deep uterine vein may undergo contraction, which poses a risk of clamp slippage. After transecting the lateral parametrial tissues, the Latzko's pararectal space and the paravesical space become continuous.

The author's team prefers not to handle the lateral parametrial nerve structures at this stage, considering that although they are located on the posterior and caudal side of the deep uterine vein, the posterior parametrial tissues have not been addressed yet, and the sacrouterine ligament cannot be adequately pulled medially. As a result, the lateral parametrial nerve structures cannot be fully exposed, and direct transection may lead to unnecessary damage and uncontrollable bleeding.

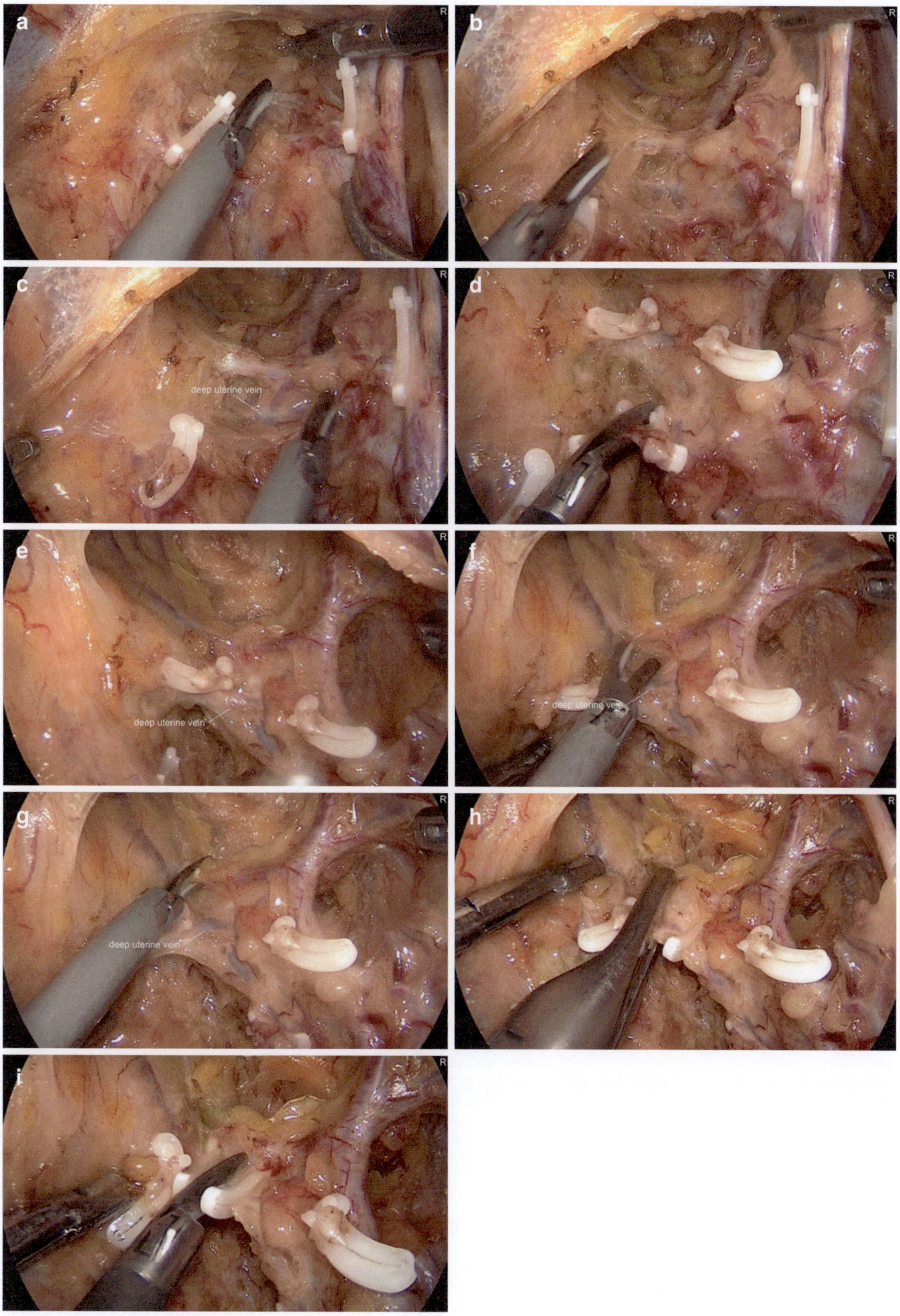

Fig. 11.18 (**a–i**) Separate and transect the deep uterine vein

11.7 Dissection and Mobilization of the Ureter

Pulling the lateral peritoneum medially and the ureter laterally exposes the fibrous tissue between the freed ureter and the lateral peritoneum (Fig. 11.19a–f). In Type C2 surgery, nerve preservation is not required. Only the ureter needs to be separated from the lateral peritoneum, and it is dissected up to 2 cm on the dorsal side of the ureter, where the mesoureter is transected and further dissected toward the caudal direction. The uterine artery and the ureter are pulled in opposite directions, and a combination of blunt and sharp dissection is used to transect the branches of the uterine artery supplying the ureter one by one (Fig. 11.20a–f), including the branches of the uterine artery that supply the bladder. The dissection can be carried out to approach or reach the entrance of the "tunnel" (Fig. 11.21a–g).

Surgical Experience and Precautions The dissection of the ureter is an essential step for all gynecologists, especially in minimally invasive surgeries where extra caution is required. The author's team adopts several methods to prevent thermal injury during this step: (1) allowing for a natural cooling of 3–5 seconds after sharp cutting; (2) utilizing the ultrasonic scalpel's coagulation function on the uterine serosa for 2–3 seconds to aid in heat dissipation, which is frequently used in robot-assisted surgeries; (3) irrigating the abdominal cavity with room temperature physiological saline for cooling, a

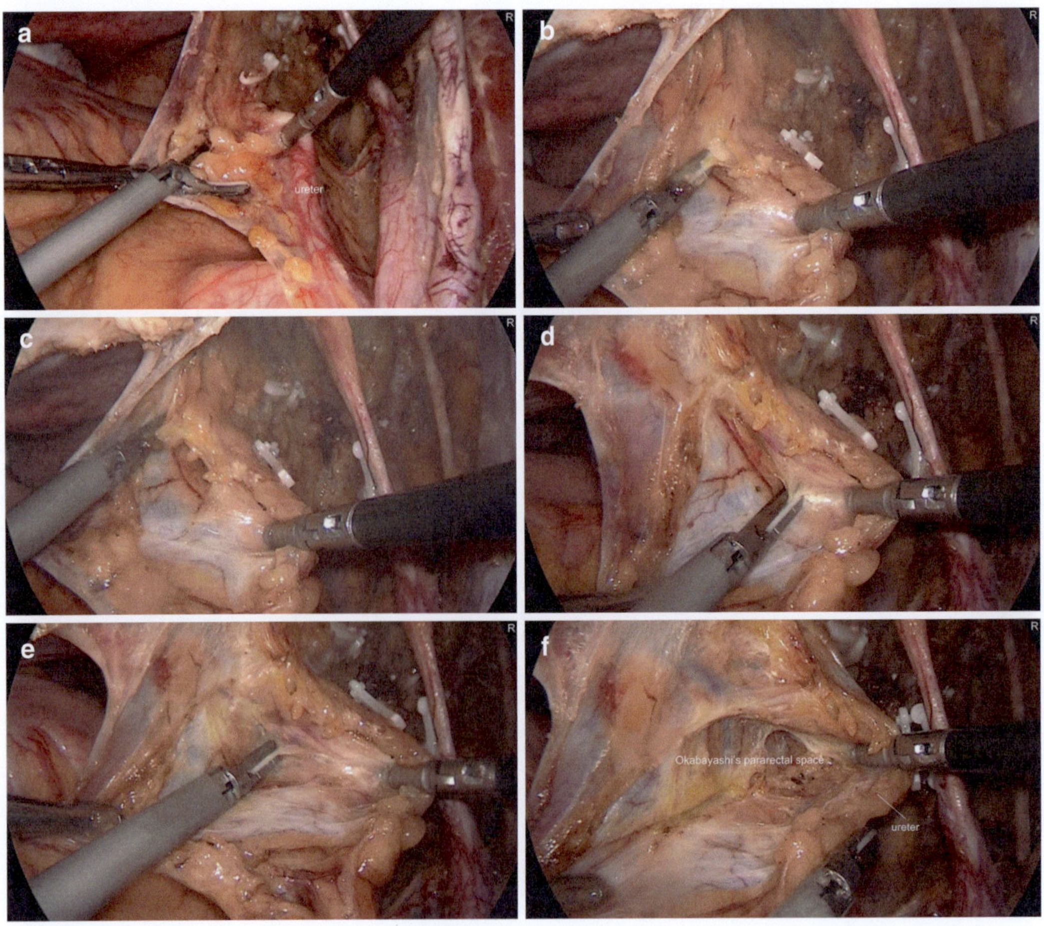

Fig. 11.19 (**a**–**f**) Expose the fibrous tissue between the freed ureter and the lateral peritoneum

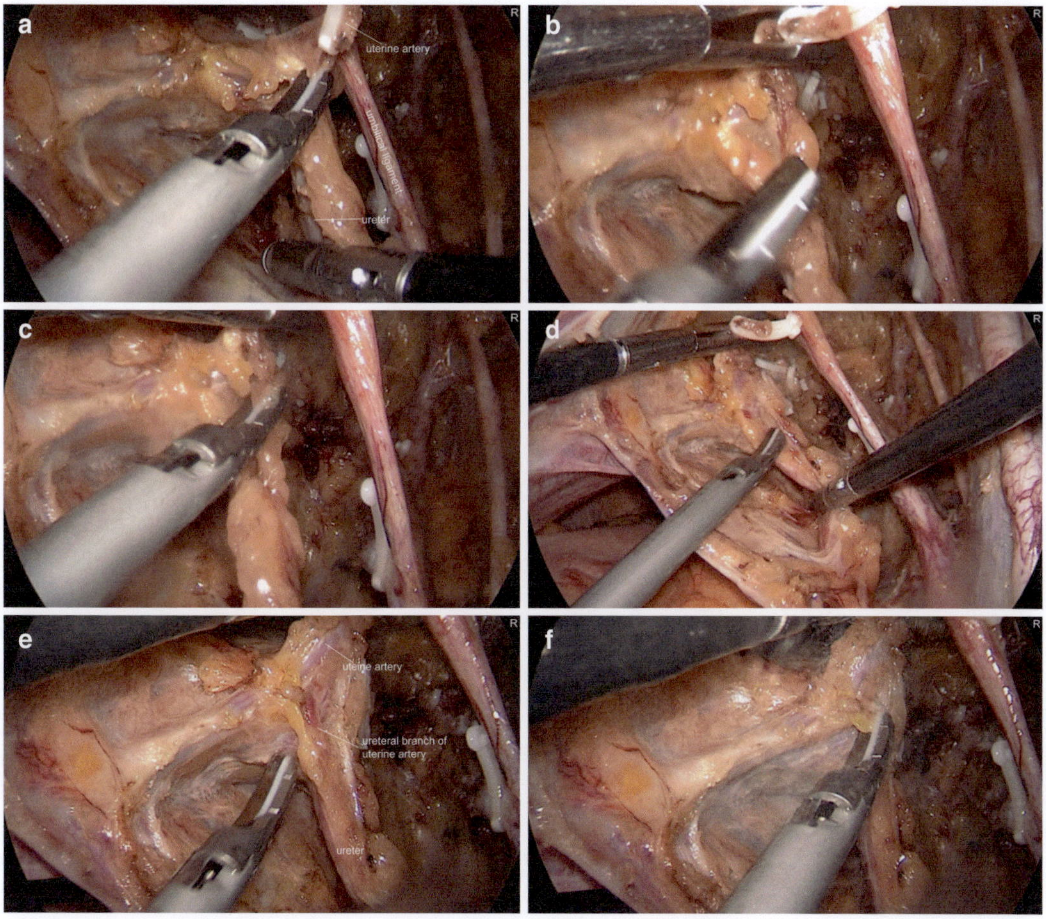

Fig. 11.20 (a–f) Bluntly and sharply transect the uterine artery ureteral branch

method commonly used in both open and laparoscopic procedures.

Ureter dissection is an essential step for all gynecologists. Minimally invasive surgery often utilizes energy devices for ureter dissection, requiring caution. The author's team adopts several methods to prevent thermal injury during this step: (1) allowing a natural cooling period of 3–5 seconds after sharp dissection; (2) using the ultrasonic scalpel in contact mode on the uterine serosa for 2–3 seconds to help dissipate heat, a method commonly used in robotic surgery; (3) irrigation with room temperature normal saline to cool the area, a technique frequently employed in open and laparoscopic surgeries.

Management of the Uterine Artery Bladder Branch In the previous description of Type C1 surgery, it was mentioned that the uterine artery bladder branch was managed from the anterior aspect of the uterine artery. However, in this case, the patient's uterine artery bladder branch was managed from the posterior aspect of the uterine artery. The author's team is accustomed to managing it from the anterior aspect of the uterine artery, as the tissue planes are relatively looser in this region.

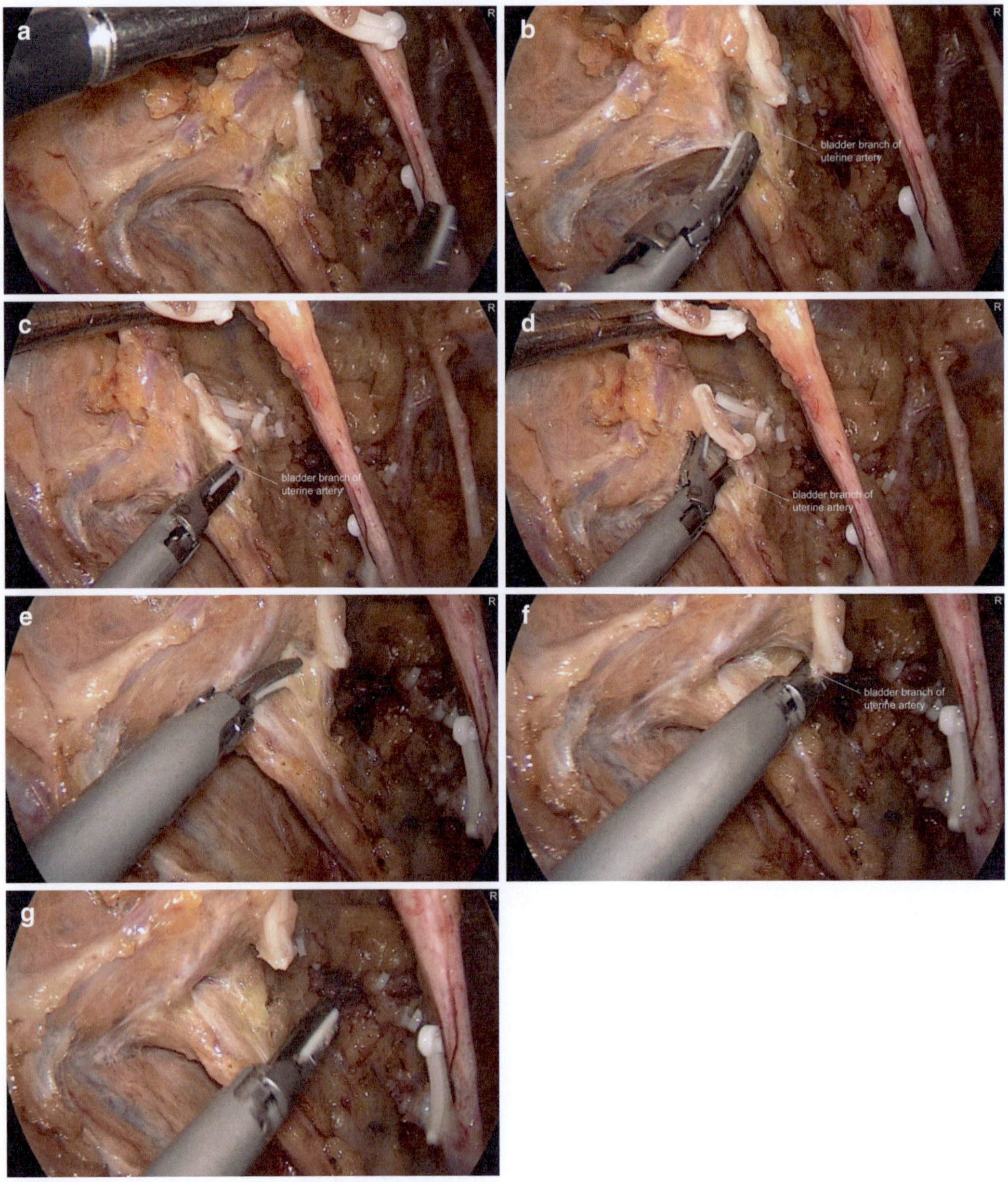

Fig. 11.21 (**a**–**g**) Separate and transect the branches of the uterine artery that supply the bladder. Dissect ureter to the entrance of the "tunnel"

11.8 Management of the Dorsal Parametrium

11.8.1 Exposure of the Dorsal Parametrium

Pull the uterus caudally and the rectum cranially to expose the peritoneal reflection of the rectum and create a sharp incision (Fig. 11.22a–f). Perform precise dissection within the white, loose fibrous tissue between the posterior wall of the vagina and the anterior wall of the rectum.

Surgical Experience and Precautions

1. Opening the vaginorectal space can be approached through various routes, and the author's team prefers the lateral approach, as

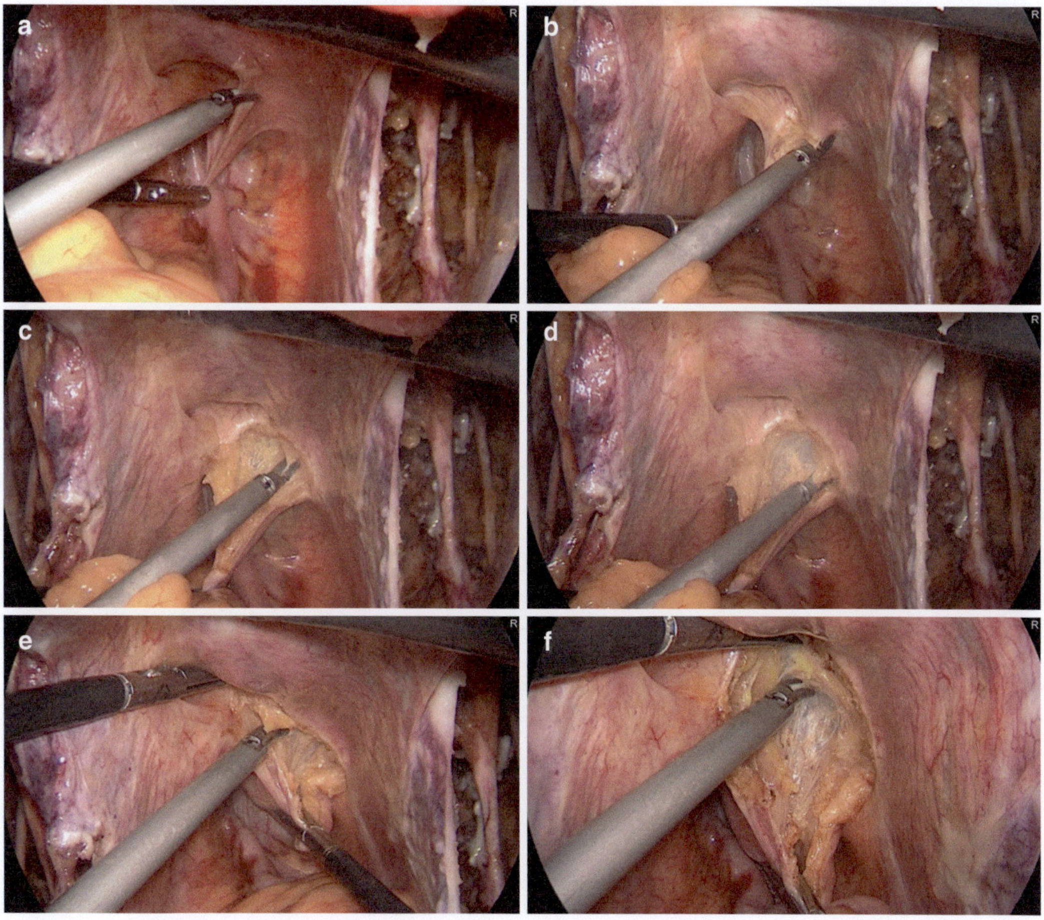

Fig. 11.22 (**a**–**f**) Expose and cut the rectal peritoneum reflection

demonstrated in Type C1 surgery. However, for a more comprehensive exposure, in this case, the patient's vaginorectal space was initially opened through a midline approach and then widened bilaterally to free the posterior parametrial tissue from the lateral rectal wall (Fig. 11.23a–f). In Type C2 surgery, unlike Type C1, the sacrouterine ligaments are excised at the level of the sacral fascia. The lateral rectal wall is usually attached to the middle segment of the sacrouterine ligament, and there is often a distinct "yellow-white" boundary in the peritoneal part. Dissecting within this space and posteriorly to the level of the sacral fascia is necessary (Fig. 11.24a–d).

2. During the process of opening and dissecting the spaces, it is beneficial to consider the concept of membrane anatomy dissection. The advantages are as follows: ①when opening the spaces, the position of the peritoneum can be identified at the "membrane bridge," which is the junction of the "yellow-white" boundary of the peritoneum at the fusion point of two embryonic compartments. ② During the separation of the spaces, sharp dissection is performed within the white, loose fibrous tissue located between two distinct embryonic compartments.

11.8.2 Transect the Dorsal Parametrial and Lateral Parametrial Nerve Plexus Tissues

Gently pull the ureter laterally to ensure its protection while transecting the lateral peritoneum and exposing the sacrouterine ligaments. Care-

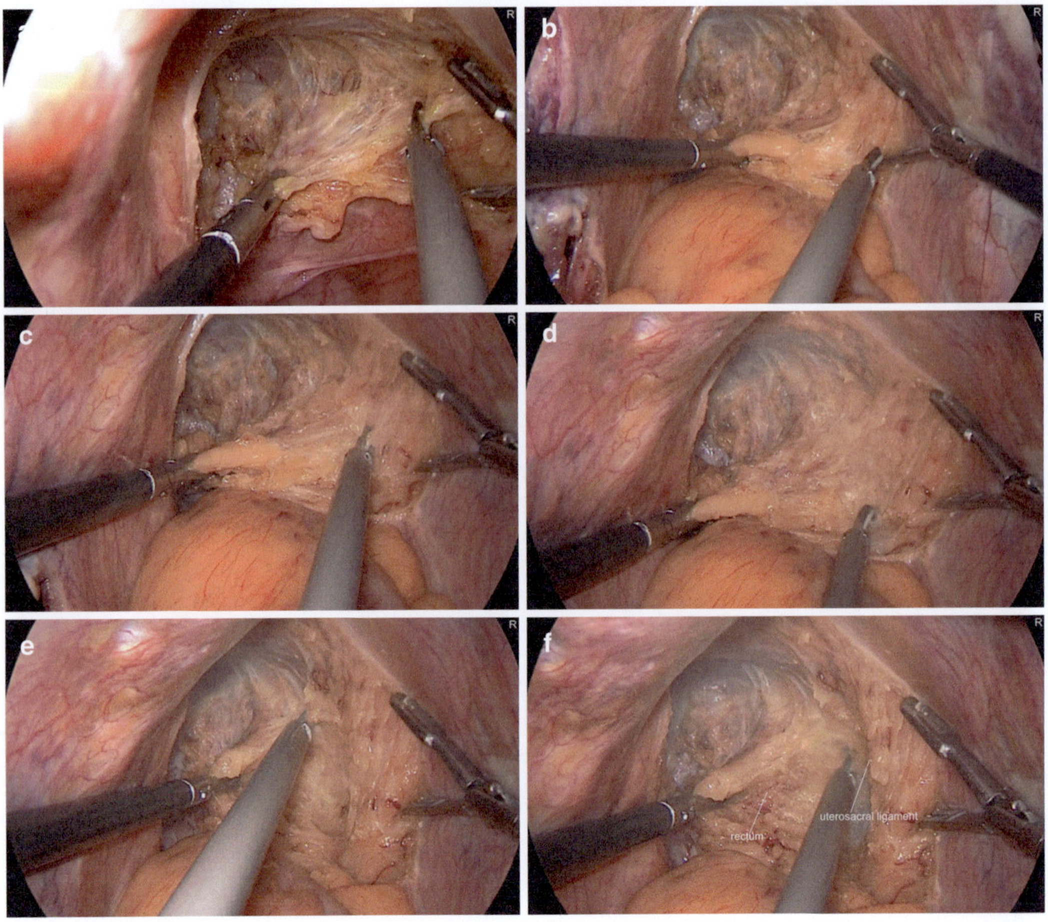

Fig. 11.23 (**a–f**) Free lateral rectal mesentery and uterosacral ligament

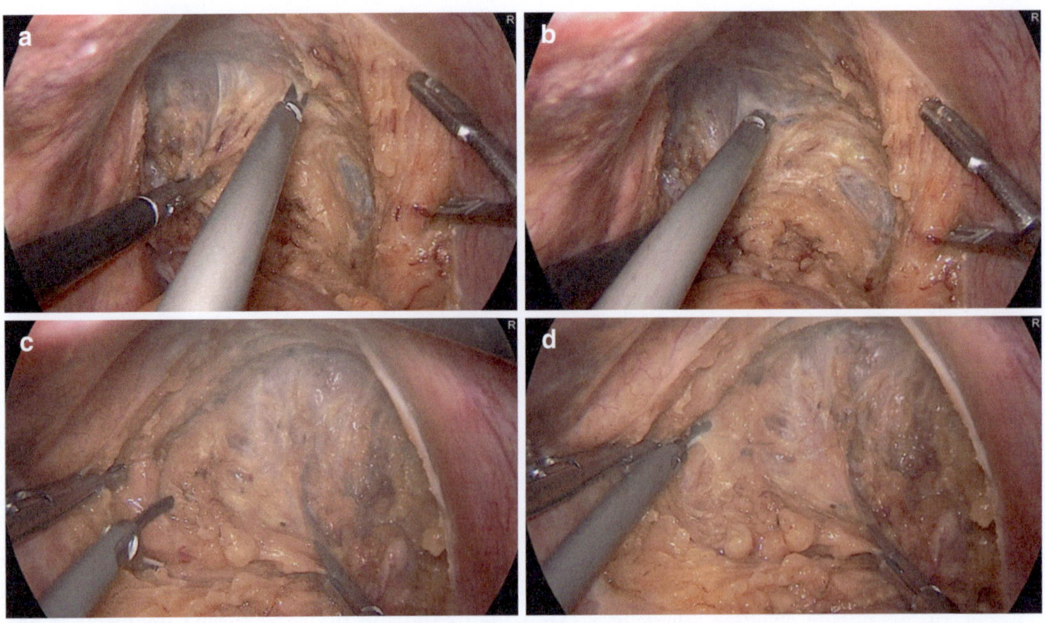

Fig. 11.24 (**a–d**) Separate the dorsal parametrium from the lateral rectal space to the sacral fascia level

fully dissect the sacrouterine ligaments along the level of the sacral fascia in a vertical direction toward the vaginal axis, and completely remove them (Fig. 11.25a–j). Pull the transected sacrouterine ligaments medially to expose the nerve plexus tissues of the lateral parametrial region, and perform precise dissection using an ultrasonic scalpel (Fig. 11.26a–c).

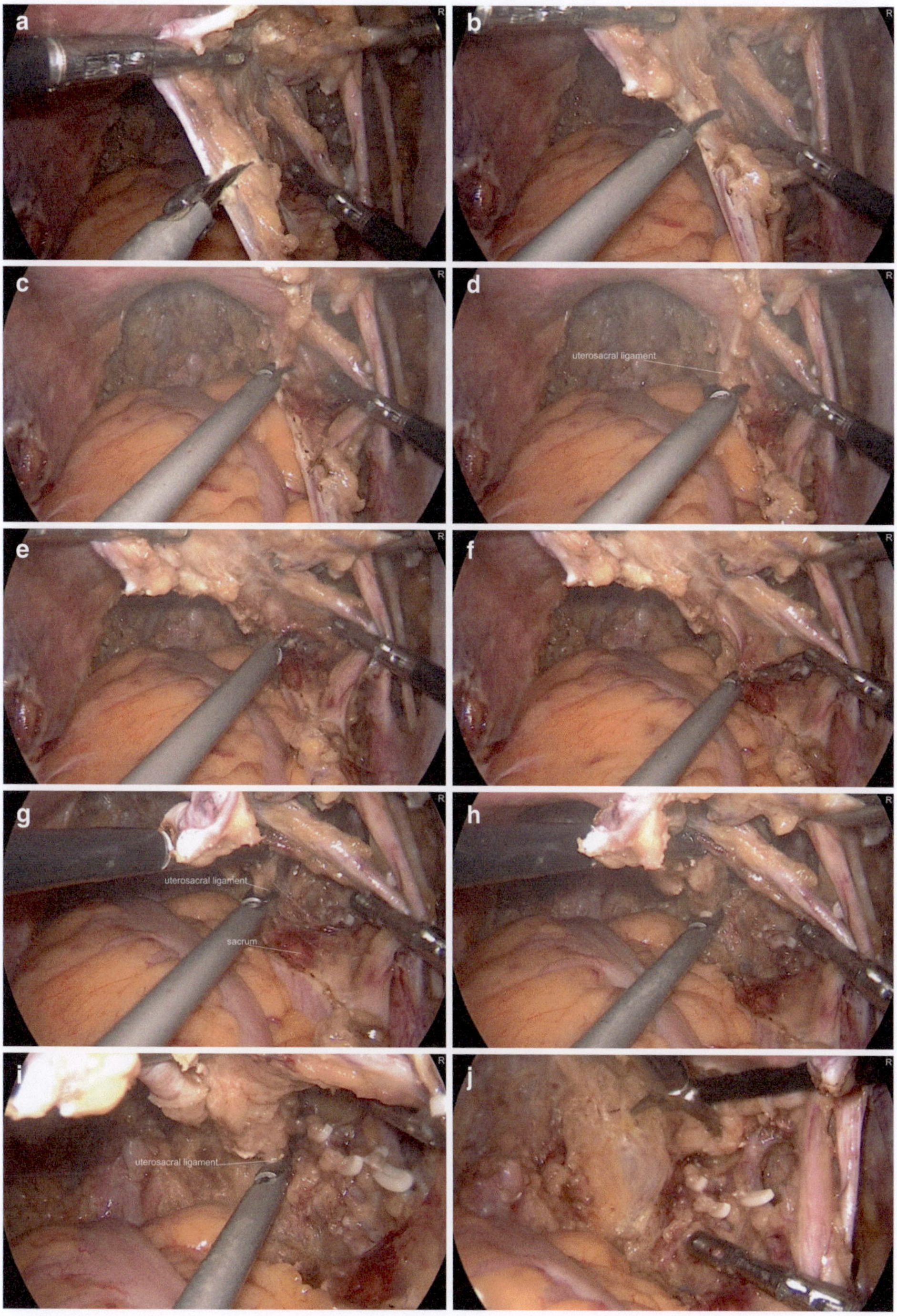

Fig. 11.25 (**a–j**) Transect the lateral peritoneum and expose the sacrouterine ligaments, then dissect the sacrouterine ligaments along the level of the sacral fascia in a vertical direction toward the vaginal axis, and completely remove them

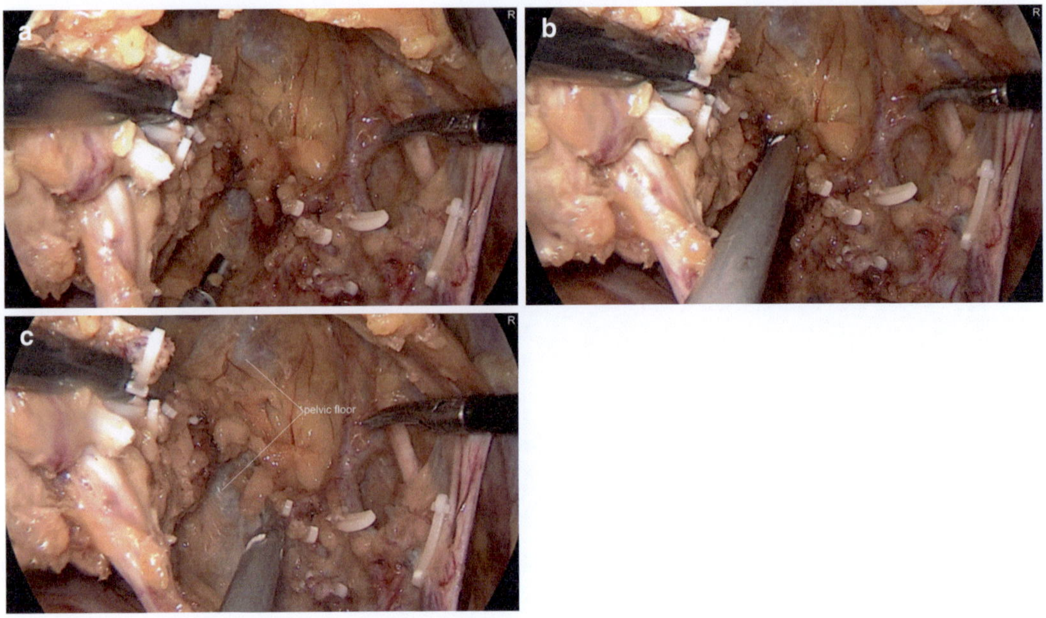

Fig. 11.26 (**a–c**) Expose the nerve plexus tissues of the lateral parametrial region

Surgical Experience and Precautions

1. When transecting the sacrouterine ligaments, it is essential to carefully identify the sacral fascia to avoid inadvertently injuring the presacral vessels near the sacrum, which could result in uncontrollable bleeding.
2. After the transection of the sacrouterine ligaments, the nerve plexus tissues of the lateral parametrial region are adequately exposed. The author's team considers this moment as the safest and most suitable time for the transection of the nerve plexus tissues of the lateral parametrial region.

11.9 Exposure of the Vesicocervical Space and the Vesicovaginal Space

After transecting the round ligaments, perform a sharp incision along the yellow-white boundary to open the vesicouterine peritoneal fold. Pull the bladder and vesicouterine peritoneal fold caudally to expose the vesicocevical space and the vesicovaginal space using an ultrasonic scalpel (Fig. 11.27a–h). The vesico-vaginal space should be further dissected toward the caudal direction and expanded laterally to facilitate the subsequent exposure of the fourth space.

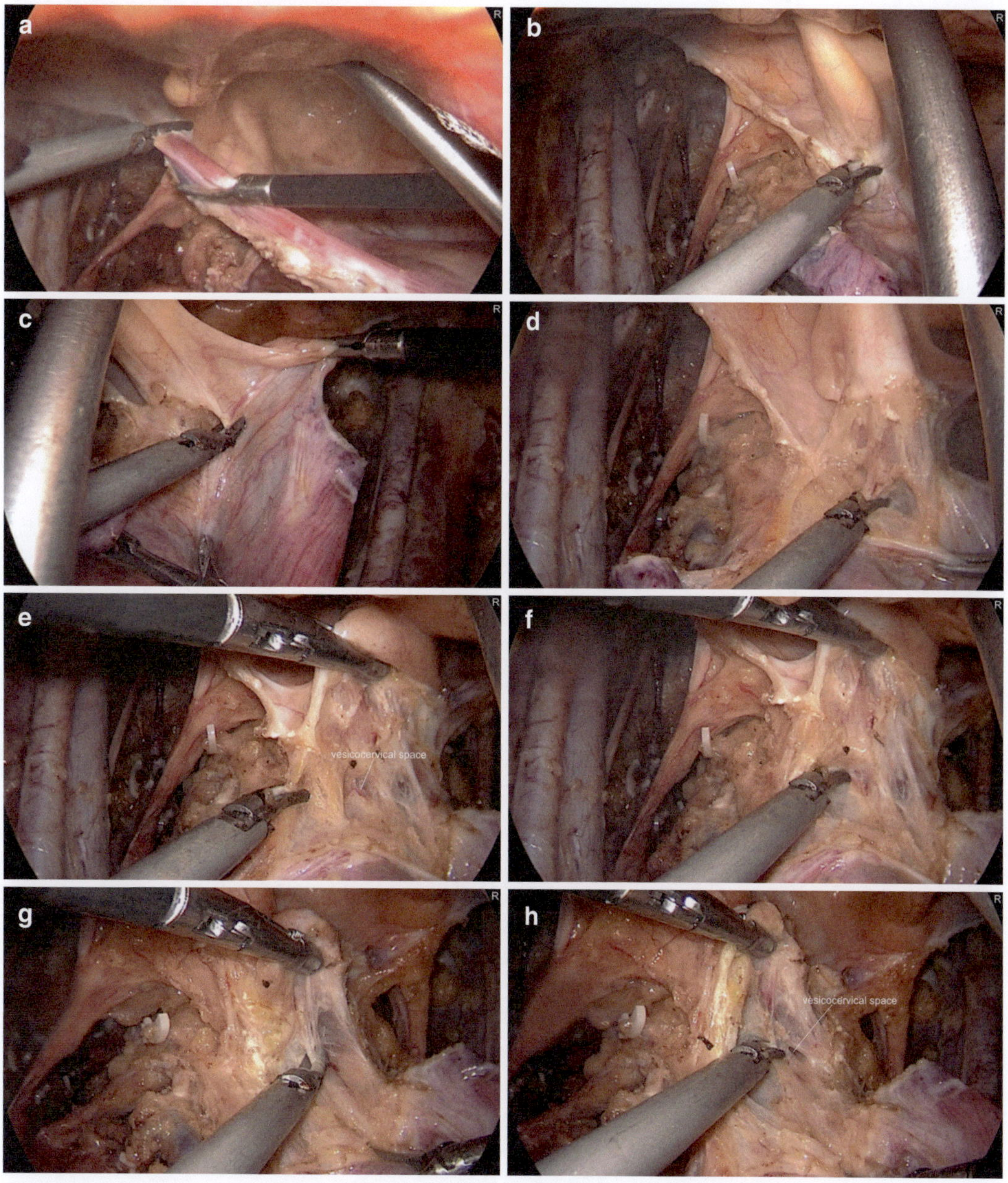

Fig. 11.27 (A–H) Expose the vesicocevical space and the vesicovaginal space

11.10 Exposure of the Fourth Space

Pull the ureter laterally, the bladder caudally and ventrally, and the uterus cranially and posteriorly to create tension. Use an ultrasonic scalpel to sharply expand the vesicovaginal space laterally. During the progressive dissection, the ureter becomes visible. Continue pulling the ureter ventrally, then employ both blunt and sharp dissection to separate the space between the ureter, bladder, and parametrium, revealing the fourth space (Figs. 11.28, 11.29, 11.30, and 11.31).

Surgical Experience and Precautions

1. This step is particularly critical and depends on the safe management of the vesicocevical ligament. The author's team is accustomed to utilizing this space for handling the vesico-cervical ligament, which allows for safe transection of the ligament while maintaining a clear view of the entrance and exit of the "ureter tunnel." Even if there is bleeding during the transection process, we can calmly perform suturing and electrocoagulation for hemostasis without worrying about ureteral injury.
2. For patients with dense spaces, exposing the fourth space can be challenging, and it may be difficult to directly visualize during the process of widening the vesicovaginal space. In such cases, thinning the vesico-cervical ligament medially can facilitate the exposure of the fourth space and the subsequent transection of the vesicocevical ligament.

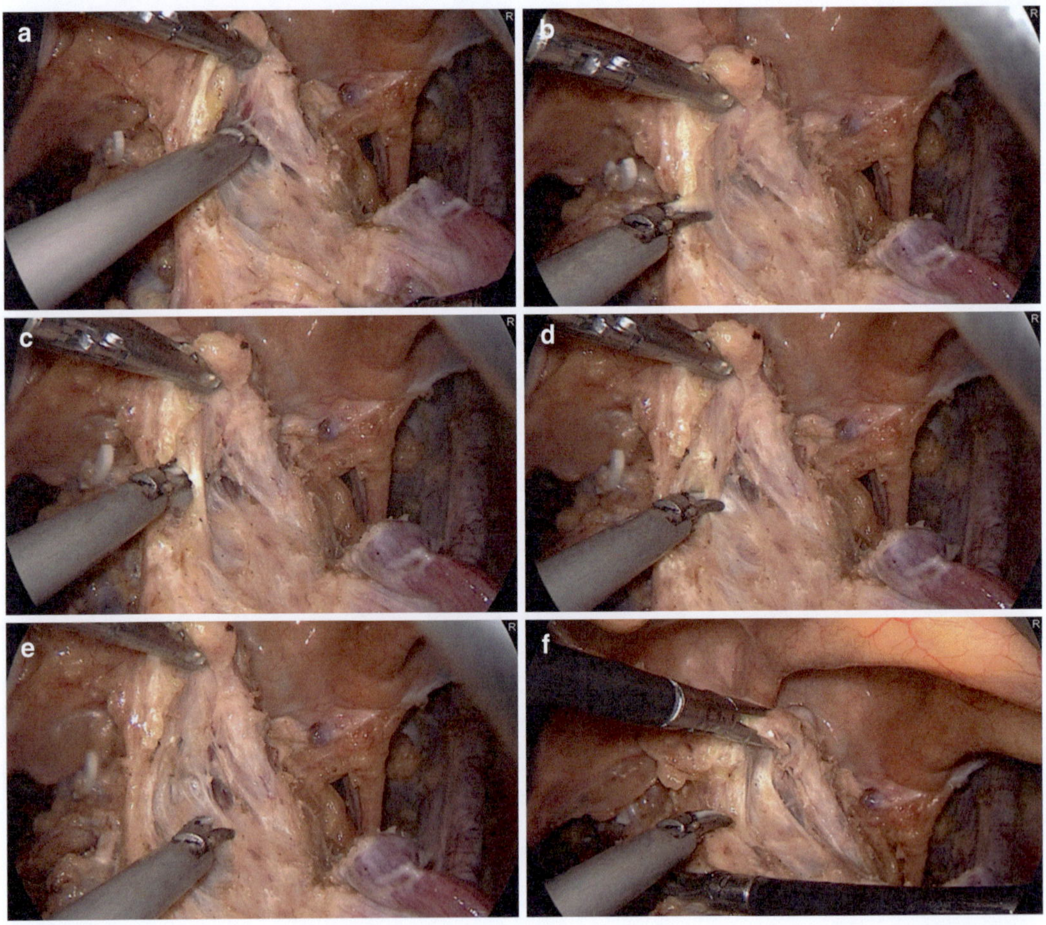

Fig. 11.28 (**a**–**f**) Expose the fourth space

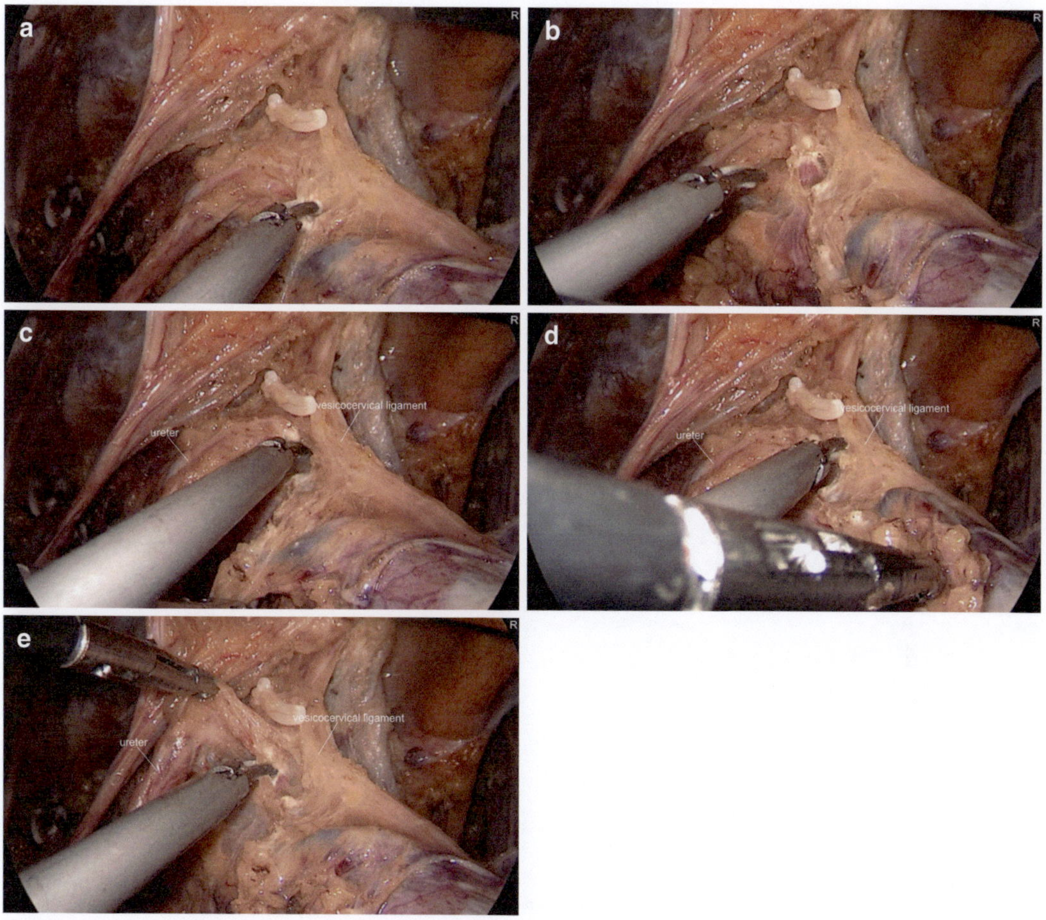

Fig. 11.29 (**a**–**e**) Both blunt and sharp dissection to separate the space between the ureter, bladder, and paracolpium, revealing the paravaginal space

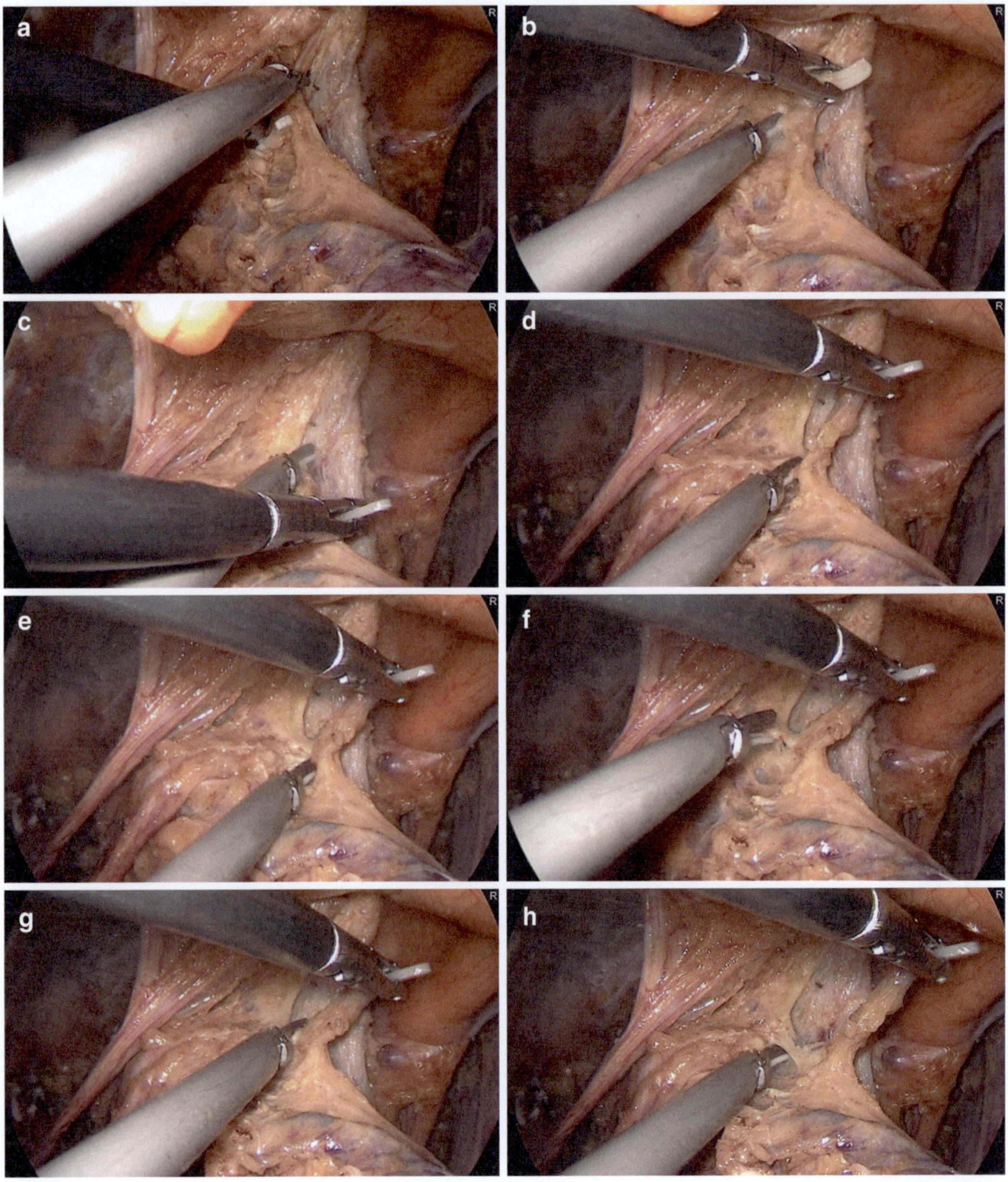

Fig. 11.30 (**a**–**h**) Separate the ureter and uterine artery

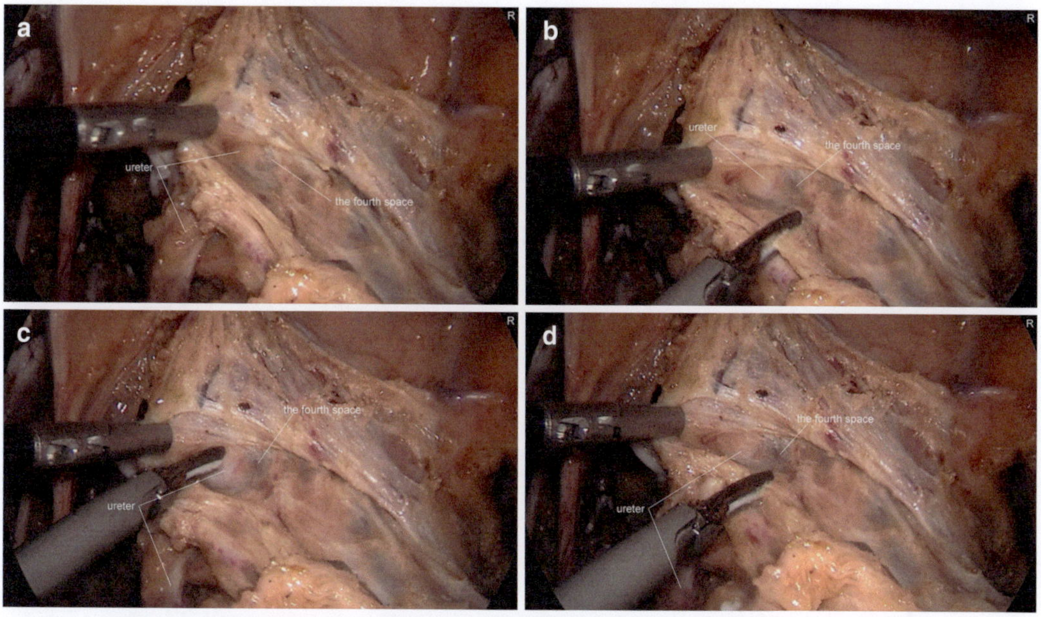

Fig. 11.31 (**a**–**d**) Thinning the vesicocevical ligament medially, exposing the fourth space

11.11 Management of the Vesicocervical Ligament and Vesicovaginal Ligament

After achieving adequate exposure of the fourth space, pull the ureter laterally and ventrally. Use an ultrasonic scalpel to sharply transect the vesicocevical ligament (Fig. 11.32a–d). Continue pulling the ureter laterally and ventrally, and progressively transect the vesico-vaginal ligament using the ultrasonic scalpel (Fig. 11.33a–h).

Surgical Techniques and Precautions During this surgical procedure, meticulous dissection is crucial due to the presence of vesical veins and their tributaries, which mostly drain into the deep uterine vein and are commonly found within these ligaments. Throughout the dissection process, the ureter can be observed to be located between the vesicocevical ligament and the vesicovaginal ligament.

For the transection of the vesicovaginal ligament, adhering to the en bloc resection principle is considered the optimal approach. The author's team experience involves performing meticulous dissection of the paravaginal space deep to the level of the pelvic floor, ensuring continuity with the paravesical space, and subsequently transecting it near the posterior bladder wall. In cases where the intravesical venous plexus tributaries are significantly enlarged, careful dissection and exposure are conducted, followed by precise clamping near the bladder for further management.

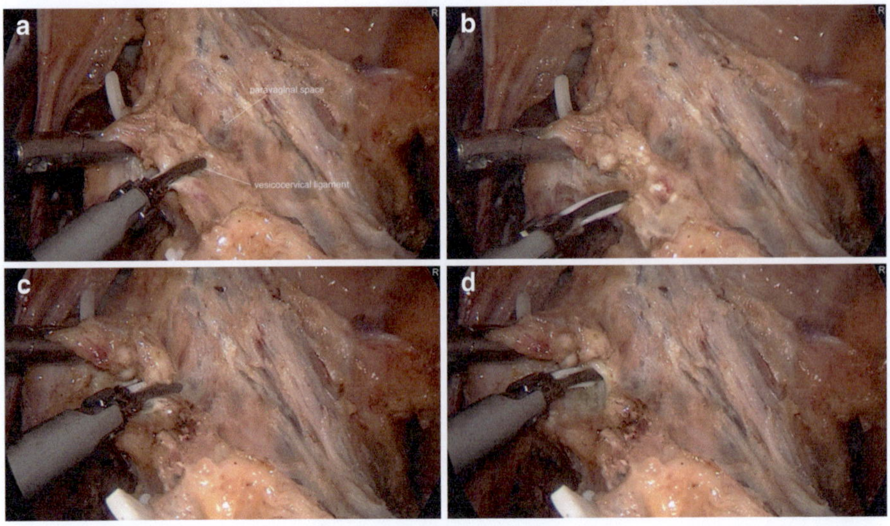

Fig. 11.32 (**a**–**d**) Sharply transect the vesicocevical ligament

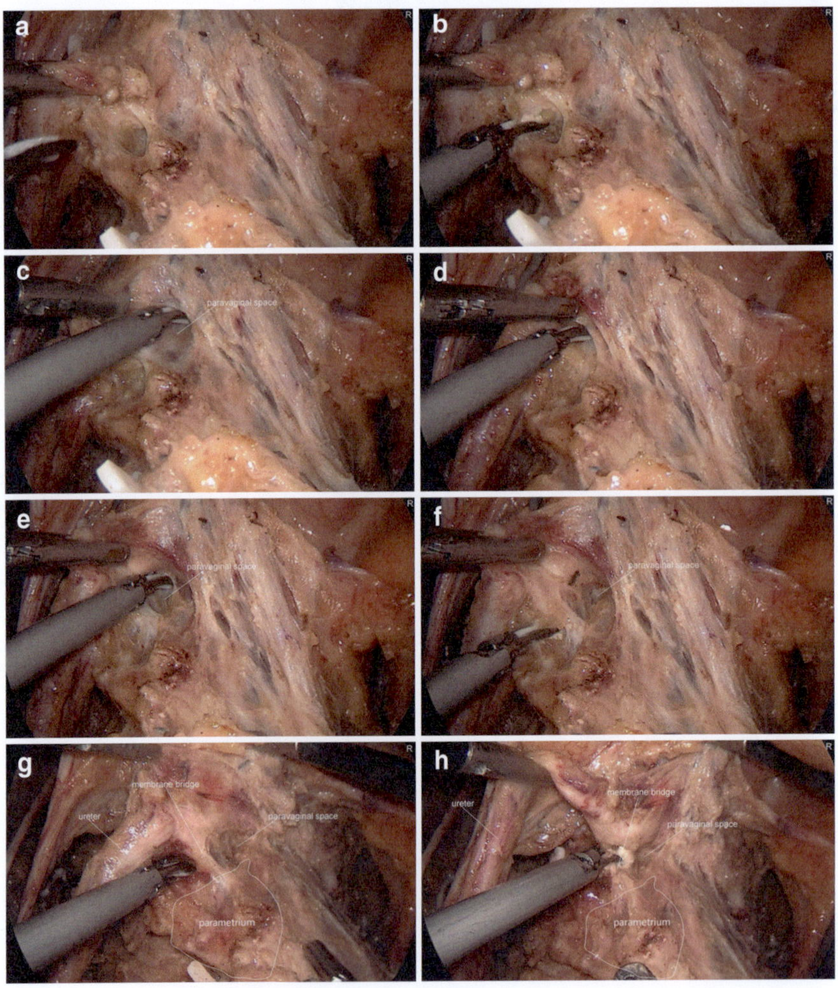

Fig. 11.33 (**a**–**h**) Transect the vesicovaginal ligament

11.12 Exposure of the Paracolpium

After transecting the vesicovaginal ligament, the posterior bladder wall can be pulled medially and laterally to expose the space between the bladder and the paracolpium. Sharp dissection with an ultrasonic scalpel is then performed (Fig. 11.34a–g) to fully expose the paracolpium down to the level of the pelvic floor fascia (Fig. 11.35a–h).

Surgical Experience and Precautions The main emphasis here is on identifying the space between the posterior bladder wall and the paracolpium. Our team is experienced in applying opposing traction by pulling the bladder wall ventrally and laterally while simultaneously pulling the paracolpium dorsally. This approach ensures sufficient tension, leading to a full exposure of the space between the two structures.

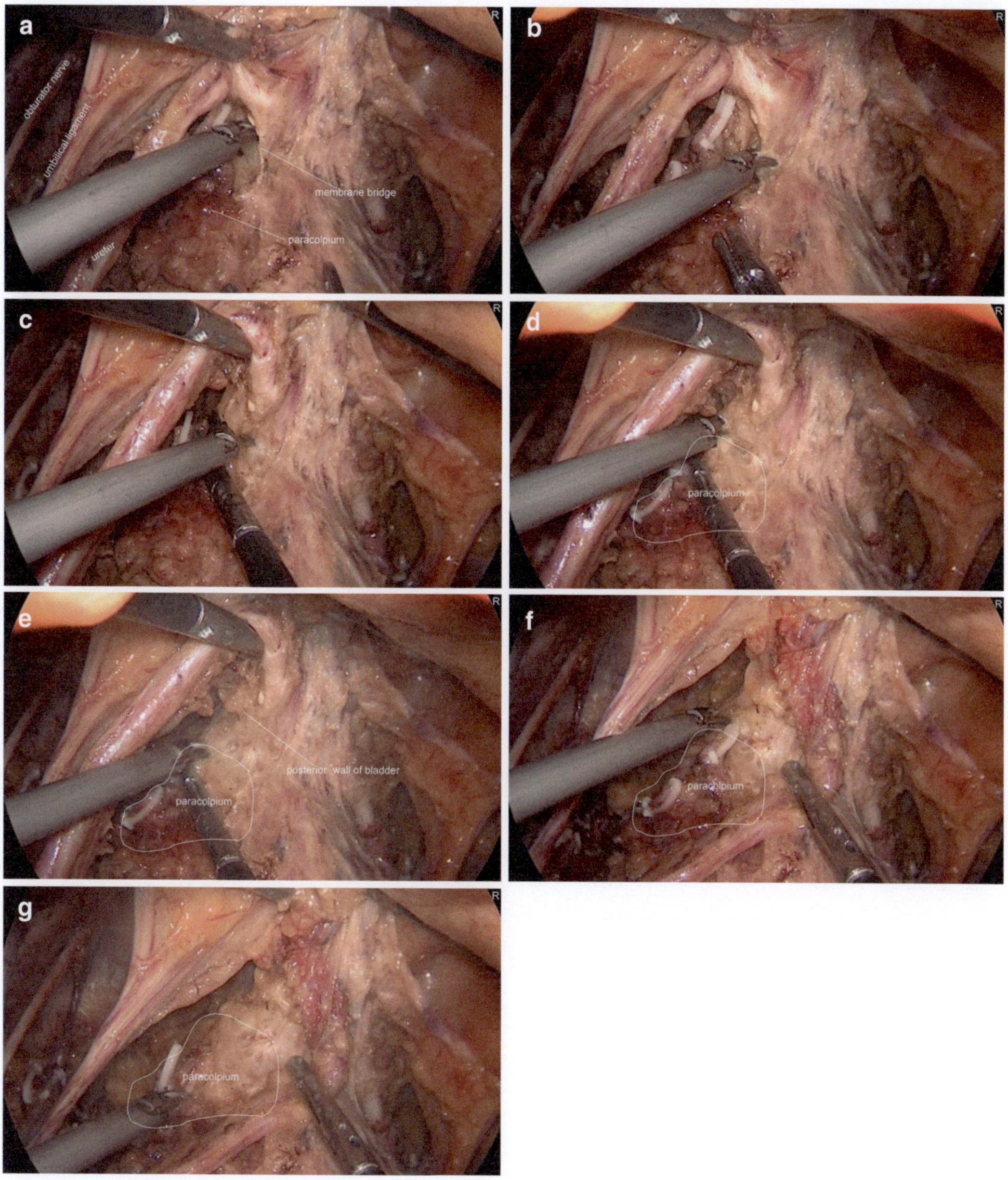

Fig. 11.34 (**a–g**) Expose the space between the posterior bladder wall and the paracolpium

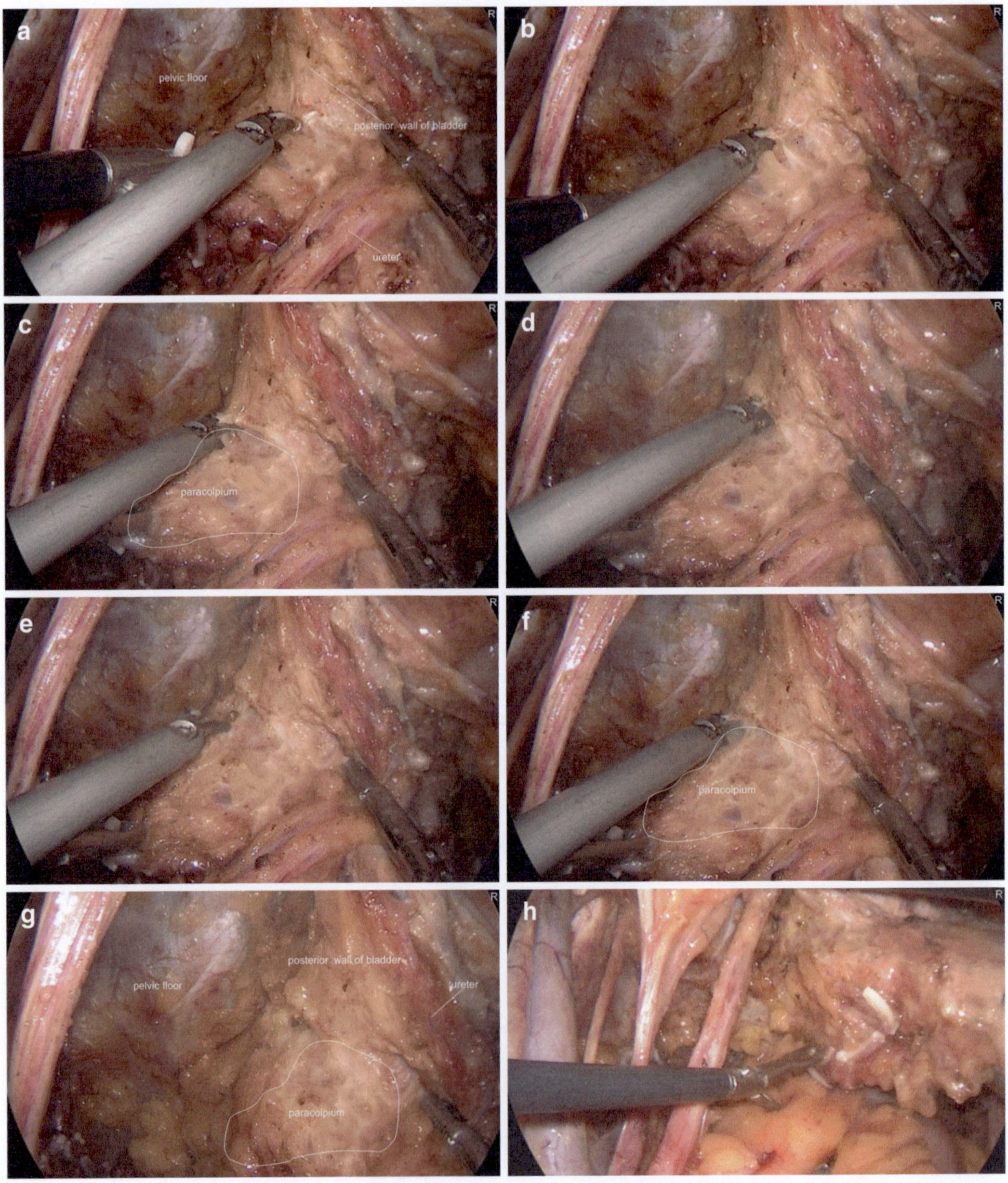

Fig. 11.35 (**a**–**h**) Fully expose the paracolpium down to the level of the pelvic floor fascia

11.13 Transection of the Paracolpium

Pull the paracolpium and parametrial tissues medially and transect the paracolpium in a vertical direction toward the vaginal axis, detaching it in its entirety to the proximity of the vagina (Fig. 11.36a–l).

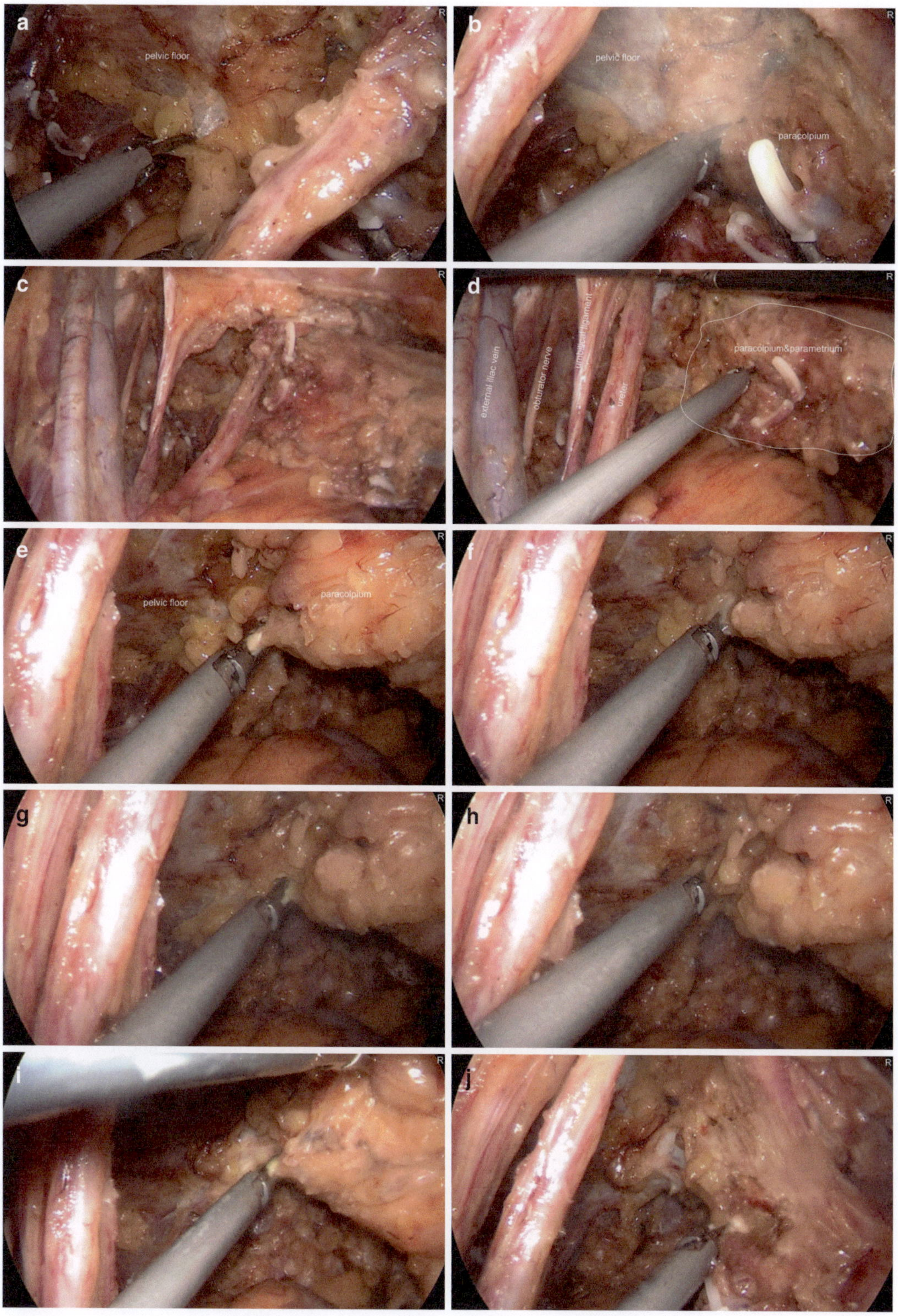

Fig. 11.36 (**a**–**l**) Transect the paracolpium in a vertical direction toward the vaginal axis, detaching it in its entirety to the proximity of the vagina

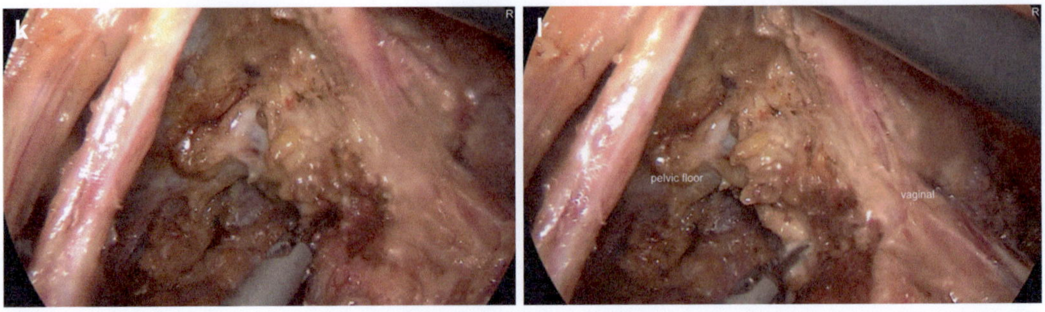

Fig. 11.36 (continued)

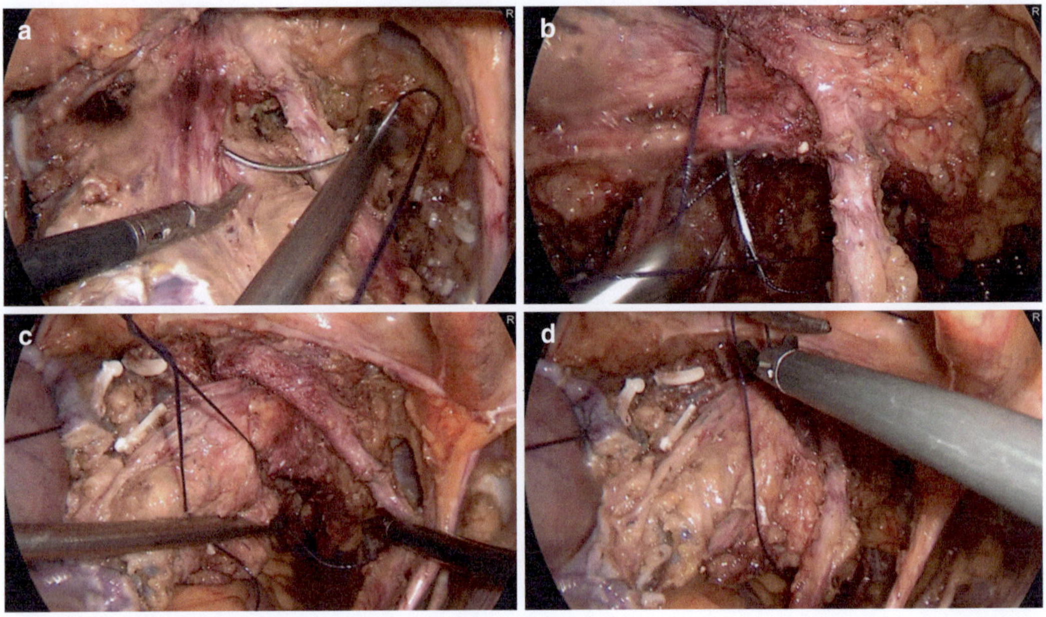

Fig. 11.37 (**a–d**) Close the vagina using absorbable sutures

11.14 Management of the Vagina

Closure of the vagina (Fig. 11.37a–d), followed by excision of the uterus through the vagina after the circular incision.

The vagina is closed with an absorbable suture in a circular fashion. The closed vagina is then repeatedly irrigated with 42 °C sterilized distilled water (Fig. 11.38a, b). Subsequently, a circular incision is made in the vagina at a location 2 cm below the cervix or lesion (Fig. 11.39a, b).

Surgical Experience and Precautions The closed vaginal cavity is repeatedly irrigated with sterilized distilled water at 42 °C. Subsequently, the vagina is transected and sutured (Fig. 11.40a, b). During the process of removing the uterus through the vagina, utmost care is taken to preserve the integrity of the uterus and avoid any cutting or damage. In Type C surgery, the requirement for the length of vaginal wall resection is 2 cm from the lower margin of the lesion. Our team understands that this 2 cm measurement refers to the natural state of the vagina, not the length of the vagina when stretched. The vaginal surface does not have specific anatomical landmarks for localization. Typically, after handling the vesicovaginal ligament, the paracolpium is already exposed, and it is in this state that we proceed with the vertical transection of the paracolpium. The corresponding length of vaginal wall resection can be achieved in

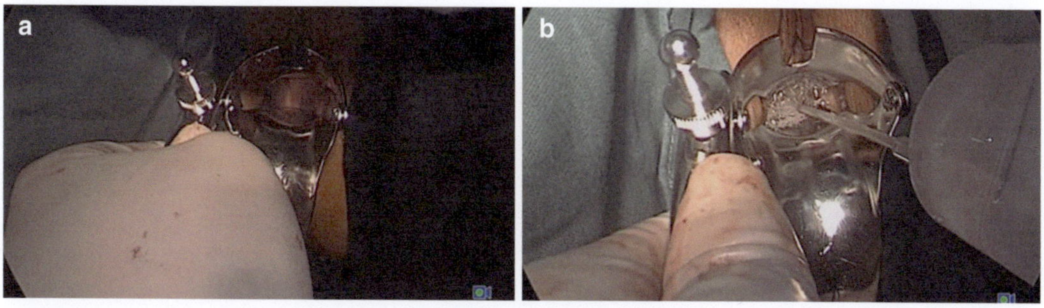

Fig. 11.38 (**a**, **b**) Repeatedly irrigate the sealed vagina with sterilized distilled water

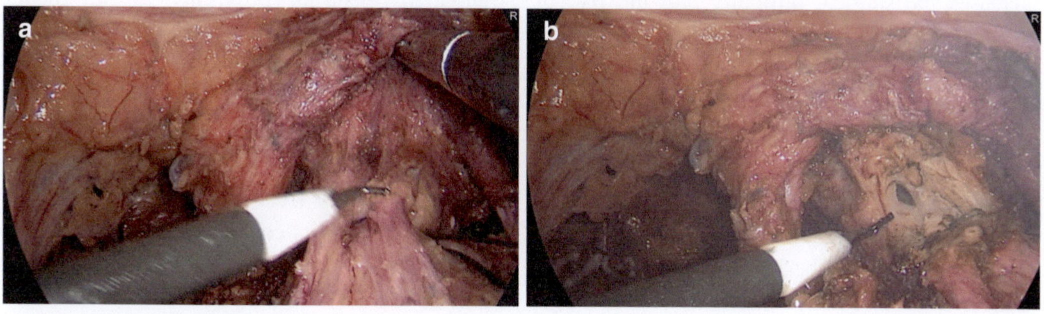

Fig. 11.39 (**a**, **b**) Circumferentially cut vagina

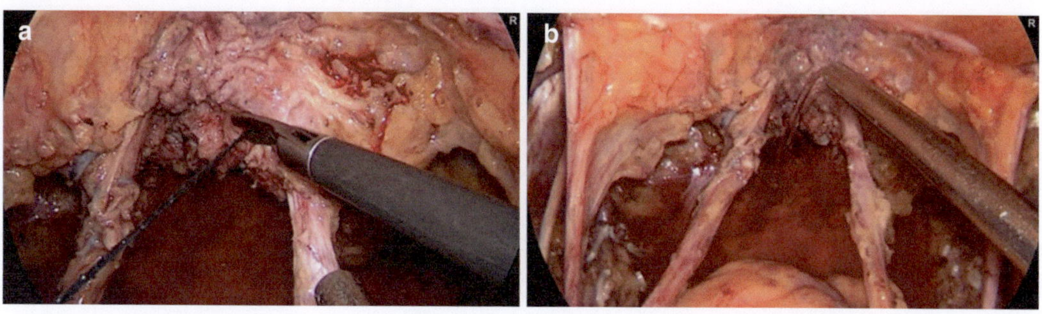

Fig. 11.40 (**a**, **b**) Suture the vaginal stump, irrigate the pelvic wound with 42 °C sterilized distilled water

this manner, measuring 2–2.5 cm in the postoperative specimen in its natural state.

11.15 Specimen Presentation after QM-C2 Type Radical Hysterectomy

The QM-C2 type radical hysterectomy (laparoscopic) is shown in Video 11.1. The QM-C2 type radical hysterectomy (open surgery) is shown in Video 11.2. Surgical Specimen Presentation (Fig. 11.41).

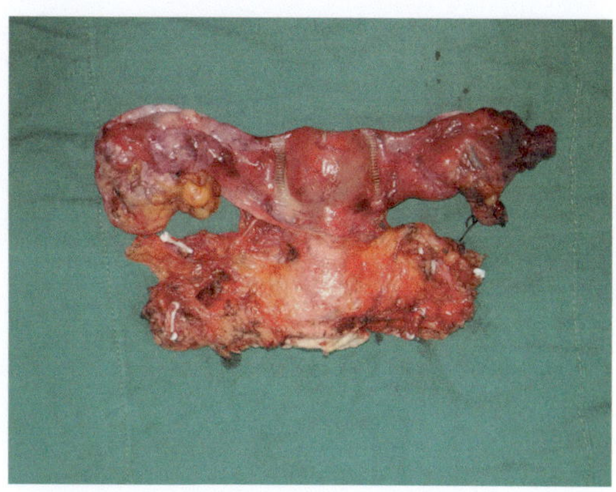

Fig. 11.41 Surgical specimen presentation (i)

Appendix Radical Excision of Residual Cervix

The treatment of residual cervical cancer is similar to that of general cervical cancer, mainly involving surgery and radiation therapy. However, due to the previous removal of the uterus, the adhesion between the bladder, rectum, and the cervical stump, as well as the formation of surgical scars, can lead to increased adhesion of surrounding tissues, especially the parauterine tissues. This increases the surgical difficulty and the risk of bladder and ureteral injuries during the procedure.

During the surgery, particular attention is given to the anatomical dissection of the spaces and embryonic-derived "membrane anatomy" planes to ensure a standardized resection of the parametrial tissues while minimizing the risk of damaging adjacent organs. The surgical steps are similar to those conducted in open radical hysterectomy.

Management of the Lateral Parametrial Vascular Tissues

Exposure of the Latzko's pararectal space and the paravesical space (Fig. 11.42a, b).

Transection of the lateral parametrial vascular tissues (Fig. 11.43a, b). At this stage, the Latzko's pararectal space and the paravesical space have been successfully opened, providing full exposure of the lateral parametrial vascular tissues. The lateral parametrial vascular tissues are meticulously transected, ensuring proximity to the medial aspect of the internal iliac vessels (Fig. 11.44a, b).

Dissection of the ureter in relation to the lateral peritoneum. In C2-type surgery, nerve preservation is not required, and only the ureter needs to be mobilized from the lateral peritoneum. The ureter is carefully freed down to approximately 2 cm posterior to its course, where the mesoureter is transected, followed by further mobilization in the caudal direction.

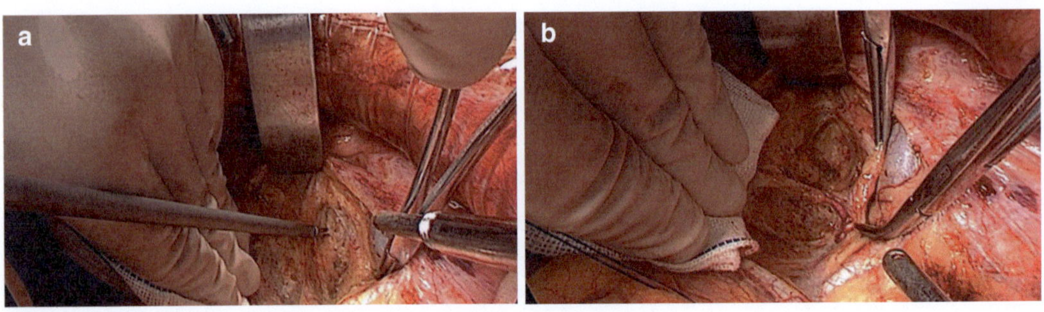

Fig. 11.42 (**a**, **b**) Separate the Latzko's pararectal space and paravesical space

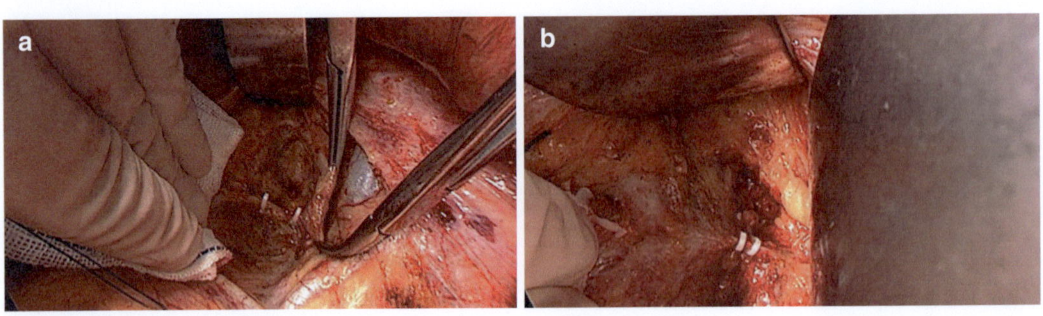

Fig. 11.43 (**a**, **b**) Transect the lateral parametrial vascular tissues

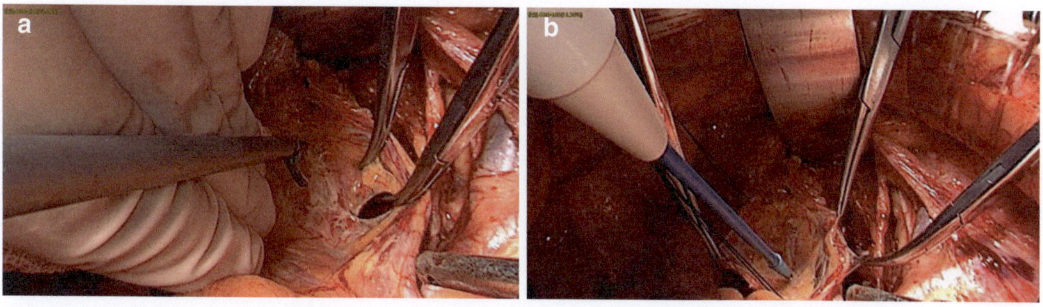

Fig. 11.44 (**a**, **b**) Free ureter and lateral peritoneum

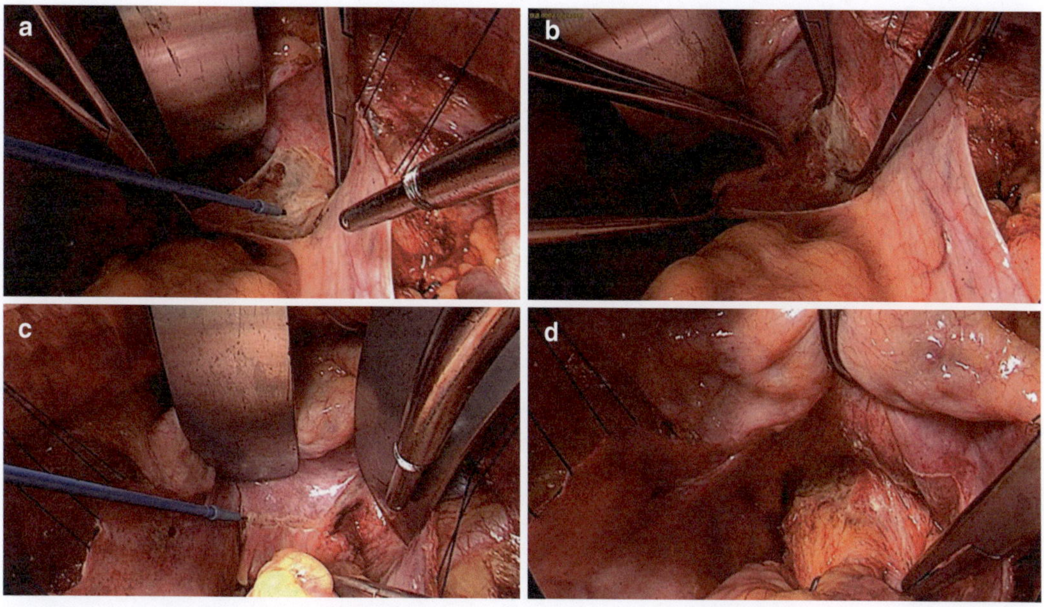

Fig. 11.45 (**a–d**) Expose the dorsal parametrium

Management of the Dorsal Parametrium

Exposure of the Dorsal Parametrium Pull the lateral peritoneum laterally and the rectal sidewall medially, perform sharp dissection with an ultrasonic scalpel until the level of the sacral fascia. Pull the rectum cranially, the uterus ventrally, and the rectouterine fold laterally. Sharply open the peritoneum covering the rectum and separate the rectovaginal space (Fig. 11.45a–d).

Transection of the Dorsal Parametrium (Fig. 11.46a, b).

Management of the Ventral Parametrial

Exposure of the Vesicocevical Space and Vesicovaginal Space Using a right-angle clamp, grasp the cranial aspect of the cervix and gently pull it cranially. Make a precise incision along the yellow-white boundary to open the fold of vesicouterine peritoneum. Carefully pull the fold of bladder and vesicouterine peritoneum caudally and ventrally, and continue the meticulous dissection with an ultrasonic scalpel to progressively expose the vesicocevical space and the vesicovaginal space (Fig. 11.47a–d). The vesicovaginal space should not only be dis-

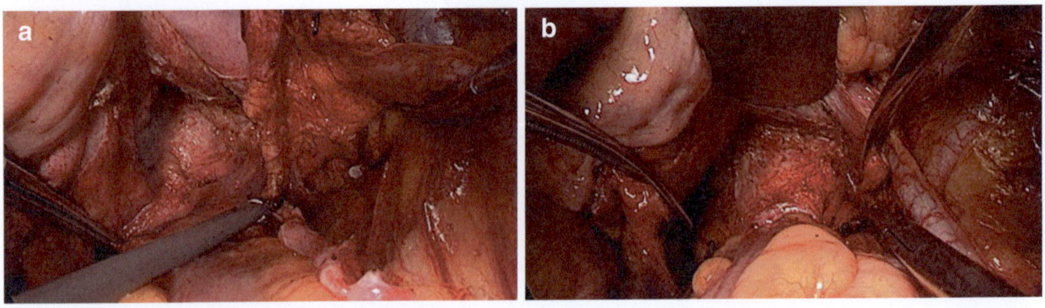

Fig. 11.46 (**a**, **b**) Transect the dorsal parametrium

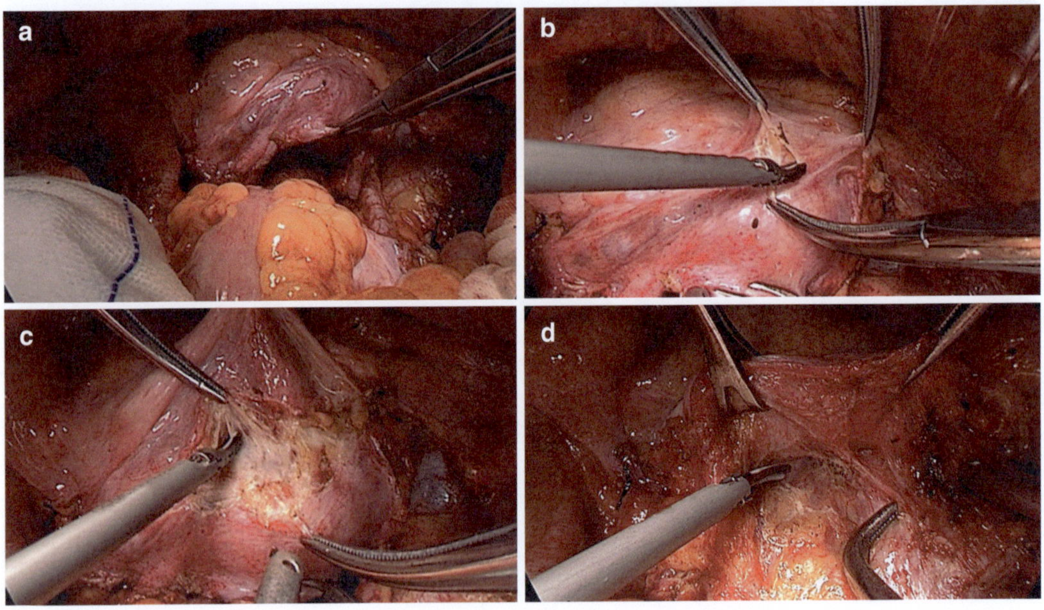

Fig. 11.47 (**a–d**) Expose the vesicocevical space and vesicocevical space

sected deeply toward the caudal direction but also expanded laterally to provide a foundation for subsequent the fourth space exposure.

Exposure of the Fourth Space (Fig. 11.48a, b).

Management of the Vesicocevical and Vesicovaginal Ligaments (Fig. 11.49a–c).

Management of the Paracolpium and Vagina These steps are consistent with the procedures of QM-C2 type radical hysterectomy.

Surgical Specimen Presentation of Residual Cervical Cancer Residual cervical cancer surgical specimen (Fig. 11.50).

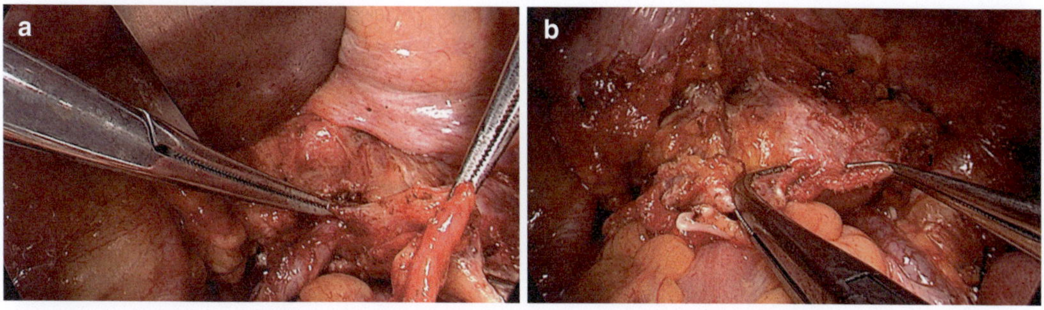

Fig. 11.48 (**a**, **b**) Expose the fourth space

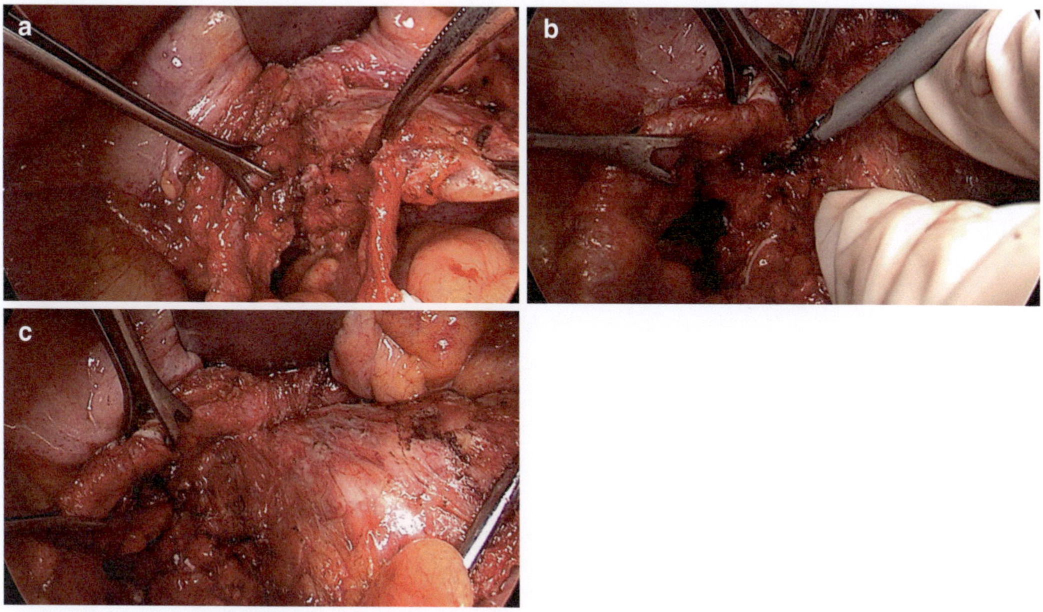

Fig. 11.49 (**a**–**c**) Management of the vesicocevical and vesicovaginal ligaments

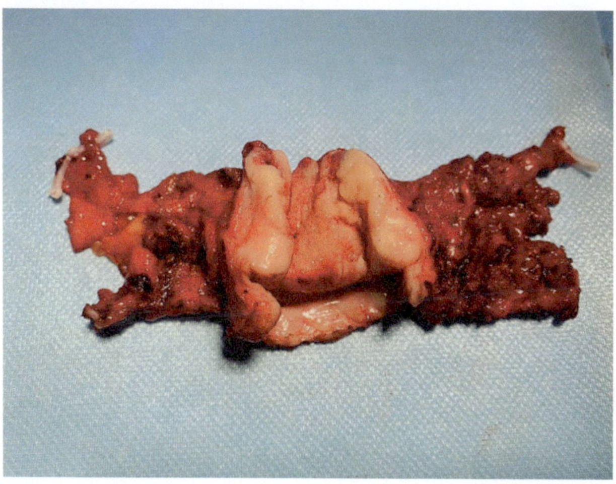

Fig. 11.50 Surgical specimen presentation (ii)

Reference

1. NCCN. NCCN clinical practice guidelines in oncology—cervical cancer. (2022-12-23) [2023-03-15]. https://www.nccn.org/professionals/physician_gls/pdf/cervical.pdf

Fertility-Sparing Radical Trachelectomy for Cervical Cancer

12

Shichao Han, Jun Wang, Jing Na, Ya Li, and Xinyou Wang

Surgical indications: For stage IA1 cervical cancer without lymphovascular space invasion (LVSI), transvaginal cervical conization procedure is recommended. For stage IA1 cervical cancer with LVSI, stage IA2, stage IB1, and a small portion of stage IB2, a fertility-preserving radical trachelectomy can be performed either via laparotomy or transvaginally (Recommended by the 2022 Chinese Expert Consensus on Fertility-Sparing Treatment of Cervical Cancer) [1].

Surgical Experience and Precautions In our team's practice of radical trachelectomy, we always preserve the bilateral ascending branches of the uterine arteries to minimize the impact on uterine blood supply. Adhering to the principle of tumor-free resection, we ensure that the vaginal cuff and cervix are brought out of the body during the dissection. In cases of fertility-sparing radical trachelectomy via a vaginal approach, it is necessary to perform either sentinel lymph node biopsy or systematic lymphadenectomy under laparoscopic guidance. However, the laparoscopic approach for fertility-sparing radical trachelectomy is not recommended in the Chinese Expert Consensus on Fertility-Sparing Treatment of Cervical Cancer. When dividing the cervix via the laparoscopic approach, it is crucial to carefully pull the uterus from the vagina toward the vaginal cuff to prevent inadvertent rupture of the preserved ascending branches of the uterine arteries. Therefore, our team opts for the abdominal route to perform fertility-sparing radical trachelectomy.

12.1 Uterine Suspension

Using absorbable sutures, perform a two-stitch figure-of-eight suture at the fundus of the uterus, securing the sutures with a needle holder to lift the uterus (Fig. 12.1).

Supplementary Information The online version contains supplementary material available at https://doi.org/10.1007/978-981-97-7687-0_12.

S. Han (✉) · J. Wang · J. Na · Y. Li · X. Wang
Department of Gynecology and Obstetrics, Second Affiliated Hospital of Dalian Medical University, Dalian, China

S. Han, J. Wang (eds.), *Open, Laparoscopic, and Robotic Surgery for Cervical Cancer*, https://doi.org/10.1007/978-981-97-7687-0_12

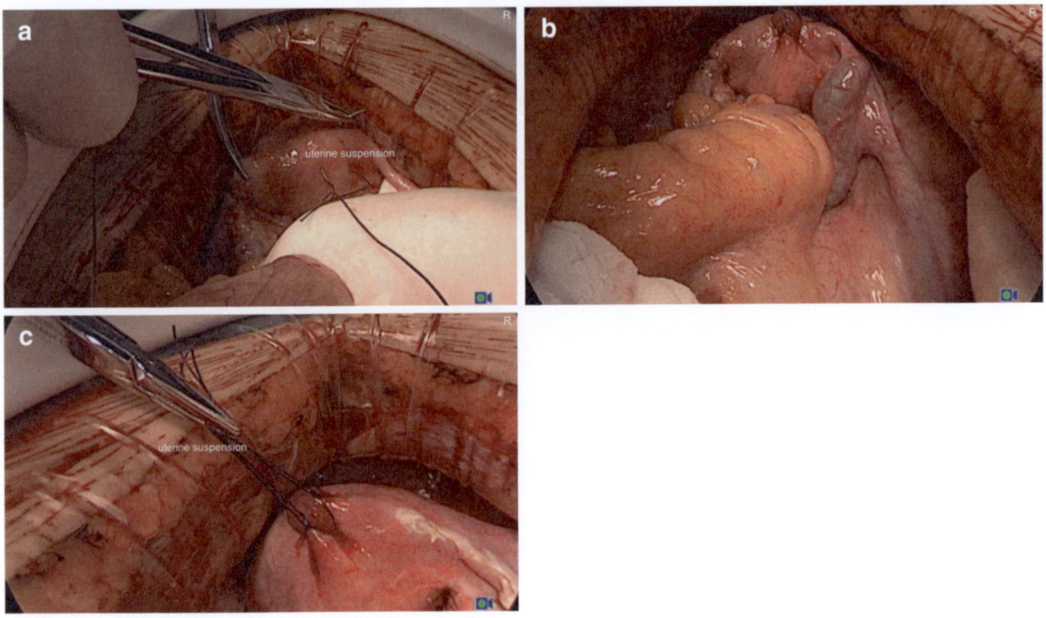

Fig. 12.1 (**a–c**) Suspend uterus

12.2 Management of the Fallopian Tubes

For cases with organic lesions of the fallopian tubes (such as adhesions or hydrosalpinx), a multidisciplinary consultation with a reproductive medicine center is essential before the surgery. If necessary, the recommendations of the reproductive specialist are followed, and informed consent is obtained from the patient. During the surgery, salpingectomy (removal of the fallopian tubes) is performed (Fig. 12.2) according to the agreed-upon plan.

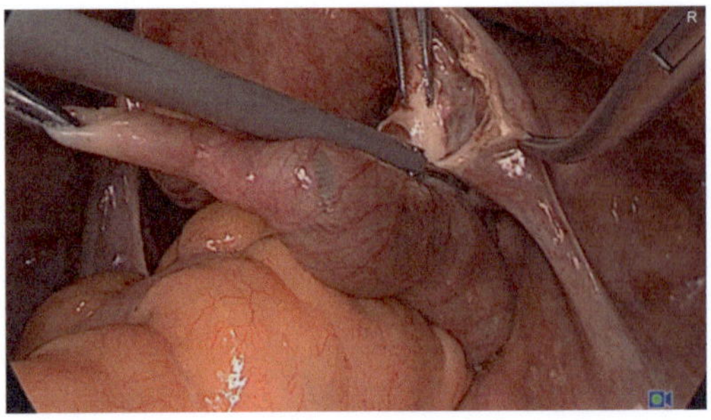

Fig. 12.2 Salpingectomy

12.3 Lymph Node Dissection

For patients with stage IA1 cervical cancer accompanied by LVSI, stage IA2, or with stage IB1 detected after conization with negative margins, our team usually adopts sentinel lymph node mapping. For cases with clearly identified lesions of stage IB1 and IB2, systematic pelvic lymph node dissection is performed, and intraoperative frozen section pathology examination is conducted. If the results are negative, the procedure continues with radical trachelectomy. However, in cases of positive findings, the extensive radical trachelectomy is abandoned, and only bilateral ovarian transposition is performed, followed by adjuvant chemotherapy and radiotherapy. For patients with positive pelvic lymph nodes during surgery, our team also informs them beforehand that they have the option to undergo lower para-aortic lymph node dissection. If the pathology indicates metastasis, postoperative extended-field radiation therapy is required. However, if the pathology does not show lymph node involvement, postoperative extended-field radiation therapy is not necessary. Additionally, our team is currently conducting clinical research on surgical staging of cervical cancer at stage IIICr involving lymph nodes.

In cases of positive pelvic lymph nodes during surgery, our team informs the patient preoperatively about the option of low para-aortic lymph node dissection. If pathology indicates metastasis, postoperative extended-field radiation therapy is required. If pathology does not indicate lymph node metastasis, postoperative extended-field radiation therapy is not necessary. Our team is also currently conducting a clinical study on lymph node staging in stage IIICr cervical cancer.

12.4 Management of Lateral Parametrium

Sharp incision is made to open the lateral peritoneum (Fig. 12.3a–d). The adnexa is pulled medially, and sharp dissection using an ultrasonic scalpel is performed to identify the paravesical space and the Latzko's pararectal space (Fig. 12.4a–d).

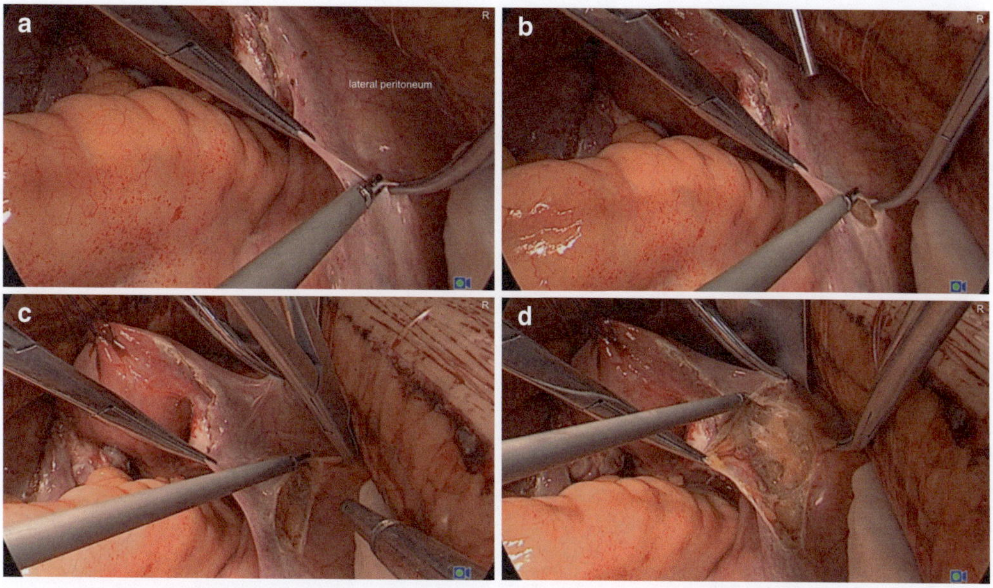

Fig. 12.3 (**a–d**) Sharply open the lateral peritoneum

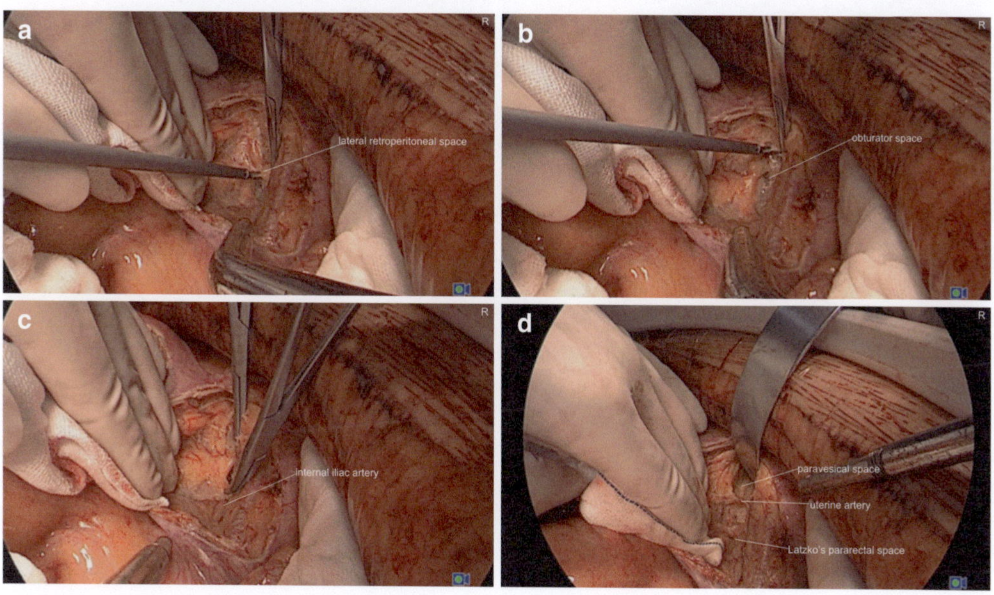

Fig. 12.4 (**a–d**) Sharply dissect the paravesical space and the Latzko's pararectal space

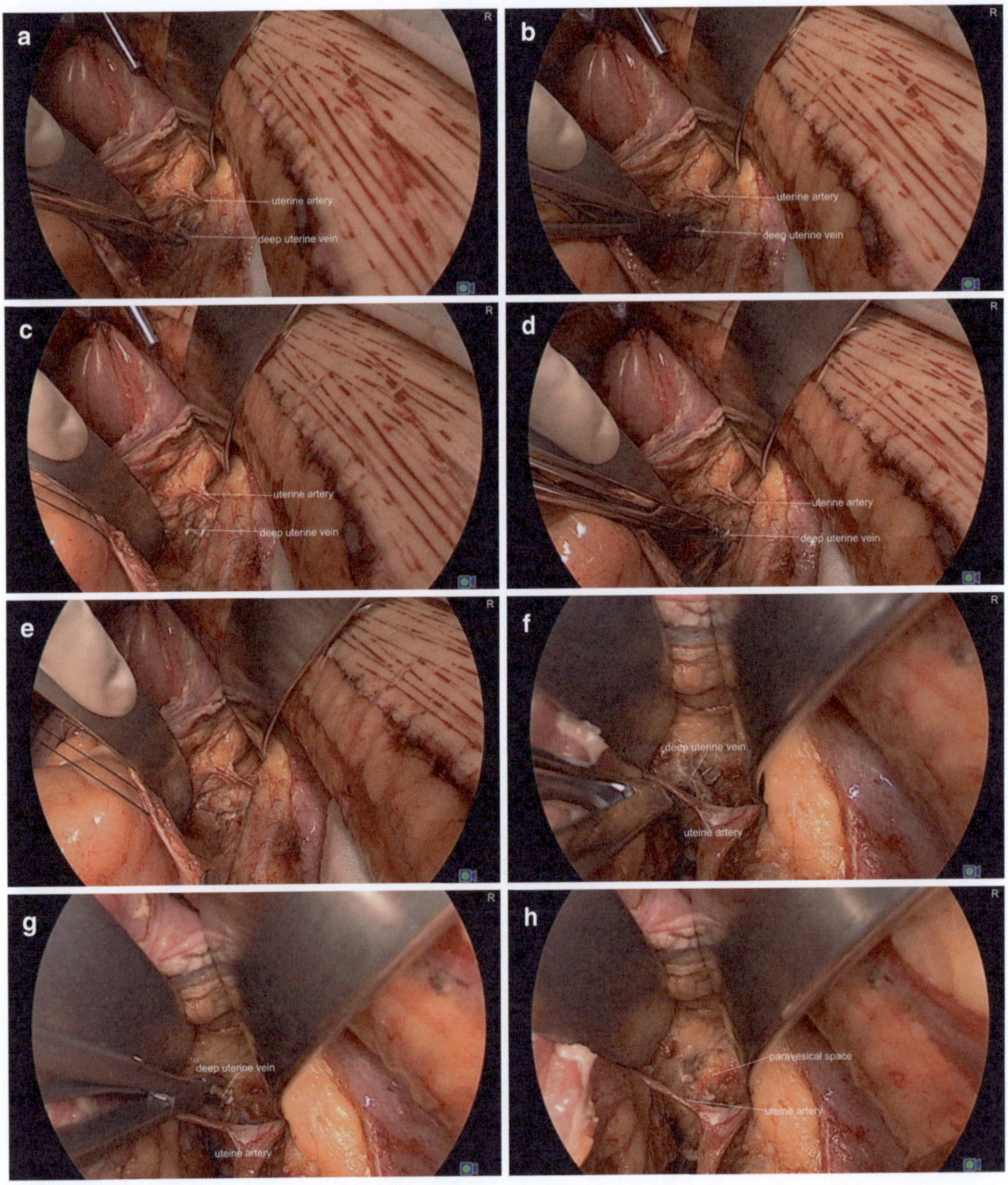

Fig. 12.5 (**a**–**h**) Separate the deep uterine vein

Subsequently, the uterine artery, superficial uterine vein, and deep uterine vein are separated. The uterine artery is preserved, while the superficial uterine vein and deep uterine vein are individually transected near the inner edge of the internal iliac vein (Fig. 12.5a–h).

12.5 Mobilization of the Ureter

Pull the lateral peritoneum medially and the ureter laterally, separating the ureter from the lateral peritoneum. Continue the dissection caudally until approaching the entrance of the ureteral tunnel (Fig. 12.6a, b).

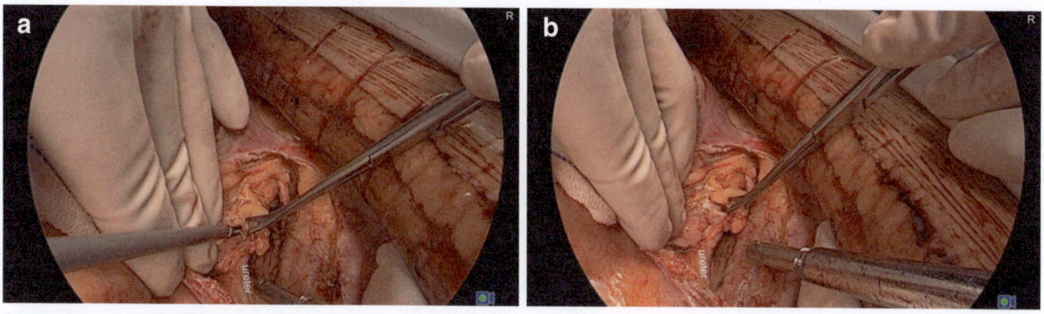

Fig. 12.6 (**a**, **b**) Separate the ureter

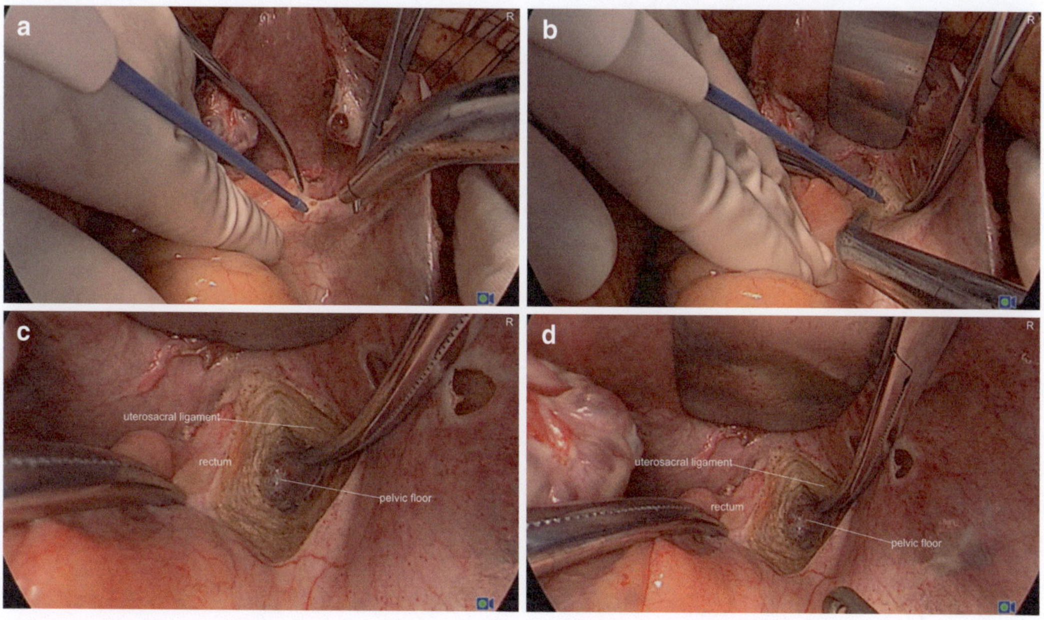

Fig. 12.7 (**a**–**d**) Open the peritoneum from the lateral side to expose the rectovaginal space

12.6 Exposure of the Dorsal Parametrium

The team's preferred approach involves first opening the peritoneum from the lateral side to expose the rectovaginal space (Fig. 12.7a–d). Then, the dissection proceeds toward the posterior direction, reaching the level of the sacral fascia. Next, the peritoneal reflection of the rectum is opened from the midline, exposing the rectovaginal space (Fig. 12.8a–d). These two dissections are then merged and connected, ensuring a complete exposure of the dorsal parametrium.

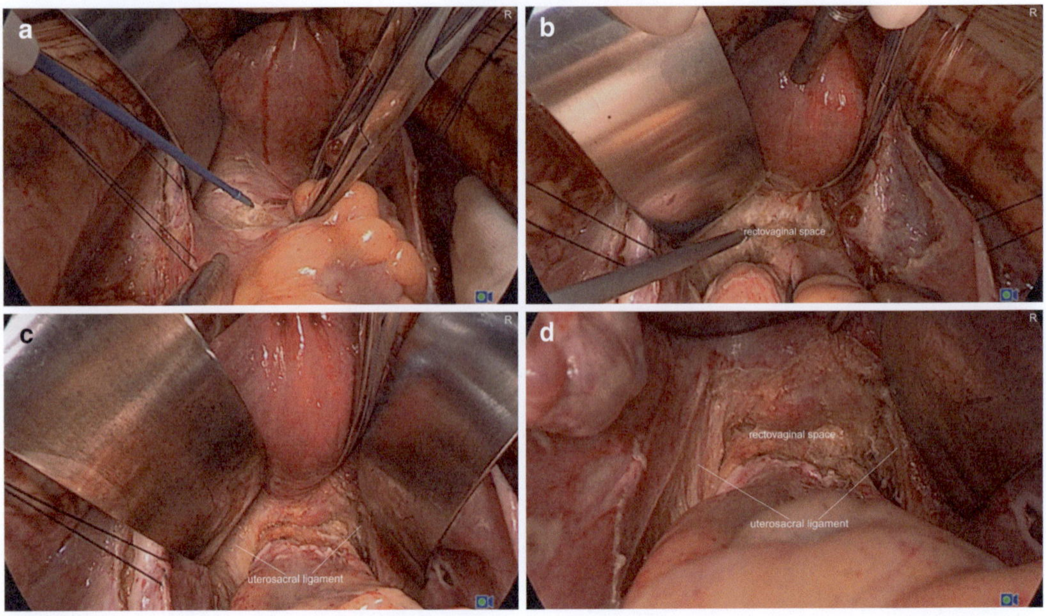

Fig. 12.8 (**a**–**d**) Expose the rectovaginal space

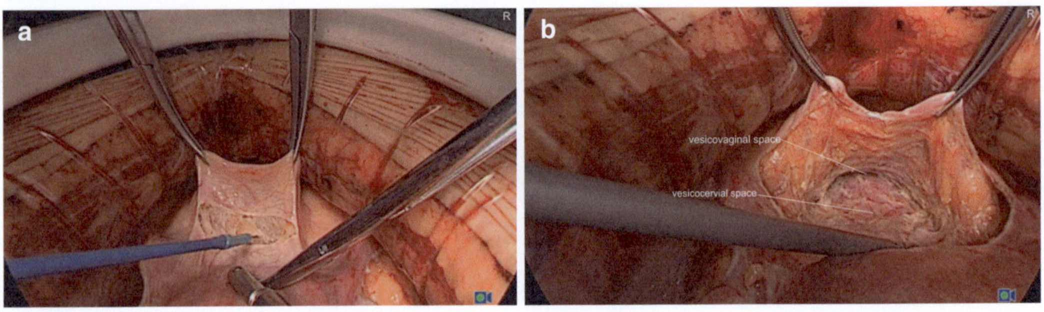

Fig. 12.9 (**a**, **b**) Expose the vesicocevical space and vesicovaginal space

12.7 Exposure of the Vesico-Cervical Space and Vesico-Vaginal Space

During this process, when expanding the transverse incision of the peritoneal reflection of the bladder on both sides, it is important not to transect the round ligaments to ensure the support and blood supply of the uterus (Fig. 12.9a, b).

12.8 Dissection of the Uterine Arteries

Separate the ascending and descending branches of the uterine artery, and then transect the descending branch (Fig. 12.10a, b).

Surgical Experience and Precautions The key to preserving the ascending branch of the uterine artery lies in performing a bloodless dissection during the exposure of the uterine artery. Our team's practice involves first handling the lateral parametrium to expose the main trunk of the uterine artery. Then, the relationship between the uterine artery and the ureter is freed, and the ureter is further mobilized circumferentially. Particularly, the ureter is mobilized both internally and externally to clearly expose the nourishing branches of the uterine artery to the ureter. Each branch is carefully transected, starting with the nourishing branches of the uterine artery to the ureter, followed by the ascending and descending branches of the uterine artery. Finally, the descending branch of the uterine

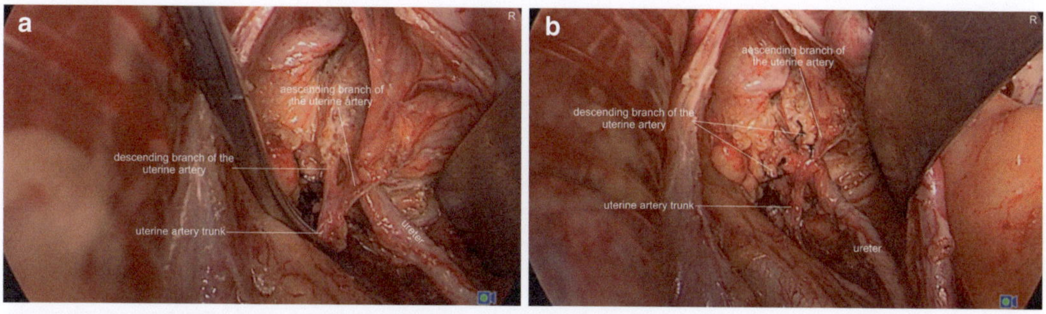

Fig. 12.10 (**a**, **b**) Separate the ascending and descending branches of the uterine artery

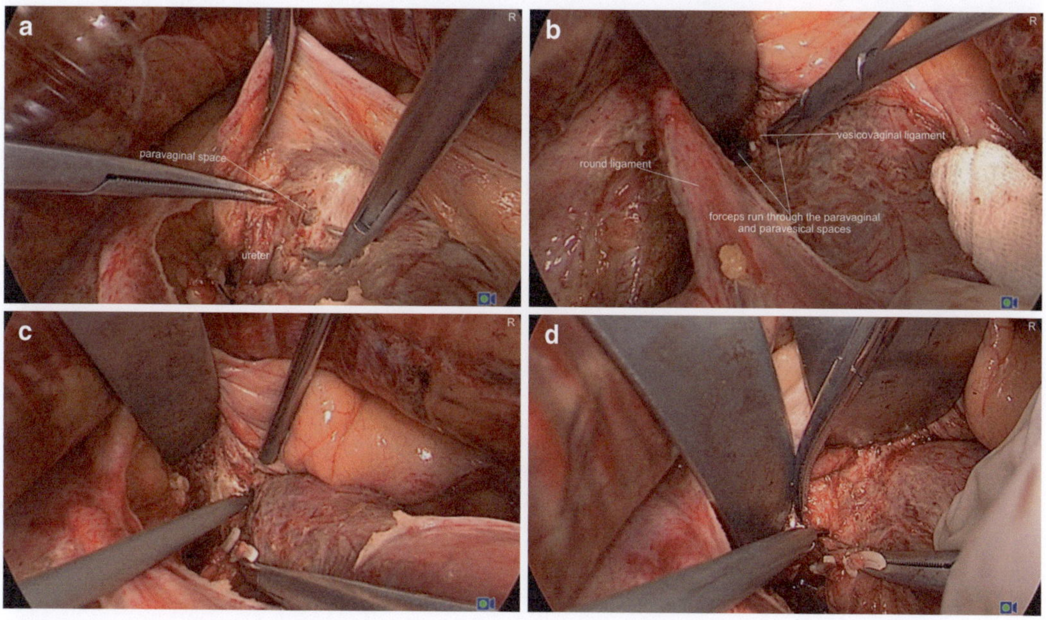

Fig. 12.11 (**a**–**d**) Management of vesicocevical ligament and vesicovaginal ligament

artery is transected while preserving the ascending branch.

12.9 Management of Vesicocervical Ligament and Vesicovaginal Ligament

Surgical Experience and Precautions Using the fourth space to its full advantage, the exit of the ureteral "tunnel" is meticulously mobilized. The fourth space is carefully connected to the vesicovaginal space, and the dissection involves transecting both the vesicovaginal ligament and the vesicovaginal ligament (Fig. 12.11a–d).

12.10 Closure of the Vagina

Our team consistently utilizes absorbable sutures to perform a meticulous circular closure of the vagina or uses long angled clamps for secure clamping (Fig. 12.12a–d). To adhere strictly to the tumor-free principle, we prefer to employ long angled clamps for closure after the circular suturing is completed.

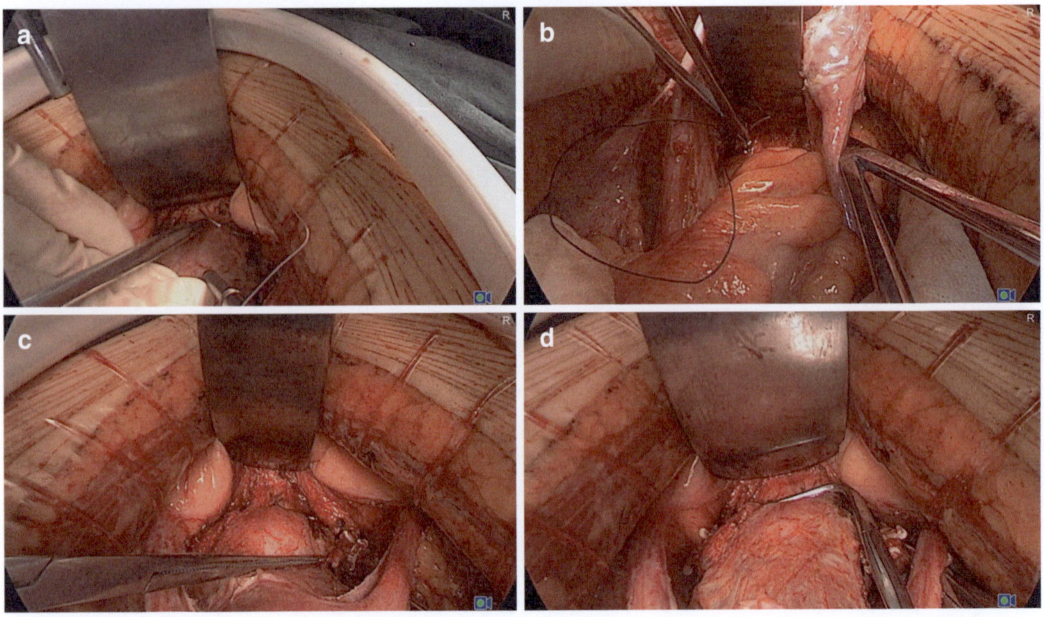

Fig. 12.12 (**a–d**) Close the vagina

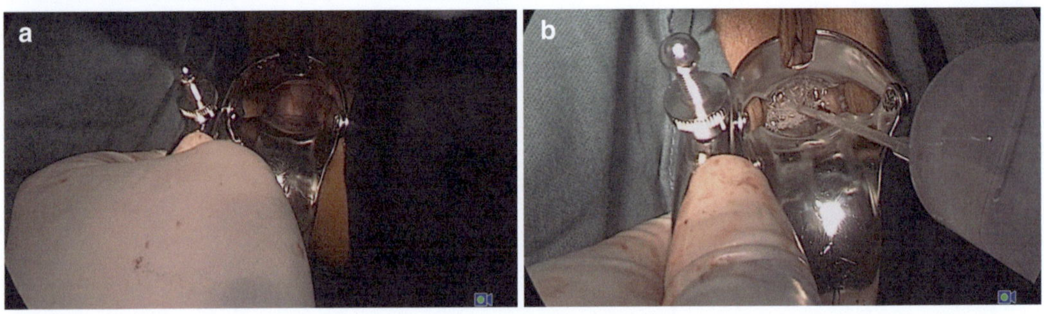

Fig. 12.13 (a, b) Repeatedly irrigate the sealed vagina with sterilized distilled water

12.11 Vaginal Irrigation

After closing the vagina, irrigate the vaginal cavity with 200 ml of sterile distilled water at 42 °C (Fig. 12.13a, b).

Transection of the uterine cervix (Fig. 12.14a–d). Reconstruction of the uterine cervix (Fig. 12.15a, b). Cervical cerclage (Fig. 12.16a, b). Peritonealization of the pelvic peritoneum (Fig. 12.17a, b).

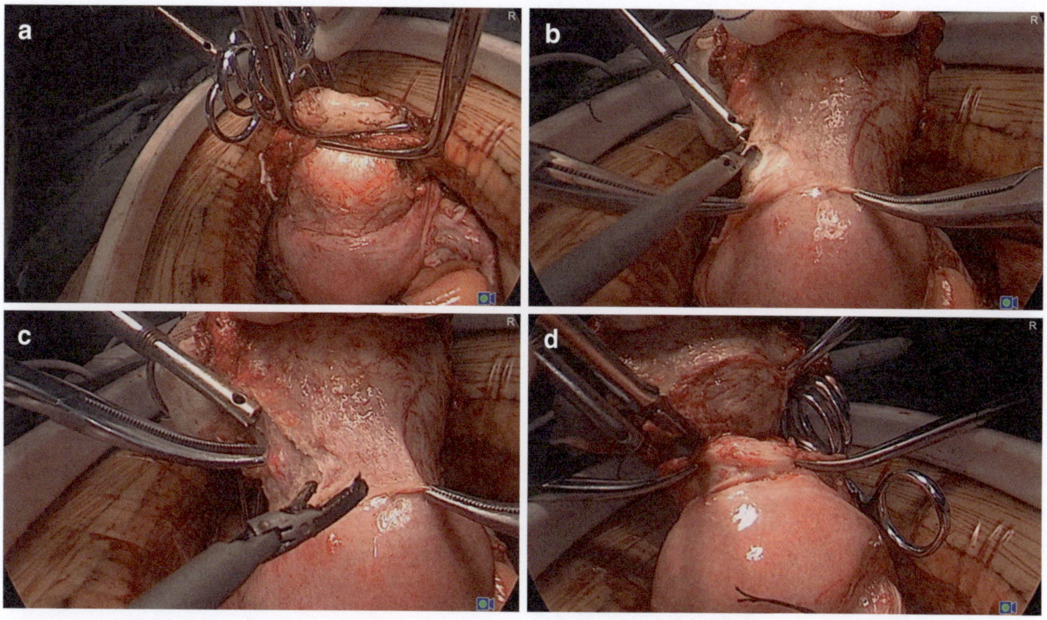

Fig. 12.14 (**a**–**d**) Transect the uterine cervix

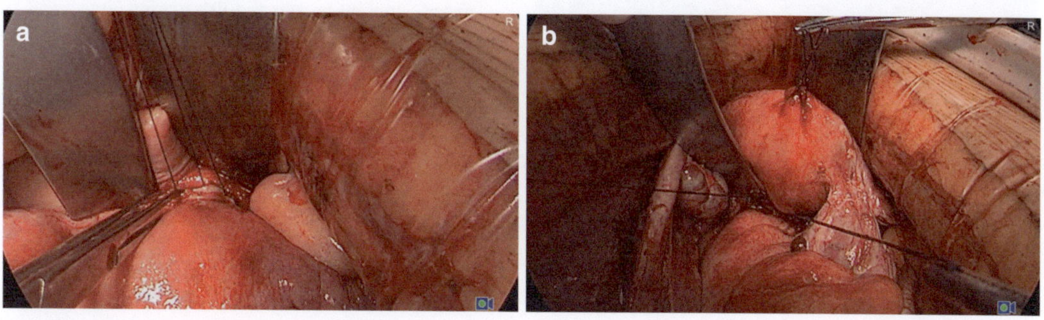

Fig. 12.15 (**a**, **b**) Reconstruct the uterine cervix

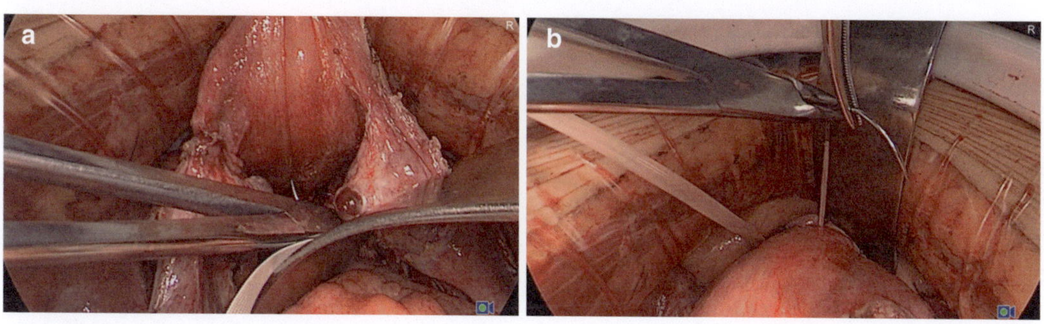

Fig. 12.16 (**a**, **b**) Cervical cerclage

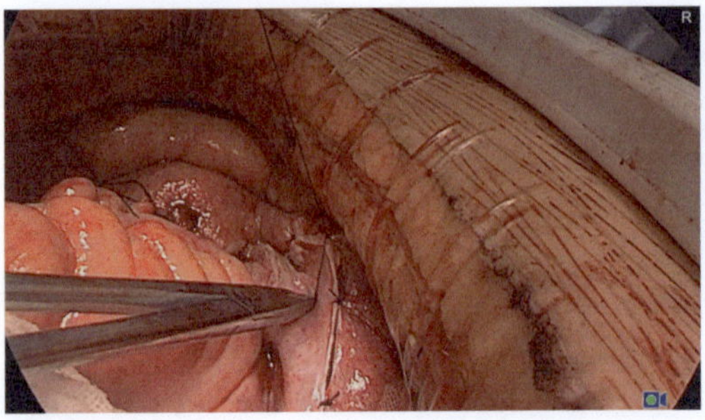

Fig. 12.17 Peritonealization of the pelvic peritoneum

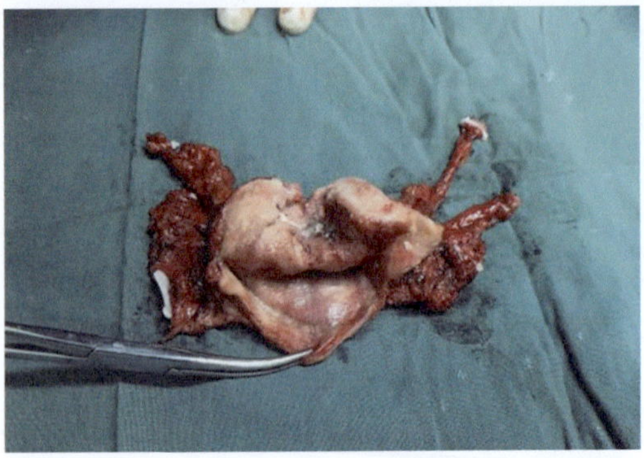

Fig. 12.18 Surgical specimen presentation

12.12 Place an Intrauterine Device for the Cervix

An intrauterine device is placed in the uterine cavity to prevent cervical duct adhesion.

12.13 Specimen Presentation after Fertility-Preserving Radical Trachelectomy

The specimen after fertility-preserving radical trachelectomy is shown in Fig. 12.18. The video of fertility-preserving radical trachelectomy for cervical cancer is available in Video 12.1.

Reference

1. Chinese Anti-Cancer Association Gynecological Tumor Professional Committee. 2022 Chinese expert consensus on fertility-sparing treatment of early-stage cervical cancer. Chin J Pract Gynecol Obstet. 2022;38(6):634–41. https://doi.org/10.19538/j.fk2022060114.

Robot-Assisted Radical Hysterectomy

13

Jun Wang, Shichao Han, Jing Na, Ya Li, and Xinyou Wang

Robot-assisted surgery offers significant advantages in performing cervical cancer surgeries, particularly in QM-C1 type cases (preserving pelvic autonomous nerve function). The main benefits lie in the magnified surgical field, which is enlarged by 10–15 times, allowing for precise and stable surgical maneuvers. Additionally, physiological tremors can be filtered out, enabling surgeons to perform delicate procedures within a highly magnified field. The system allows for accurate dissection of membrane bridges between individual embryonic compartments, precisely revealing the intermembrane spaces between these compartments. This level of precision enhances the visualization of the hypogastric nerves and the pelvic splanchnic nerves, facilitating meticulous nerve dissection. As a result, the concept of membrane dissection is fully realized and executed with utmost precision.

The bedside robotic arm system is introduced from the caudal side and can be accessed through either the right side or the midline approach.

The puncture hole layout is shown in Fig. 13.1.

Camera Arm Puncture Hole Insert a 12 mm Trocar at the midpoint between the umbilicus and the symphysis pubis, approximately 20–25 cm above the symphysis pubis and 2–3 cm to the left.

Robotic Instrument Arm Puncture Hole (Fig. 13.2)

1. Puncture site for Arm 1 (Camera Arm): 10–13 cm to the right of the camera arm puncture site, at a caudal angle of 15°–30°.
2. Puncture site for Arm 2: 8–10 cm to the left of the camera arm puncture site, at a caudal angle of 15°–30°.
3. Puncture site for Arm 3: Right side: 6–8 cm to the left of Arm 1 puncture site, at a caudal angle of 15°–30°. Left side: 6–8 cm to the left of Arm 2 puncture site, at a caudal angle of 15°–30°.

In actual practice, our team has found that positioning the puncture site for Arm 3 on the left side is more conducive to smooth operation, particularly for left-handed surgeons.

Assistant Hole The assistant hole is located on the midpoint line connecting the puncture site for Arm 1 and the camera arm puncture site, at a distance of ≥5 cm in a cephalad direction.

Supplementary Information The online version contains supplementary material available at https://doi.org/10.1007/978-981-97-7687-0_13.

J. Wang (✉) · S. Han · J. Na · Y. Li · X. Wang
Department of Gynecology and Obstetrics, Second Affiliated Hospital of Dalian Medical University, Dalian, China

S. Han, J. Wang (eds.), *Open, Laparoscopic, and Robotic Surgery for Cervical Cancer*, https://doi.org/10.1007/978-981-97-7687-0_13

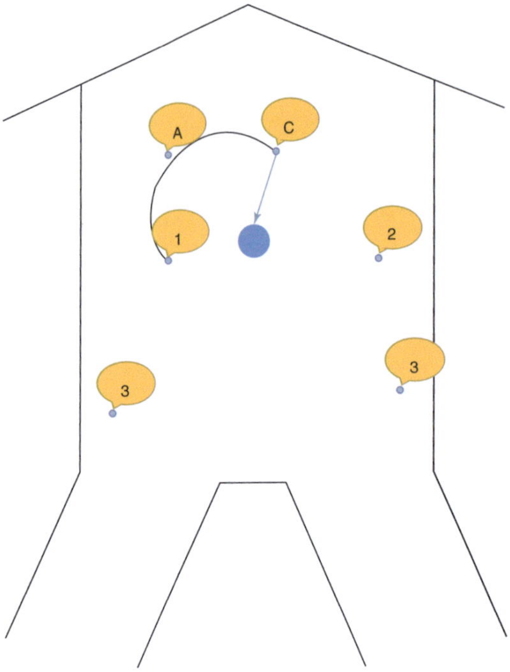

Fig. 13.1 Illustration of robotic-assisted laparoscopic abdominal wall puncture sites

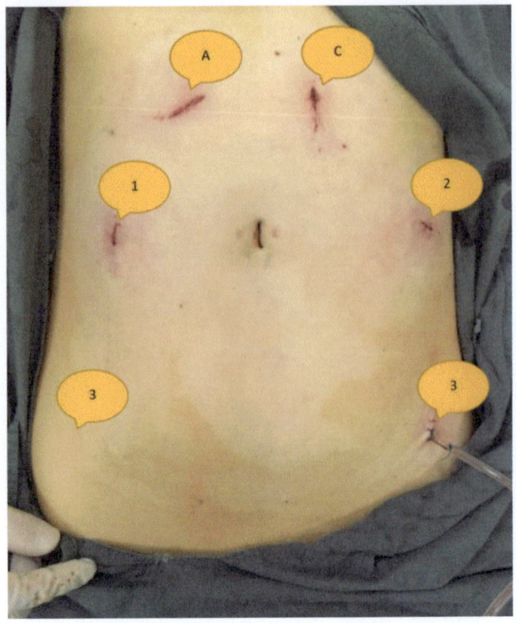

Fig. 13.2 Robotic instrument arm puncture hole

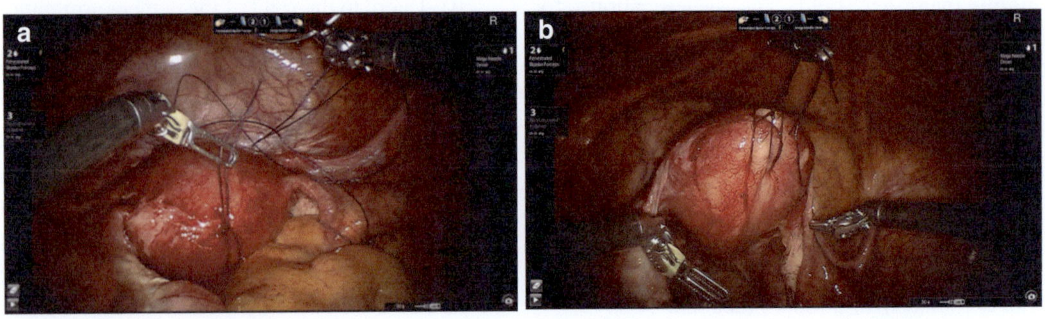

Fig. 13.3 (a, b) Suspend uterus

13.1 Uterine Suspension

The uterine fundus is sutured using 1-0 absorbable sutures. The sutures can be pulled up and suspended using Arm 3 or can be inserted into the abdominal cavity through a 0.5 cm incision placed 2–3 cm above the pubic symphysis, and then pulled up and suspended using a laparoscopic needle holder (Fig. 13.3a, b).

13.2 Opening the Lateral Peritoneum to Expose the Lateral Retroperitoneal Spaces

The uterus is pulled to the opposite side, the round ligament is pulled caudally and ventrally, the ovaries and pelvic infundibular ligaments are pulled medially, and the lateral peritoneum is

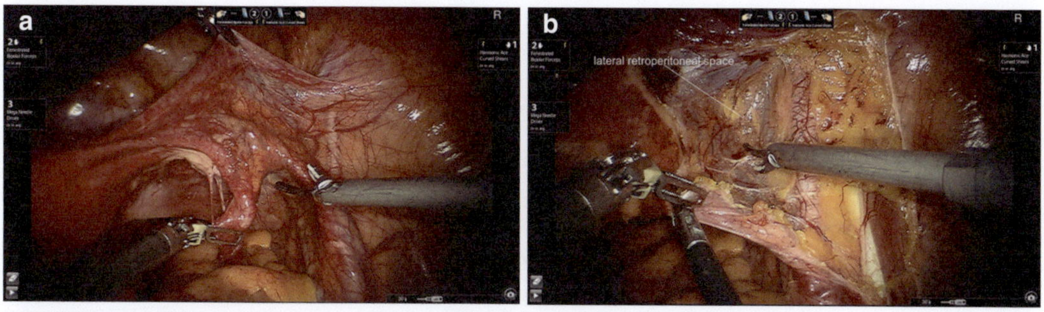

Fig. 13.4 (**a**, **b**) Dissect and expose the lateral retroperitoneal space

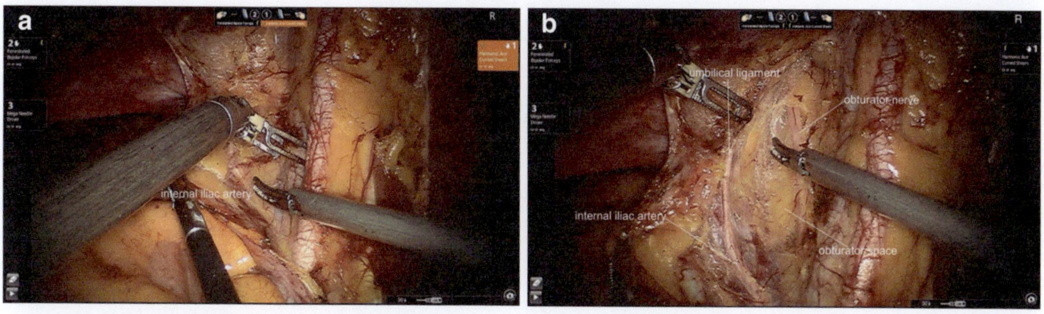

Fig. 13.5 (**a**, **b**) Expose the obturator space

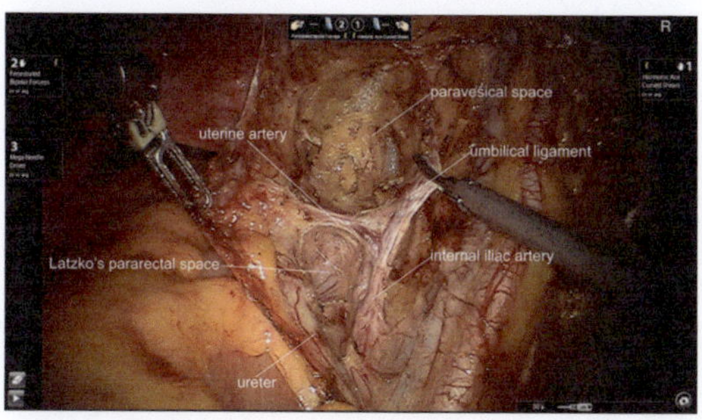

Fig. 13.6 Separate the paravesical space and the Latzko's pararectal space

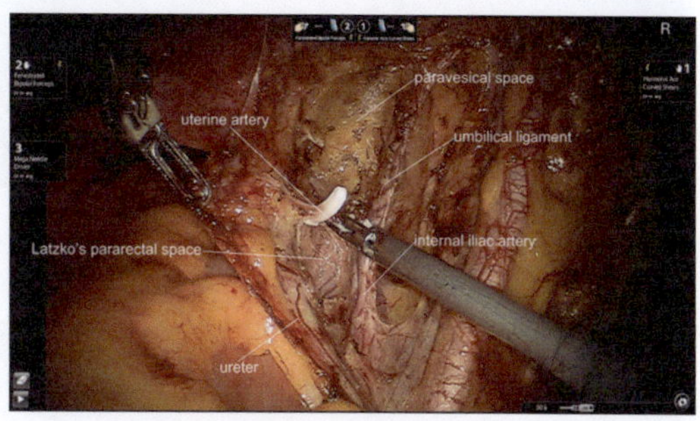

Fig. 13.7 Transect uterine artery

sharply opened to gradually separate and expose the lateral retroperitoneal spaces (Fig. 13.4a, b).

13.3 Exposure and Handling of Lateral Parametrial Structures

Further separation is performed using the lateral retroperitoneal space to meticulously dissect the obturator spaces (Fig. 13.5a, b). The internal iliac artery and the lateral umbilical ligament are pulled laterally, while the lateral peritoneum is pulled medially to separate the Latzko's pararectal space on the cranial side and the paravesical space on the caudal side (Fig. 13.6). Gradually, the blood vessels within both spaces of the lateral parametrium are clamped and transected (Figs. 13.7 and 13.8a–e), thereby completing the treatment of the lateral parametrial structures. During the nerve-sparing QM-C1 type surgery, this step also allows for simultaneous dissection of the Okabayashi's pararectal spaces, exposing the hypogastric nerve plexus, which lays the foundation for subsequent procedures aimed at preserving pelvic autonomous nerve function (Fig. 13.9a–c).

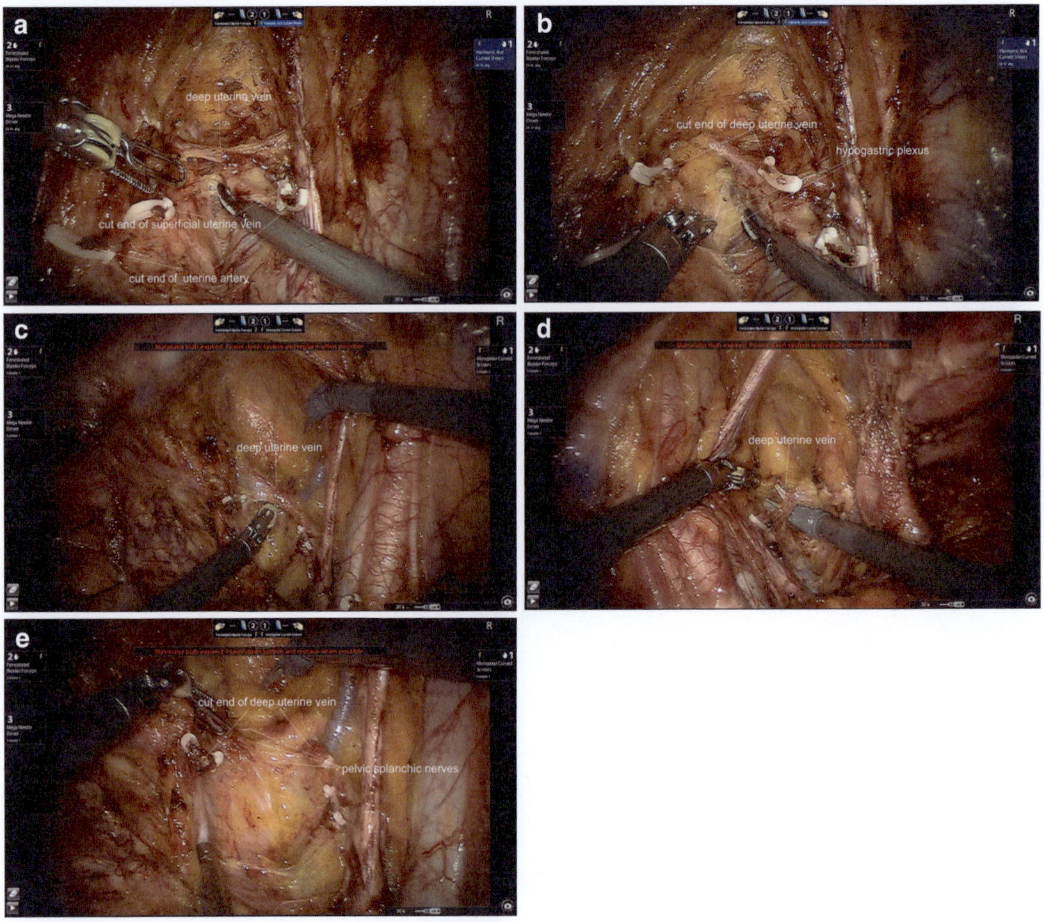

Fig. 13.8 (**a**–**f**) Separate and transect the deep uterine vein

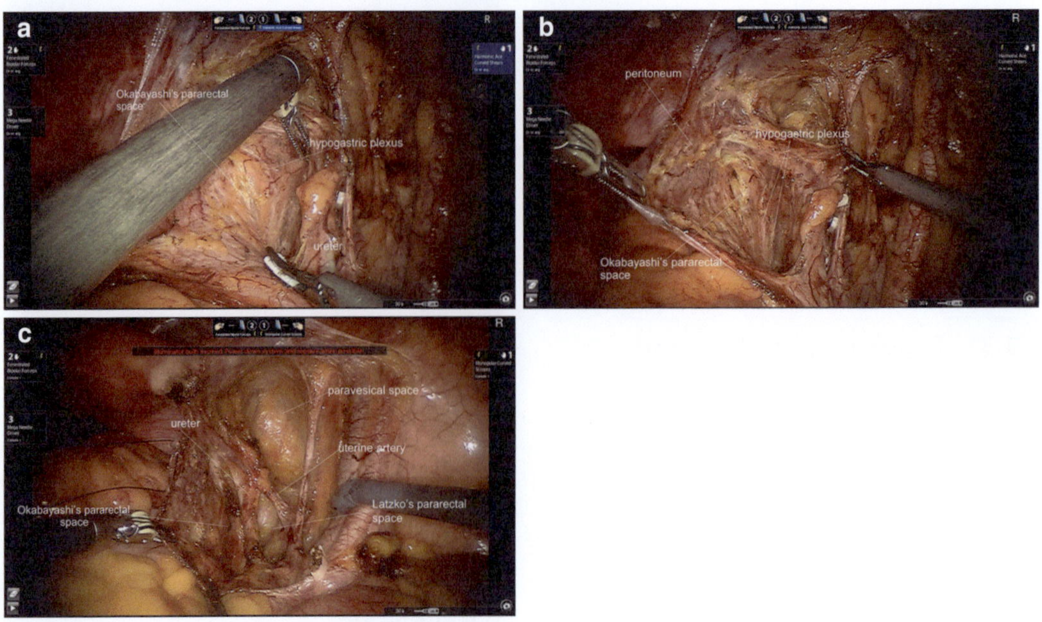

Fig. 13.9 (**a**–**c**) Expose Okabayashi's pararectal space

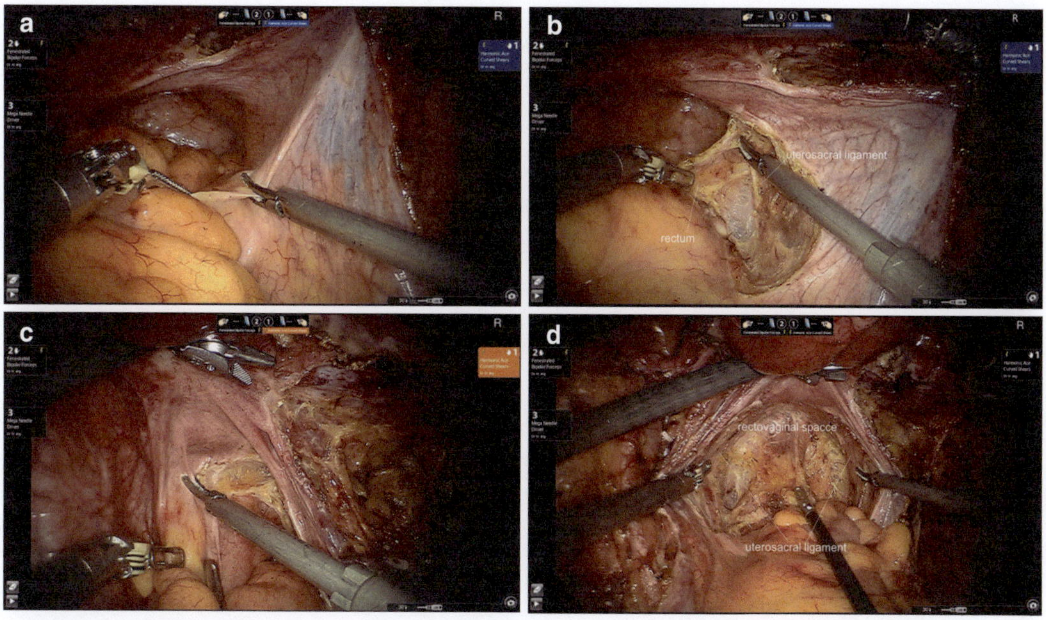

Fig. 13.10 (**a–d**) Expose the rectal peritoneum reflection and the uterosacral ligament

13.4 Exposure of the Rectovaginal Space and Sacrouterine Ligament

This process can maximize the demonstration of the essential principles of robotic surgery in membrane dissection, exposing the rectovaginal space and sacrouteral ligament, which separates the Müllerian duct embryonic compartment from the hindgut embryonic compartment.

Firstly, we need to open the peritoneal reflection of the rectum. The precise selection of the location is indeed challenging to achieve directly in one step. However, with the high magnification of the robotic system, we can clearly visualize the connection between the two embryonic compartments, known as the membrane bridge. By opening the membrane bridge, we can smoothly access the space between the two embryonic compartments. In order to better visualize the space between the two embryonic compartments, we apply appropriate countertraction to these units. By doing so, we can clearly observe that the two embryonic compartments are distinct from each other. In the Müllerian duct embryonic compartment, the vaginal wall appears reddish and smooth without any attached adipose tissue, while in the hindgut embryonic compartment, the rectum is surrounded by adipose mesentery and presents a yellowish appearance. Between the two compartments, there is a white, loose, and filamentous structure. By sharply dissecting this loose structure, we can separate the two embryonic compartments and fully and safely expose the posterior wall of the vagina, anterior wall of the rectum, inner side of the sacrouteral ligament, and the mesentery of the rectum (see Figs. 13.9a–c and 13.10a–d).

13.5 Exposure of the Vesicocervical and Vesicovaginal Spaces

This process also involves the separation of embryonic compartments, dissecting the upper part of the urogenital sinus embryonic compartment, which includes the bladder, from the Müllerian duct embryonic compartment, consisting of the cervix and vagina. This achieves the exposure of the vesicocervical space and the vesicovaginal space (Fig. 13.11a, b).

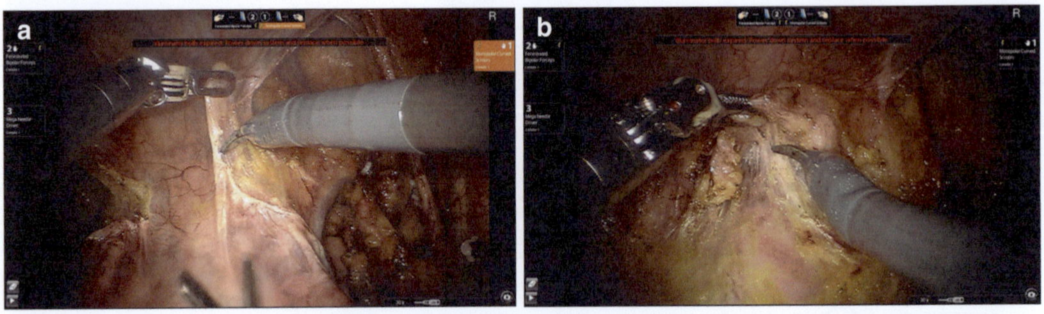

Fig. 13.11 (**a**, **b**) Expose the vesicocervical and vesicovaginal space

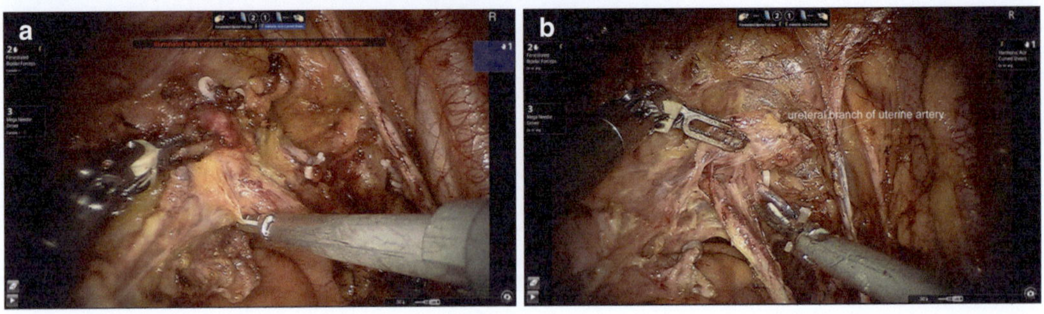

Fig. 13.12 (**a**, **b**) Dissect the uterine artery and ureter

13.6 Dissection of the Uterine Artery and Ureter

Mobilize the uterine artery and ureter (Fig. 13.12a, b).

13.7 Exposure of the Fourth Space and Paravaginal Space and Management of the Vesicocervical and Vesicovaginal Ligaments

The exposure of the fourth space involves separating the ureter from the ureteric bud embryonic compartment, the upper part of the urogenital sinus embryonic compartment (bladder), and the Müllerian duct embryonic compartment. Similarly, the first step is to identify the membrane bridge at the connection point of these embryonic compartments. During the process of widening the paravesical space laterally, dense tissues may be encountered, making it challenging to further expand the fourth space. This dense tissue represents the membrane bridge at the connection point of the embryonic compartments.

By fully lifting the bladder ventrally and pushing the uterus dorsally, the ultrasonic scalpel is used to slowly and gradually open the membrane bridge. Initially, the "tunnel" segment of the ureter is exposed, along with the ureter and bladder, which are pulled ventrally. Continuing the dissection between the posterior wall of the bladder and the paracolpium reveals the paravaginal space (Fig. 13.13a–c). The exposure of this space is crucial in C1-type surgeries as it is the key to handling the vesicovaginal ligaments (Fig. 13.14a–c). Additionally, it plays a vital role in the QM-C1 procedure for skeletonizing the superior vesical veins and exposing the pelvic plexus.

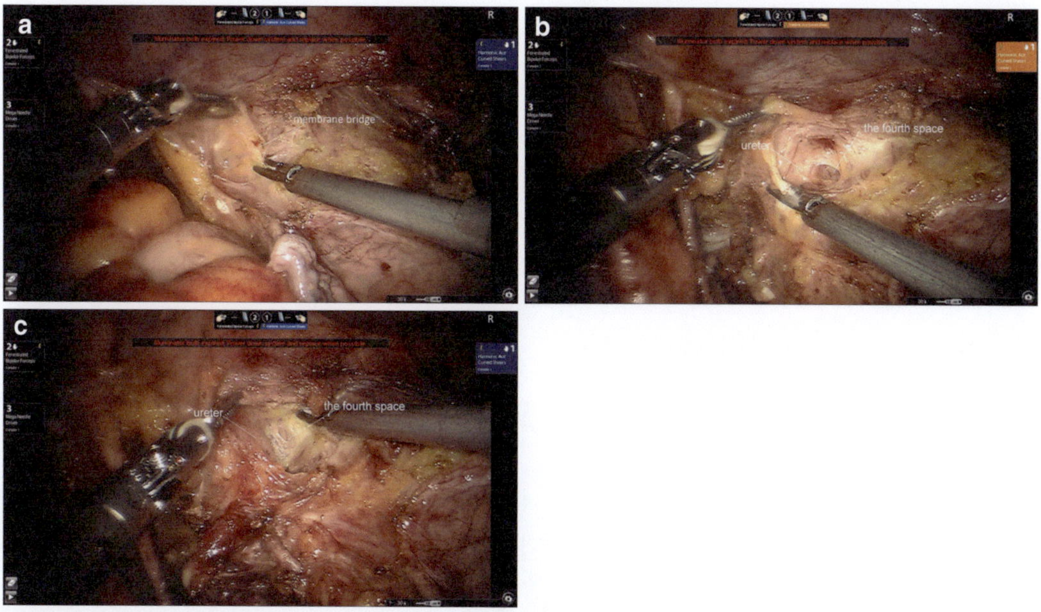

Fig. 13.13 (**a**–**c**) Separate the fourth space

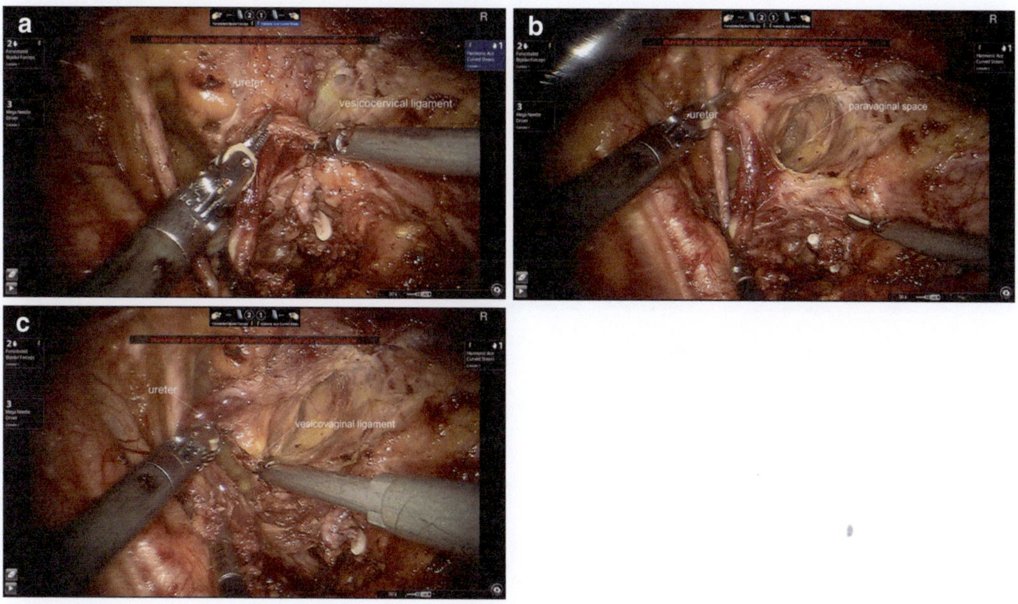

Fig. 13.14 (**a**–**c**) Transect vesicocervical ligament and vesicovaginal ligament

13.8 Exposure and Transection of the Paracolpium

After transecting the vesicovaginal ligament, the posterior bladder wall can be pulled medially and laterally to expose the space between the bladder and the paracolpium. Sharp dissection is then performed (Figs. 13.15 and 13.16).

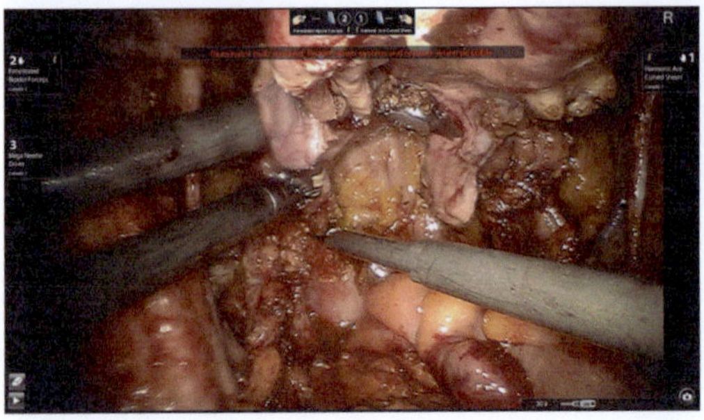

Fig. 13.15 Transect sacrospinous ligament

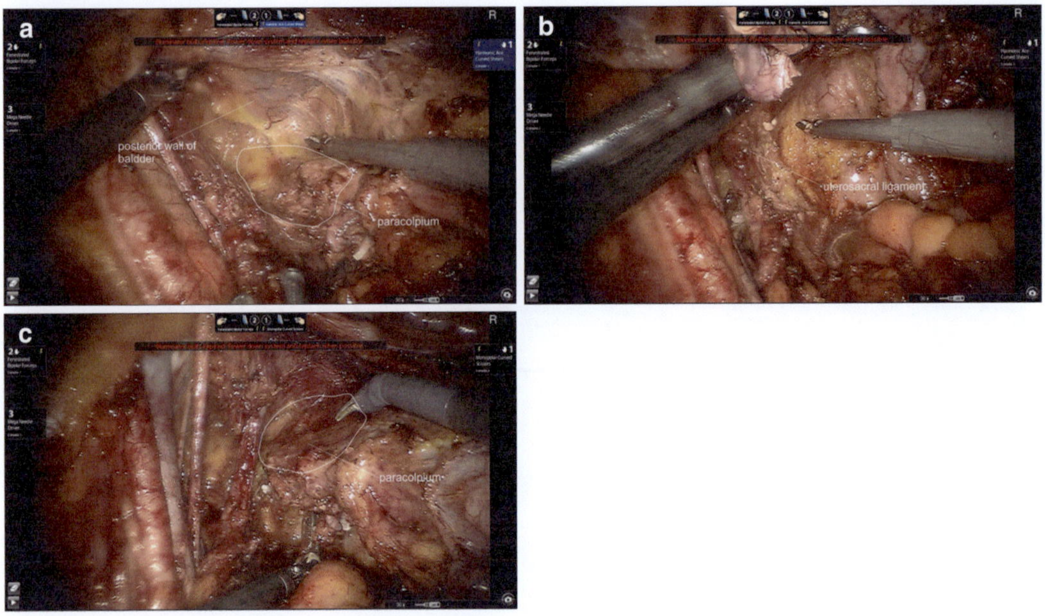

Fig. 13.16 (**a**–**c**) Expose and transect the paracolpium

13.9 Exposure of the "Crossing-Shaped IHP" in QM-C1 Procedure

Pull the uterine side of the deep uterine veins medially and the ureter laterally to fully expose the nerve junction area and its superficial fat tissue. At this point, use a push, peel, and suction technique to remove the superficial fat tissue from the nerve surface, revealing the classic "cross" structure (Fig. 13.17).

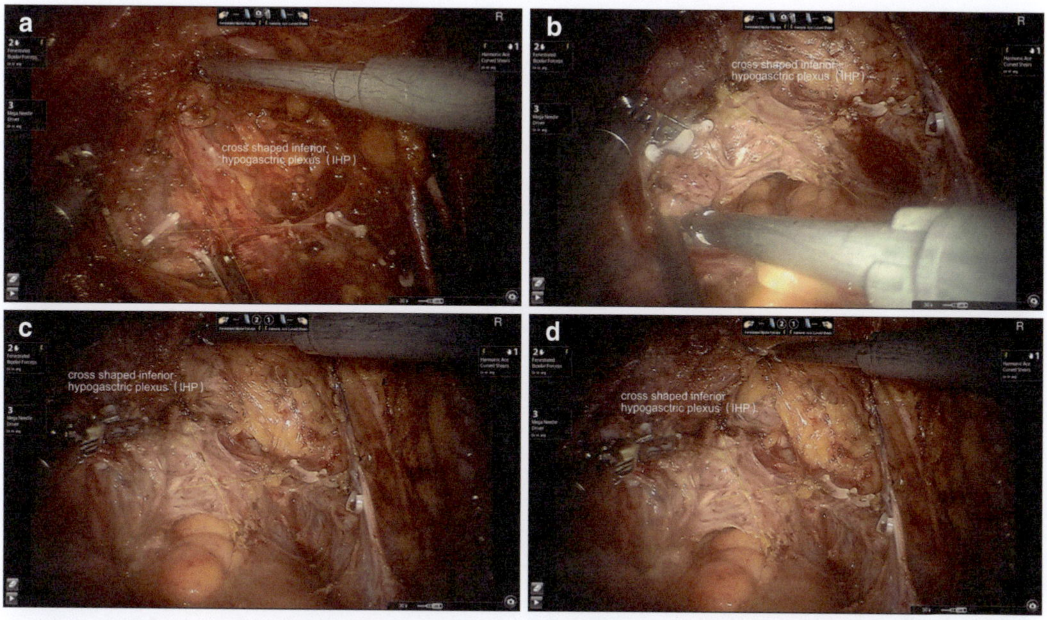

Fig. 13.17 (**a**–**d**) Expose the "Crossing-shaped IHP" in QM-C1 procedure

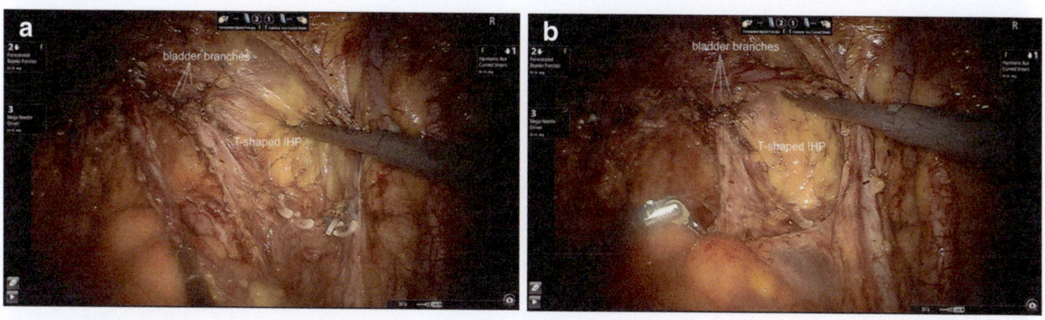

Fig. 13.18 (**a**, **b**) Expose the "T-shaped IHP" in QM-C1 procedure

13.10 Exposure of the "T-Shaped IHP" in QM-C1 Procedure

In the QM-C1 procedure, it is necessary to resect the cervix branches, uterus branches, and rectum branches of the inferior hypogastric plexus (IHP), while preserving the vesical branches, resulting in the formation of a "T-shaped anastomosis" (Fig. 13.18).

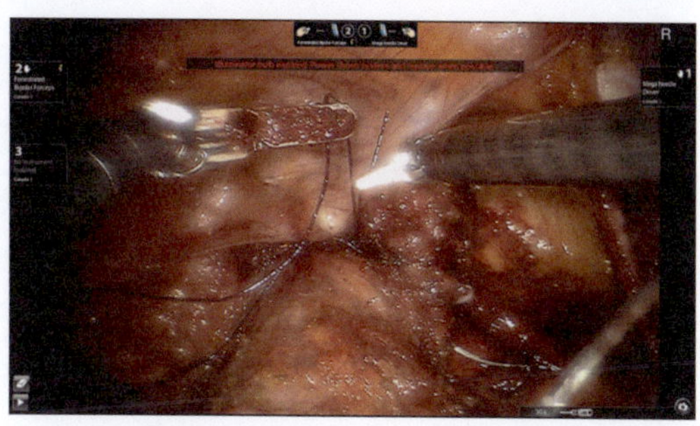

Fig. 13.19 Close the vagina

13.11 Closure of the Vagina

The vaginal cuff is closed using absorbable suture (Fig. 13.19).

13.12 Sterile Distilled Water Irrigation of Closed Vagina

Flushing the closed vagina with sterile distilled water (Fig. 13.20).

13.13 Cervical Resection, Vaginal Suturing, and Sterile Distilled Water Irrigation of the Pelvic Cavity

Suture the vaginal stump (Fig. 13.21).

Robot-assisted QM-C1, QM-C2 (Robot 1), and QM-C2 (Robot 2) radical hysterectomy procedures are demonstrated in Videos 13.1, 13.2, and 13.3, respectively.

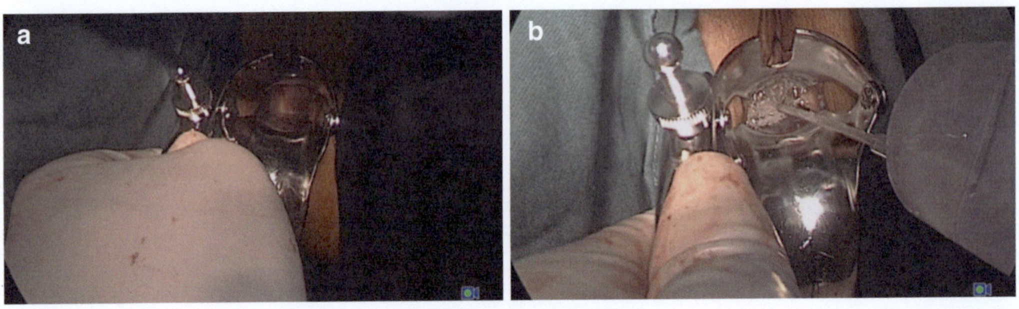

Fig. 13.20 (**a**, **b**) Repeatedly irrigate the sealed vagina with sterilized distilled water

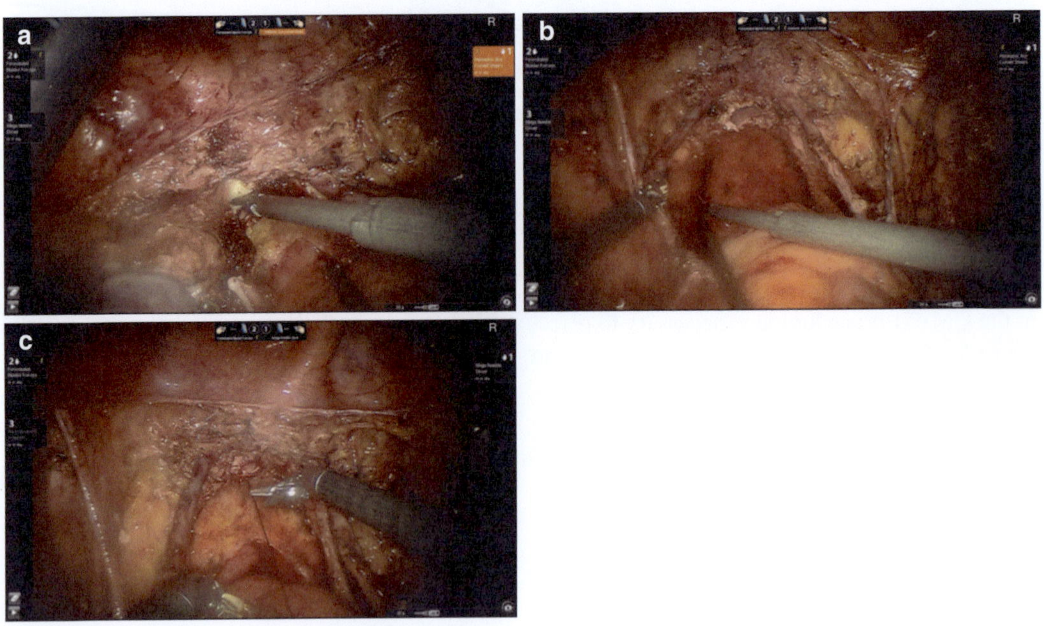

Fig. 13.21 (**a**–**c**) Suture the vaginal stump

Part III

Lymphadenectomy for Cervical Cancer

Pelvic Lymphadenectomy

14

Jun Wang and Jing Na

Cervical cancer lymphadenectomy procedure encompasses pelvic lymphadenectomy and, when indicated, low para-aortic lymphadenectomy. The pelvic lymphadenectomy encompasses comprehensive systematic lymph node dissection, sentinel lymph node biopsy, and sentinel lymph node mapping excision. The systematic pelvic lymphadenectomy procedure adheres rigorously to the cervical cancer lymphadenectomy extent as defined by the Cibula Type III classification, as executed by the author's team. Pelvic lymphadenectomy encompasses several aspects: the cranial aspect reveals the bifurcation of the common iliac vessels, the caudal aspect exposes the deep circumflex iliac vein, the dorsal aspect reveals the lymph nodes beneath the obturator nerve and pelvic floor fascia, and the lateral aspect reveals the lumbosacral trunk [1, 2]. In accordance with the findings from the LACC trial and the consensus of Chinese experts [3, 4], our team exclusively conducted minimally invasive surgery on patients with a clinical stage of ≤IB1, and preoperative imaging assessment showed no clinically positive lymph nodes. Conversely, the open surgery group encompassed patients with cervical cancer up to stage ≤IIA1. For patients exhibiting tumor diameter >2 cm, special pathological types, or intraoperative incidental detection of positive pelvic lymph nodes, routine para-aortic lymphadenectomy was performed.

Lymphadenectomy, as a standard procedure for gynecologic malignancies, is performed by surgeons with their own extensive experience. Our team follows a practice of regionalized resection when conducting lymphadenectomy procedures.

14.1 Common Iliac Lymph Node Dissection

14.1.1 Right Common Iliac Lymph Node Dissection

With the intestines positioned upward in the abdominal cavity, a precise incision is made along the surface of the right common iliac artery to access the retroperitoneum (Fig. 14.1a–e). This maneuver exposes the entire extent of the right common iliac artery, extending cranially to the bifurcation of the abdominal aorta and caudally to the bifurcation of the internal and external iliac arteries. By gently retracting and separating the lateral peritoneum on both sides, the regional lymph nodes of the right common iliac region are meticulously unveiled. Employing an ultrasonic scalpel, the space between the lateral peritoneum

Supplementary Information The online version contains supplementary material available at https://doi.org/10.1007/978-981-97-7687-0_14.

J. Wang (✉) · J. Na
Department of Gynecology and Obstetrics, Second Affiliated Hospital of Dalian Medical University, Dalian, China

S. Han, J. Wang (eds.), *Open, Laparoscopic, and Robotic Surgery for Cervical Cancer*, https://doi.org/10.1007/978-981-97-7687-0_14

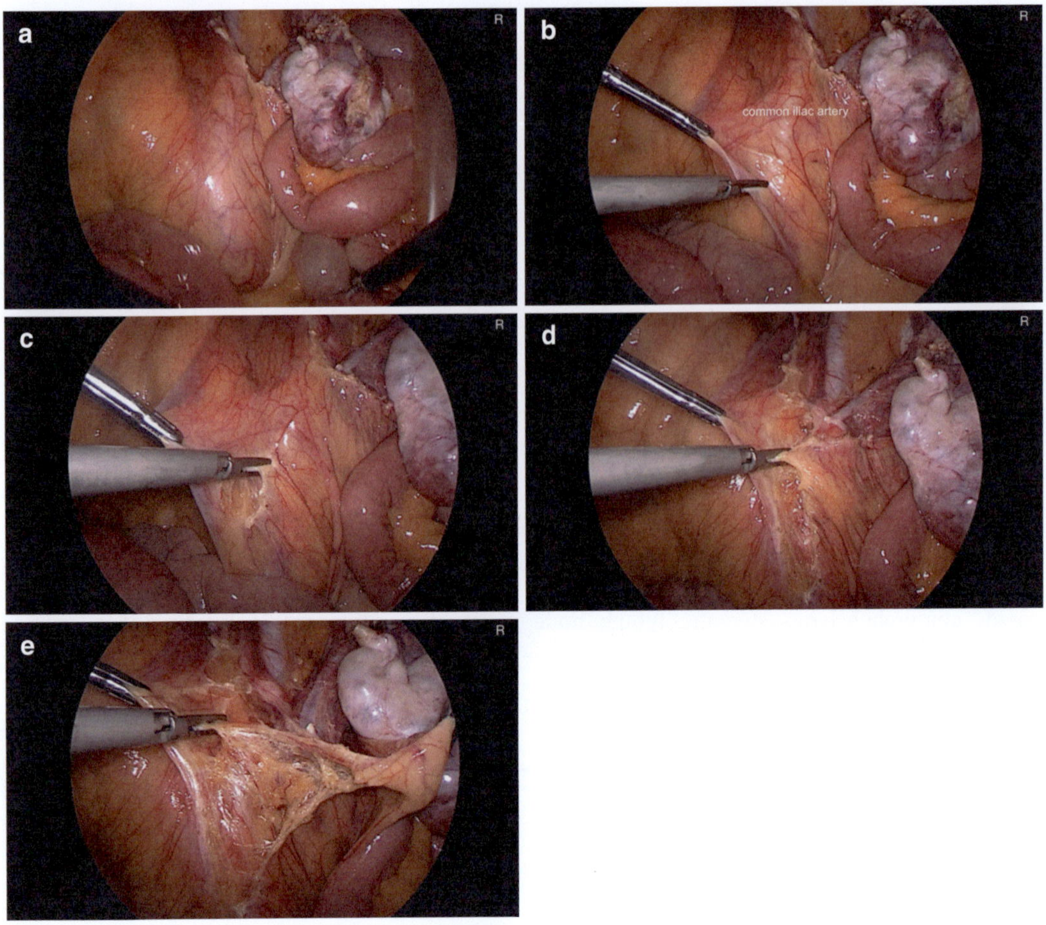

Fig. 14.1 (**a**–**e**) Along the surface of the right common iliac artery to access the retroperitoneum

and the right common iliac lymph nodes is intricately dissected. Medial dissection reveals the presence of the superior hypogastric nerves, while lateral dissection provides visibility of the right common iliac vein and the adjacent right ureter (Figs. 14.2a–e, 14.3a–d, and 14.4a–d). Using the ultrasonic scalpel, the lymph nodes are carefully dissected from the surface of the right common iliac artery, with sharp separation directed laterally. At this stage, it is crucial to meticulously identify the superior hypogastric nerves to avoid any inadvertent damage. Gradually, the space between the right common iliac artery and the right common iliac vein becomes distinctly visible (Fig. 14.5a–d). Proceeding with the dissection laterally, the right common iliac vein is further revealed (Fig. 14.6a–f). If during the separation process, enlarged lymph nodes are observed extending cranially along the surface of the right common iliac artery or vein, it is essential to completely excise these enlarged lymph nodes. Once the right common iliac vein is exposed, the lymph nodes along its surface are gradually excised from the cranial to the caudal direction. Careful attention is required when excising lymph nodes from the surface of the right common iliac vein, as there are usually 1 to 3 venous branches flowing into the vein from the lymph nodes. These branches should be delicately dissected and carefully cut using the ultrasonic scalpel (Fig. 14.7a–j). Proceed with the gradual excision of the right common iliac lymph nodes toward the bifurcation of the internal and external iliac vessels.

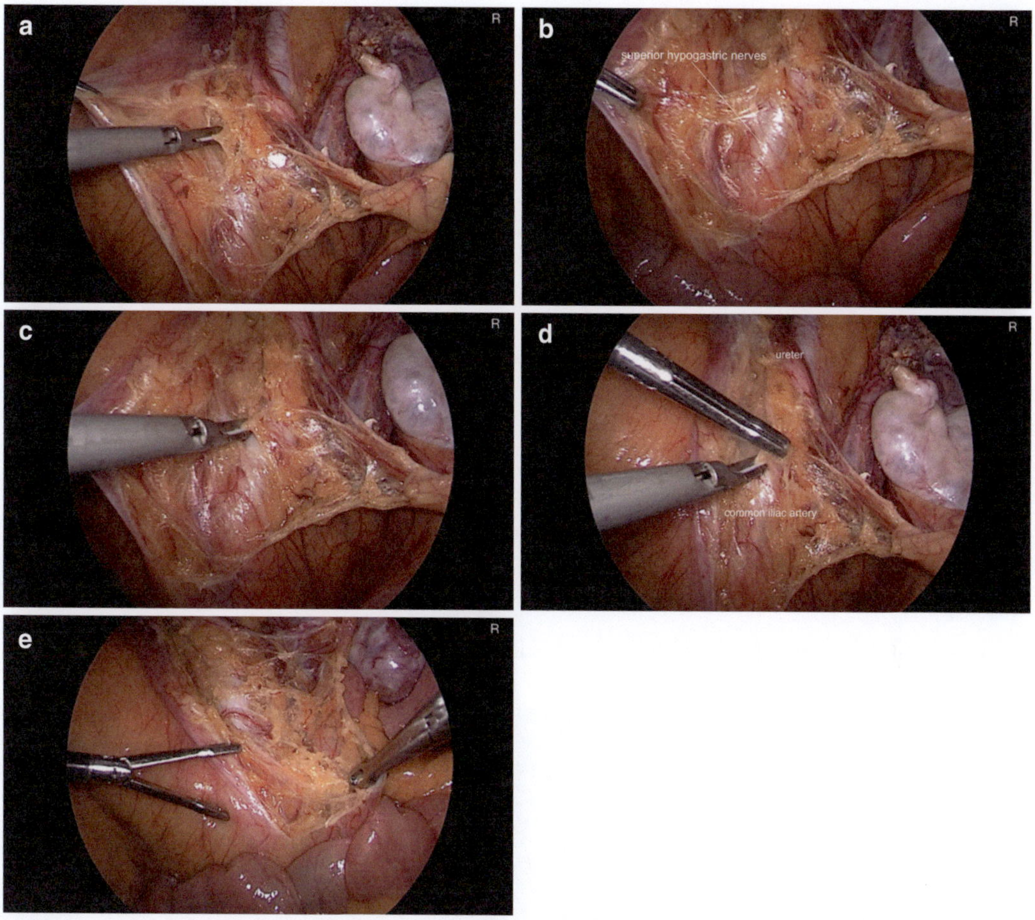

Fig. 14.2 (a–e) Open the space between the lateral peritoneum and the right common iliac lymph nodes

14.1.2 Left Common Iliac Lymph Node Dissection

Gently pulling the opened retroperitoneum of the right common iliac artery toward the ventral and lateral aspects, use the ultrasonic scalpel to meticulously separate and expose the lymph nodes in the region of the left common iliac artery and vein (Figs. 14.8, 14.9, and 14.10).

Surgical Techniques and Precautions During the exposure process, it is essential to adequately pull the peritoneum ventrally and laterally with sufficient tension to reveal the lymphatic region and the gap between the peritoneum and the intestines or ureters. In the exposure process, suspending and pulling the left peritoneum with absorbable sutures can be considered, allowing the surgeon to free their left hand instrument and facilitate field visualization (Fig. 14.10a, b).

Separate the relationship between the right common iliac artery and the lymph nodes (Fig. 14.11a, b).

Separate the relationship between the left common iliac artery and the lymph nodes (Fig. 14.12a–f).

Expose the left common iliac vein (Fig. 14.13a–h).

Separate lymph nodes along the surface of the left common iliac vein (Fig. 14.14a–d).

Expose the midline sacral vein and remove the left common iliac vein lymph nodes (Figs. 14.15, 14.16, and Fig. 14.17)

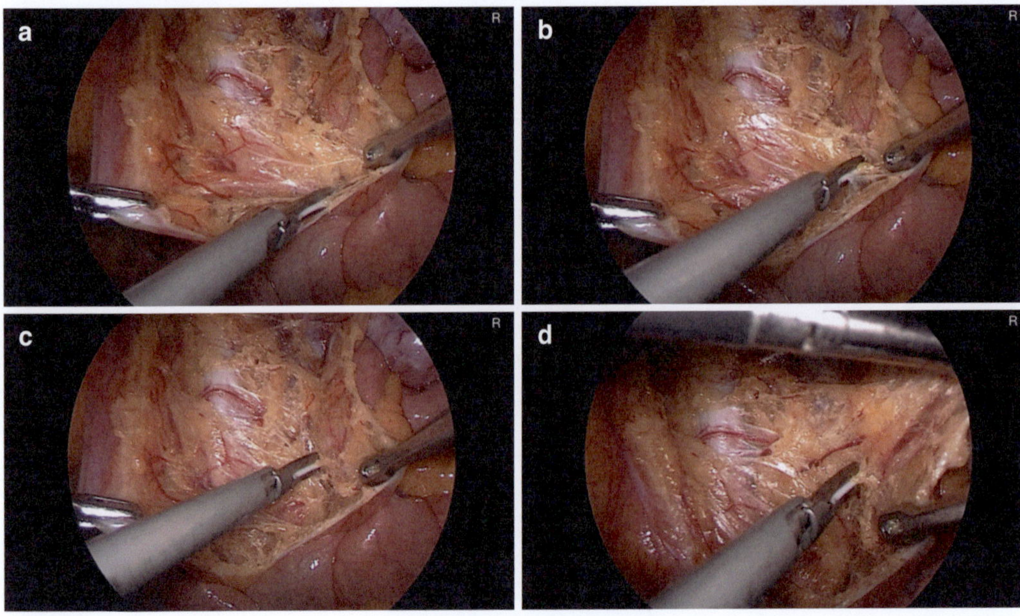

Fig. 14.3 (**a**–**d**) Dissect the space between the lateral peritoneum and the right common iliac lymph nodes

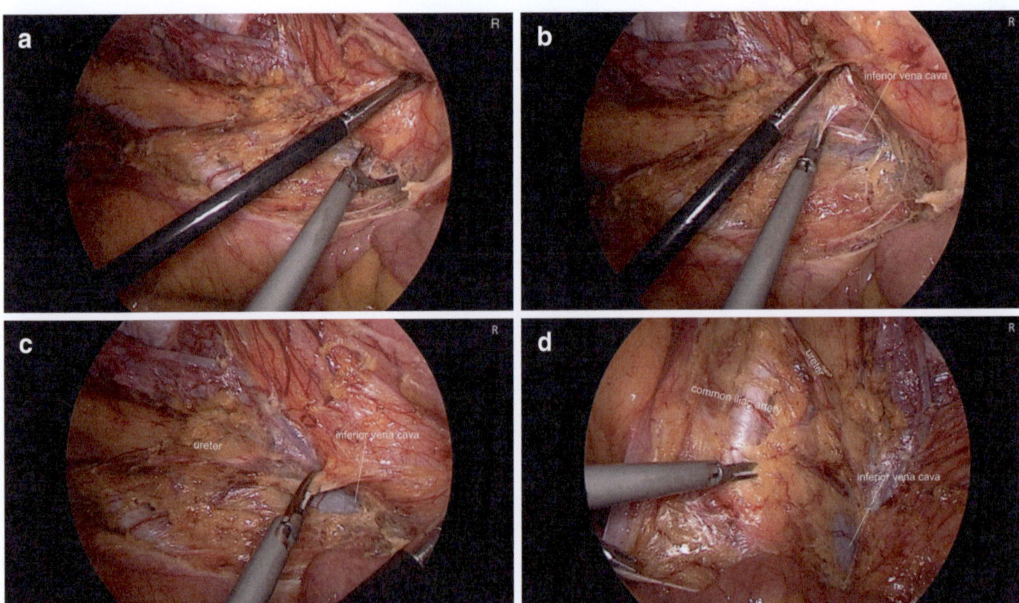

Fig. 14.4 (**a**–**d**) Expose the right common iliac lymph nodes

Expose and remove the lymph nodes on the outer side of the left common iliac artery (Figs. 14.18, 14.19, 14.20, and 14.21).

Ureter, lumbar sympathetic nerves, lumbar artery, lumbar vein.

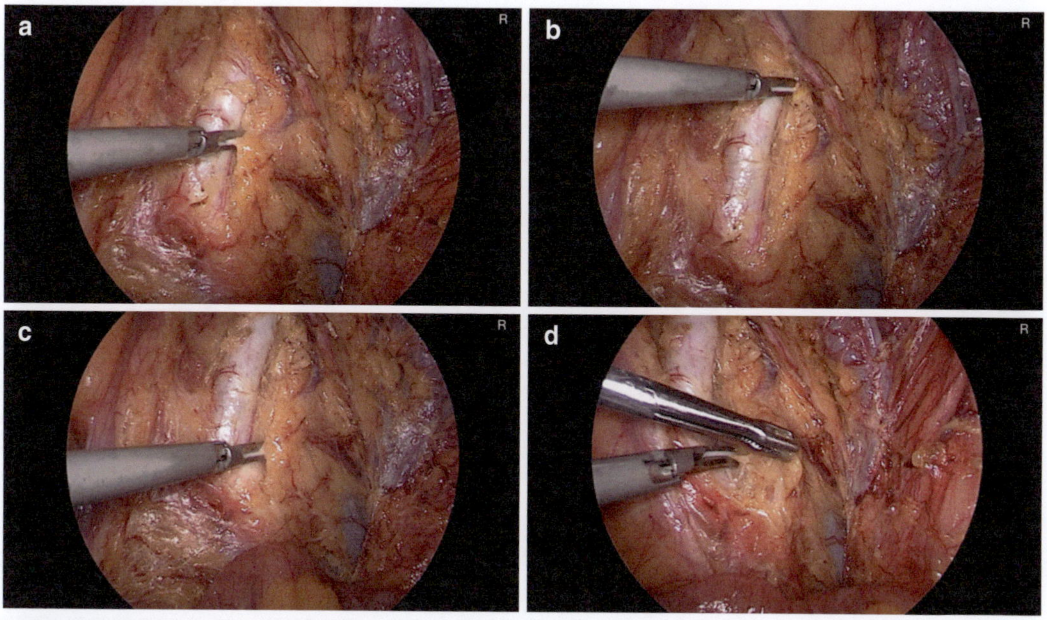

Fig. 14.5 (**a**–**d**) Expose the space between the right common iliac artery and the right common iliac vein

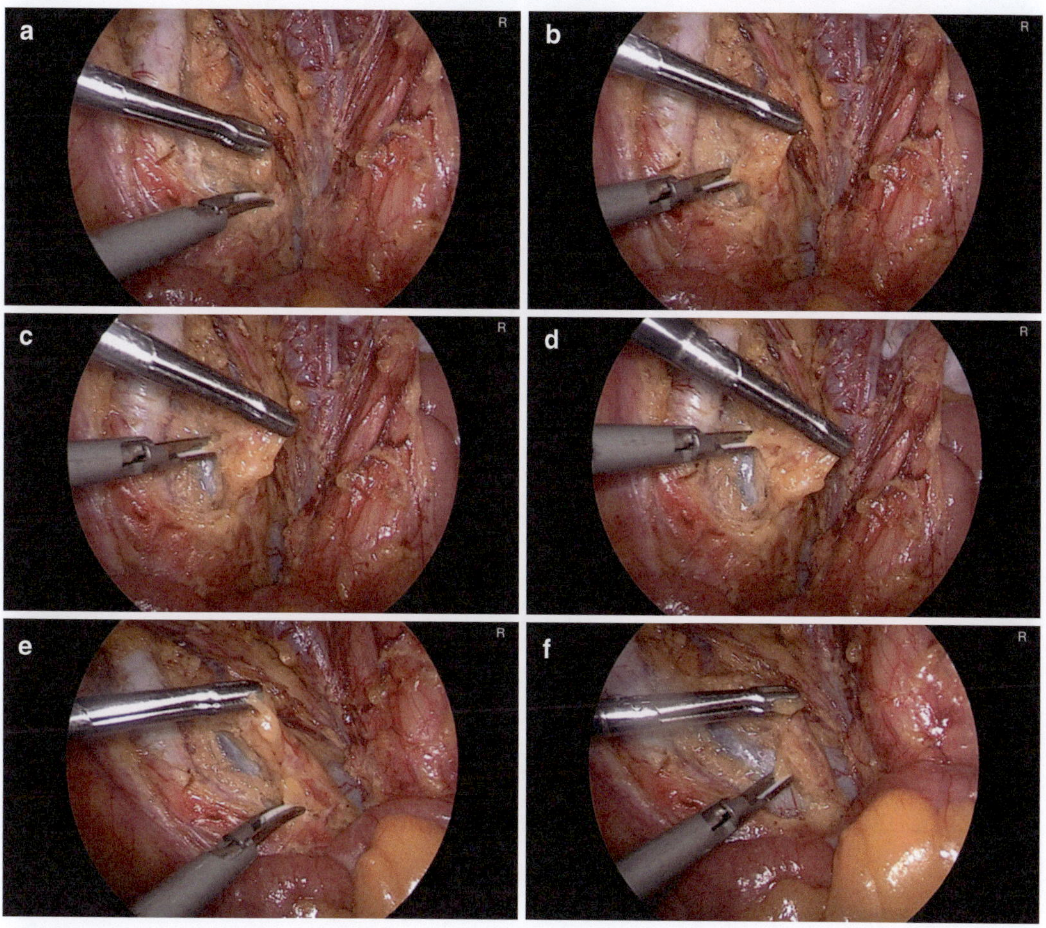

Fig. 14.6 (**a**–**f**) Expose the right common iliac vein

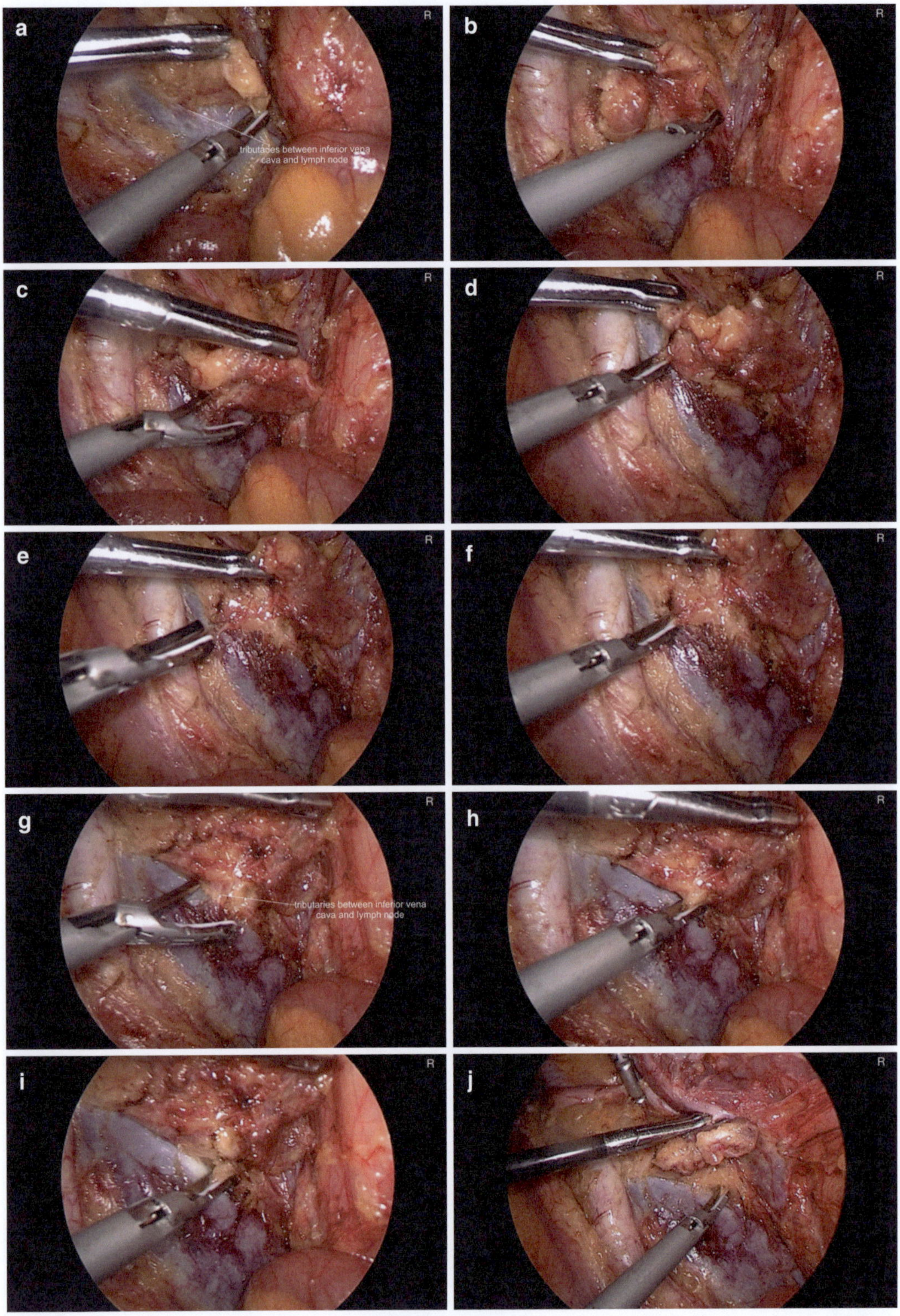

Fig. 14.7 (**a–j**) Delicately dissected and carefully separate the right common iliac vein and cut its branches

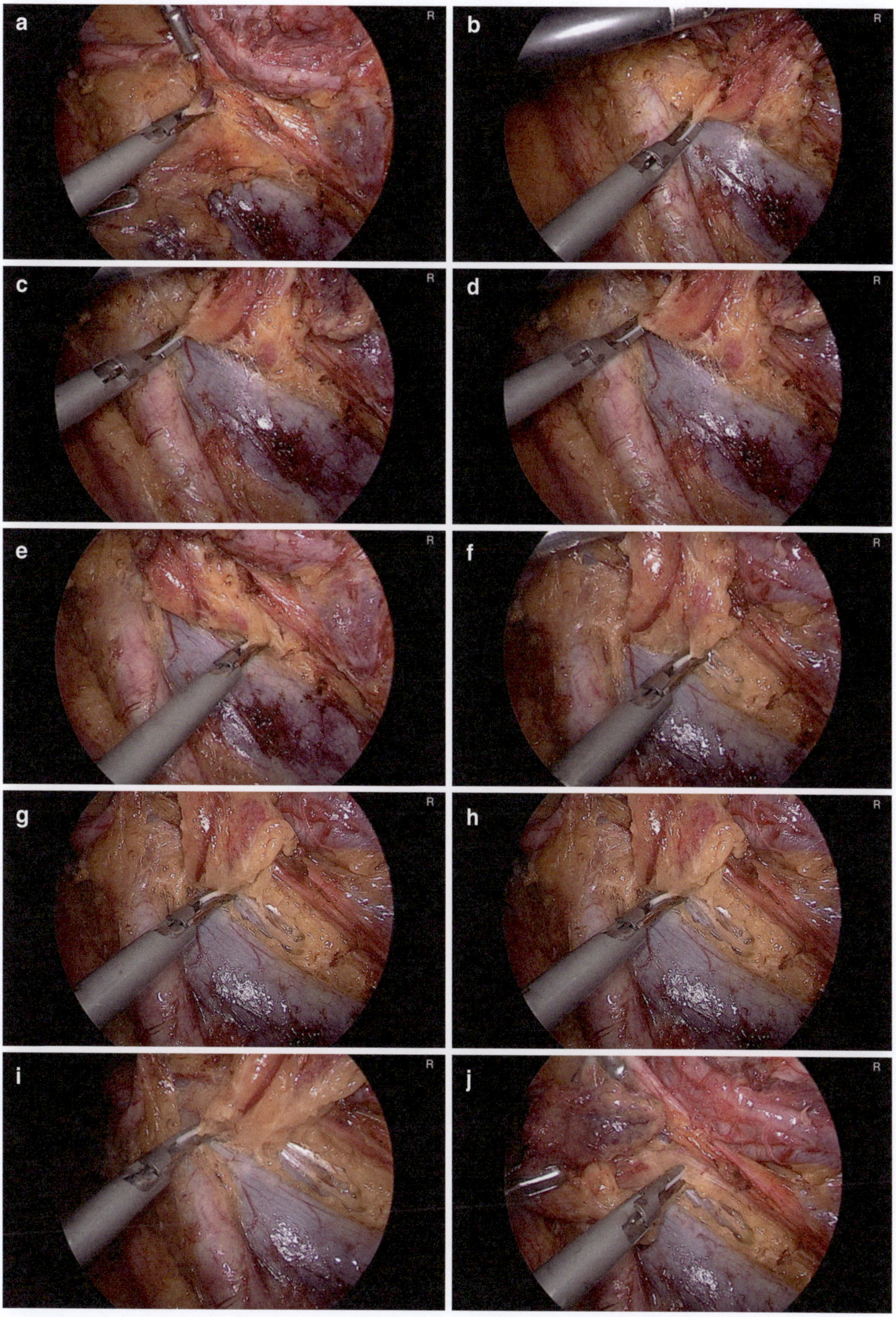

Fig. 14.8 (a–j) Transect right common iliac lymph node caudally to the bifurcation of the internal and external iliac vessels

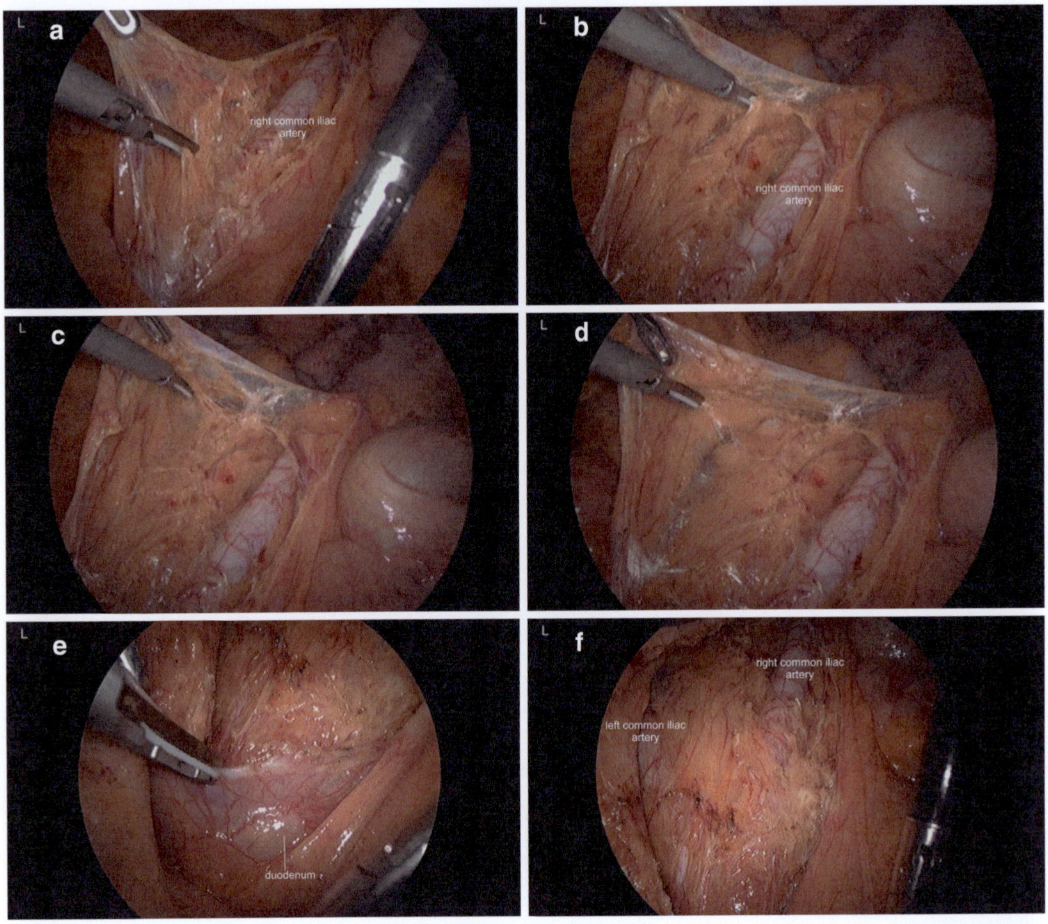

Fig. 14.9 (**a**–**f**) Separate and expose the lymph nodes in the region of the left common iliac artery and vein

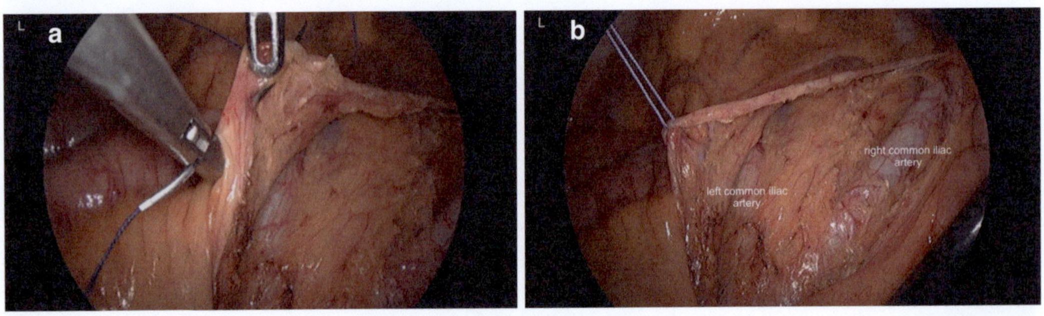

Fig. 14.10 (**a**, **b**) Suspend and pull the lateral peritoneum

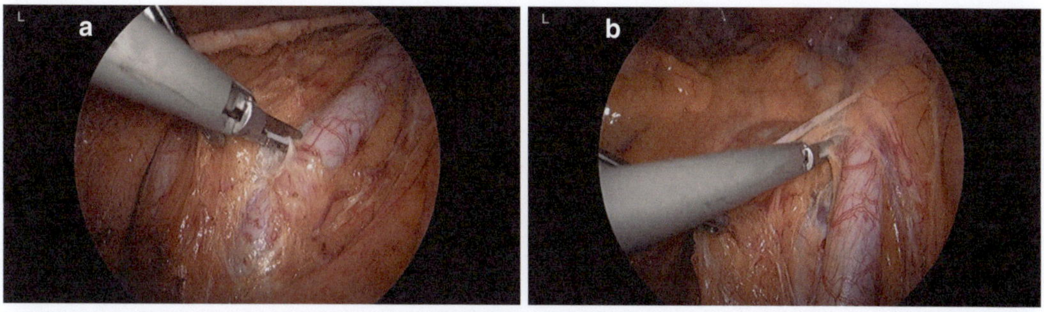

Fig. 14.11 (**a**, **b**) Separate the relationship between the right common iliac artery and the lymph nodes

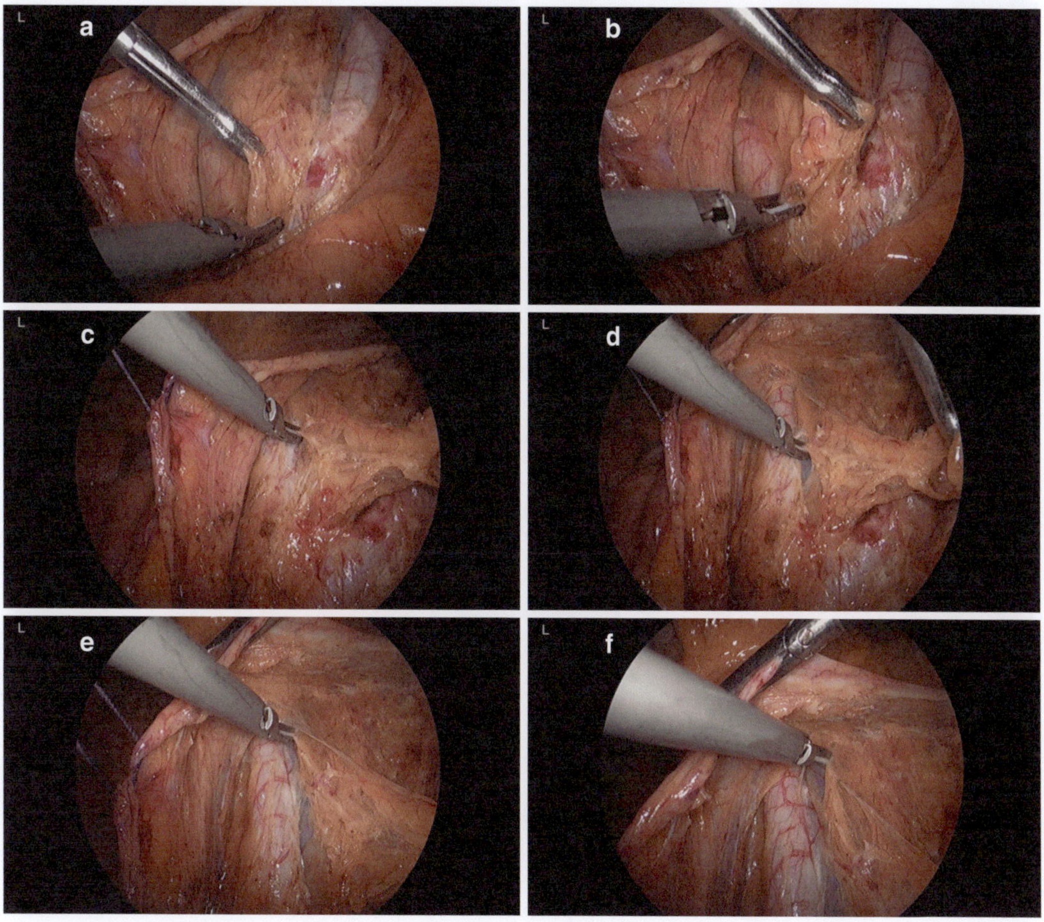

Fig. 14.12 (**a**–**f**) Separate the relationship between the left common iliac artery and the lymph nodes

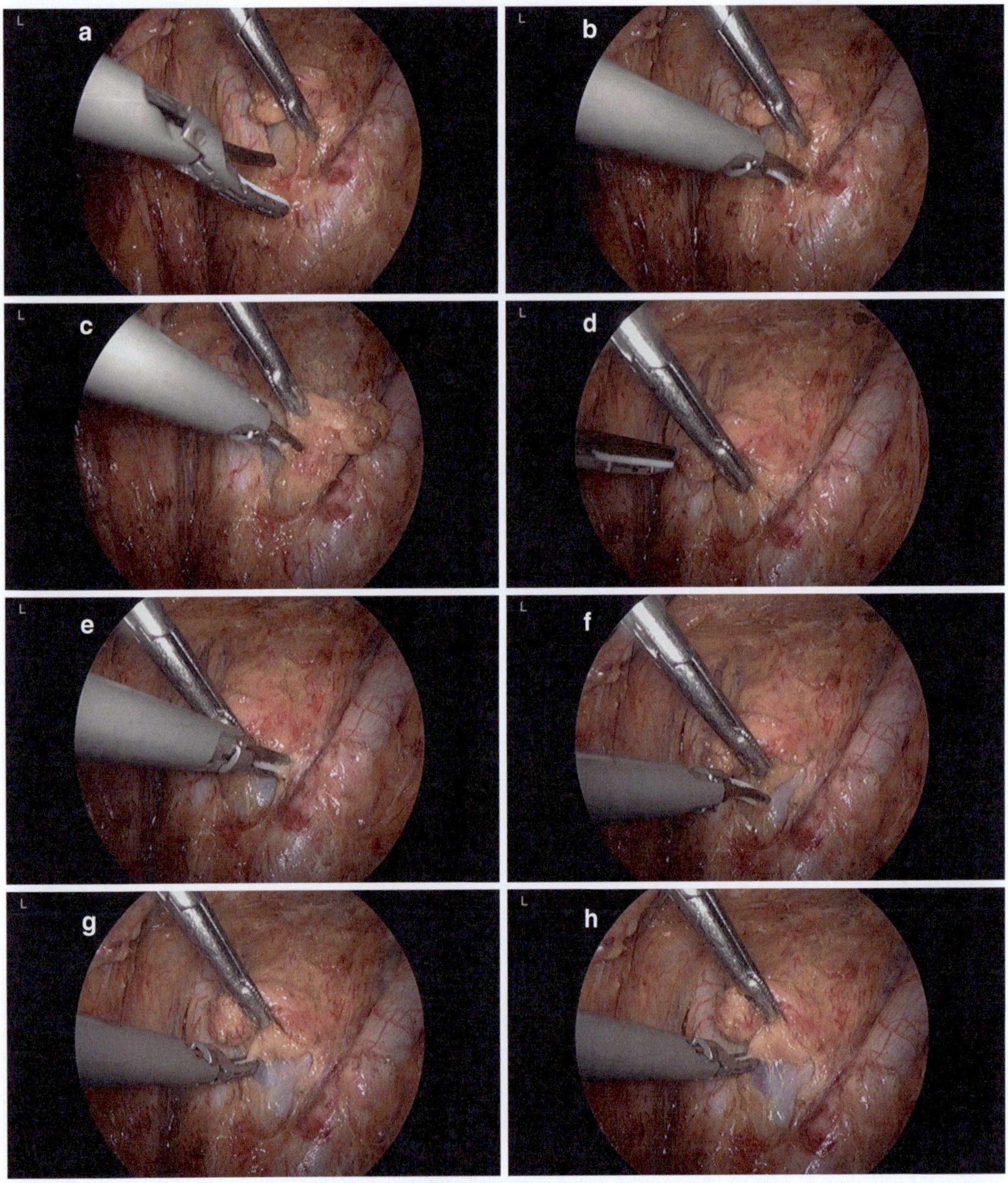

Fig. 14.13 (**a**–**h**) Expose the left common iliac vein

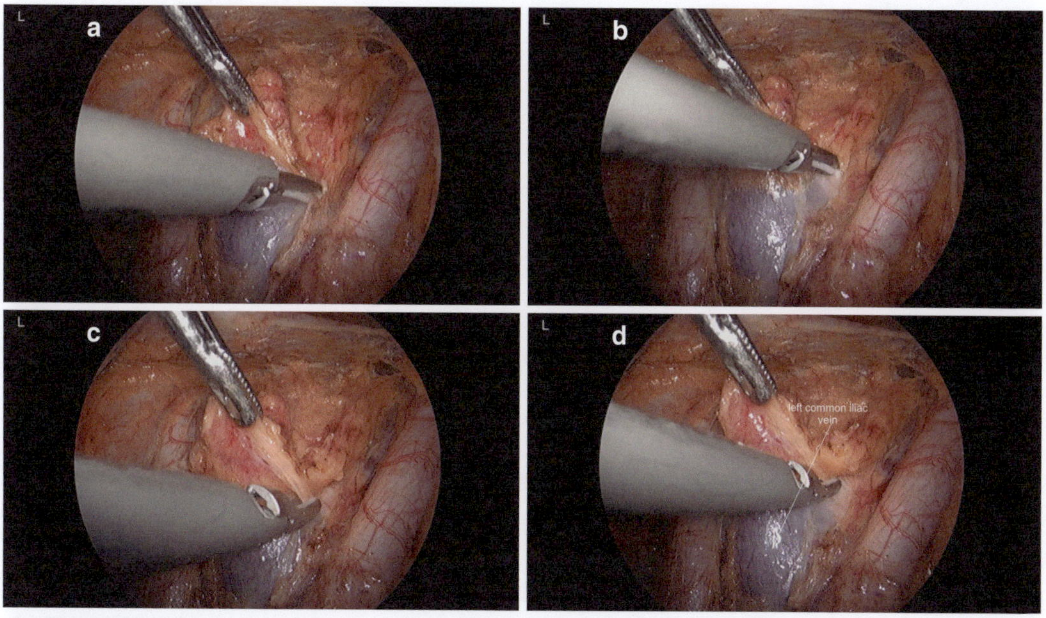

Fig. 14.14 (**a**–**d**) Separate lymph nodes along the surface of the left common iliac vein

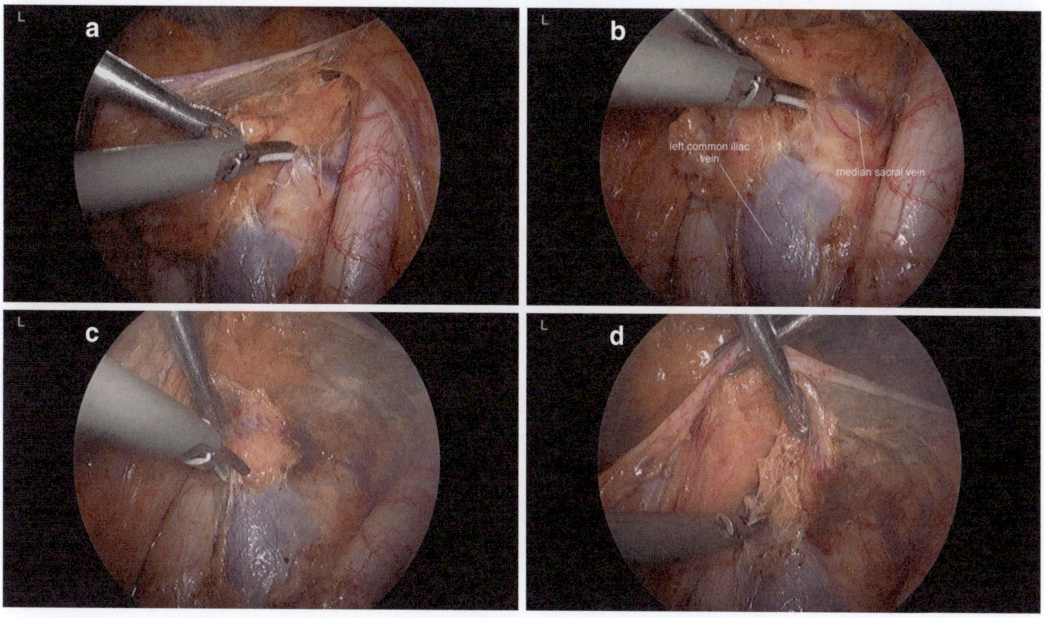

Fig. 14.15 (**a**–**d**) Recognize the midline sacral vein

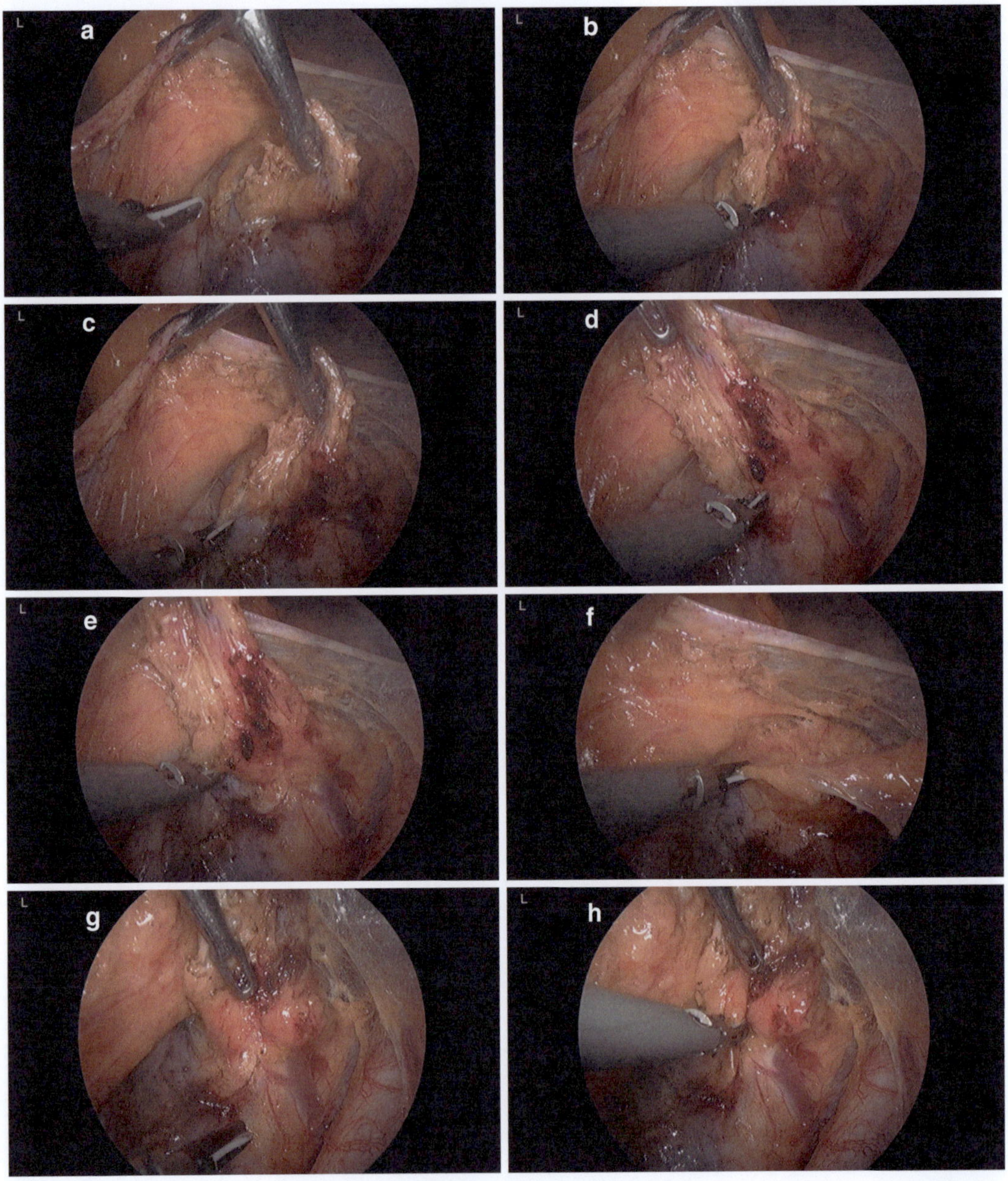

Fig. 14.16 (**a**–**h**) Separate the left common iliac vein and lymph laterally

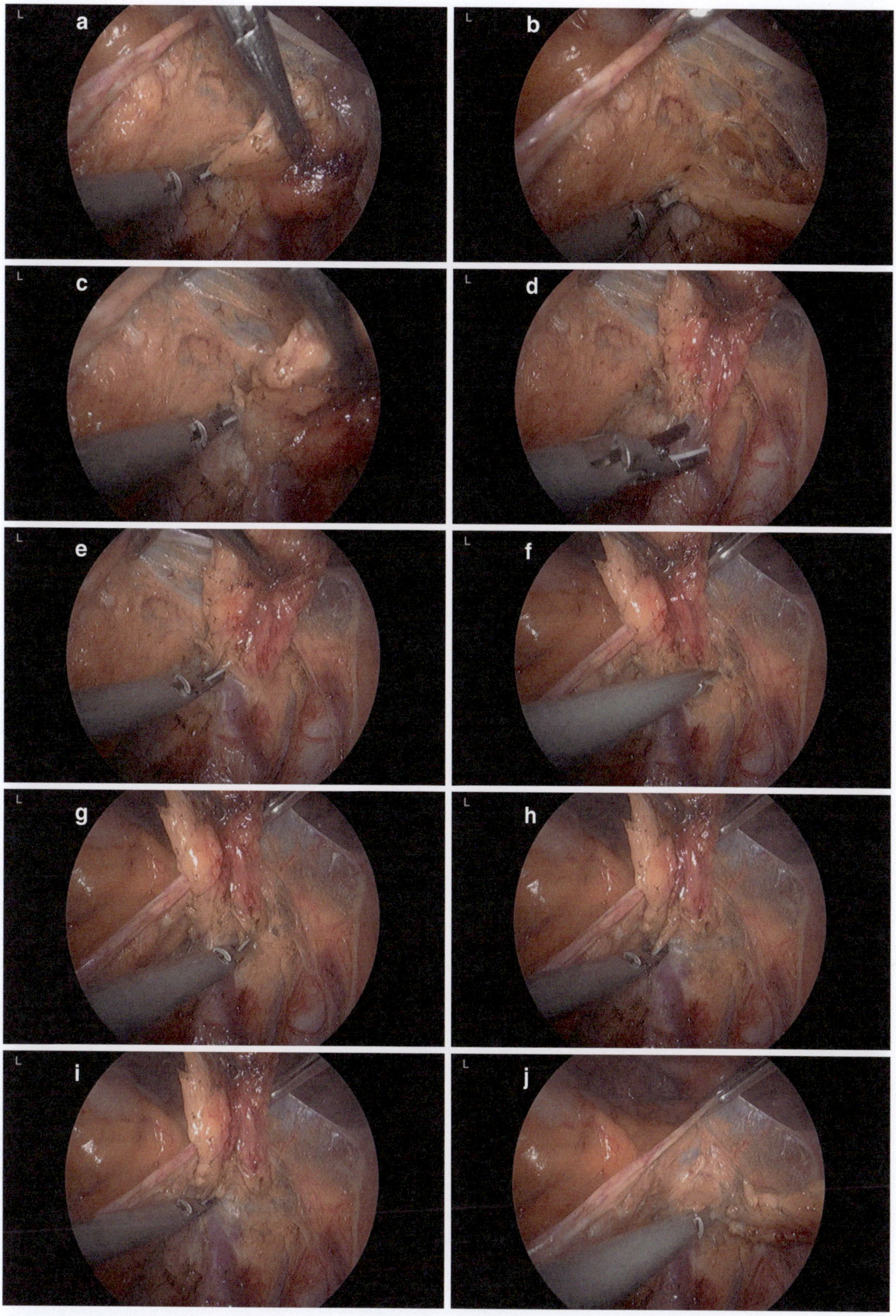

Fig. 14.17 (**a**–**j**) Expose the midline sacral vein and remove the left common iliac vein lymph nodes

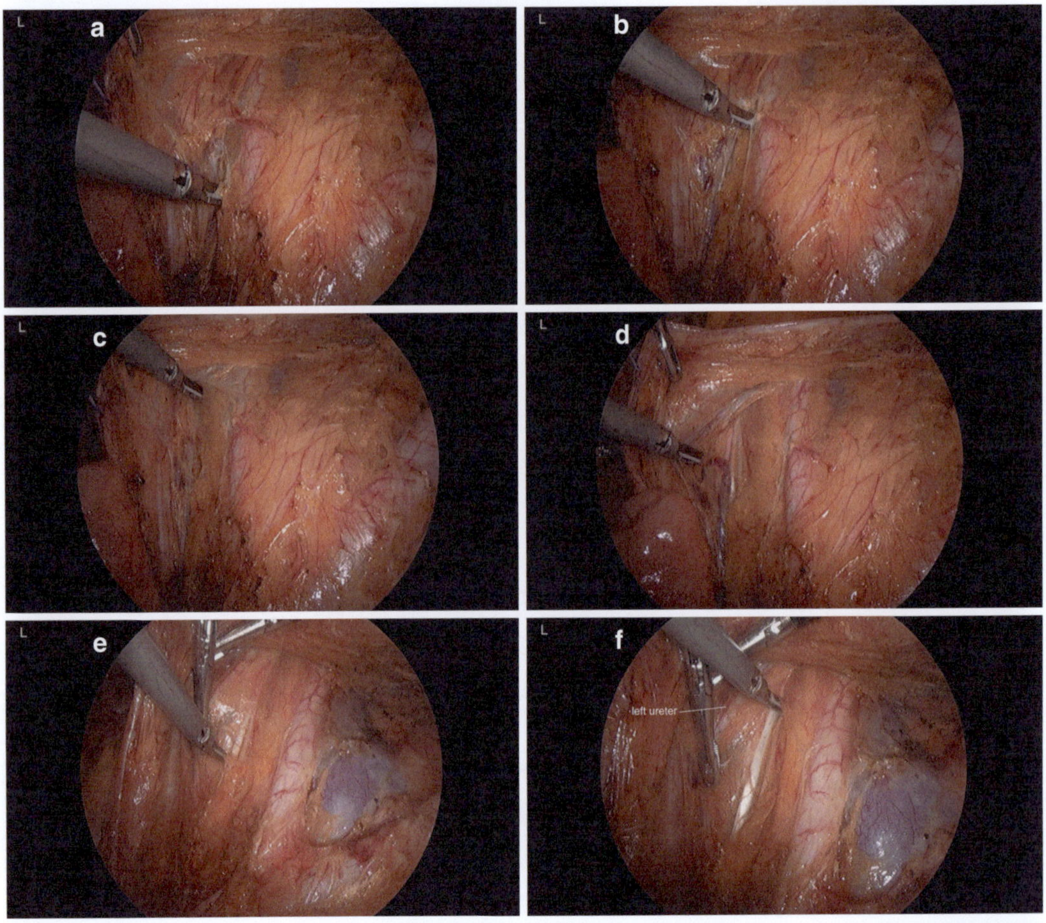

Fig. 14.18 (**a**–**f**) Separate outer boundary of lymph node of left common iliac artery (note ureter)

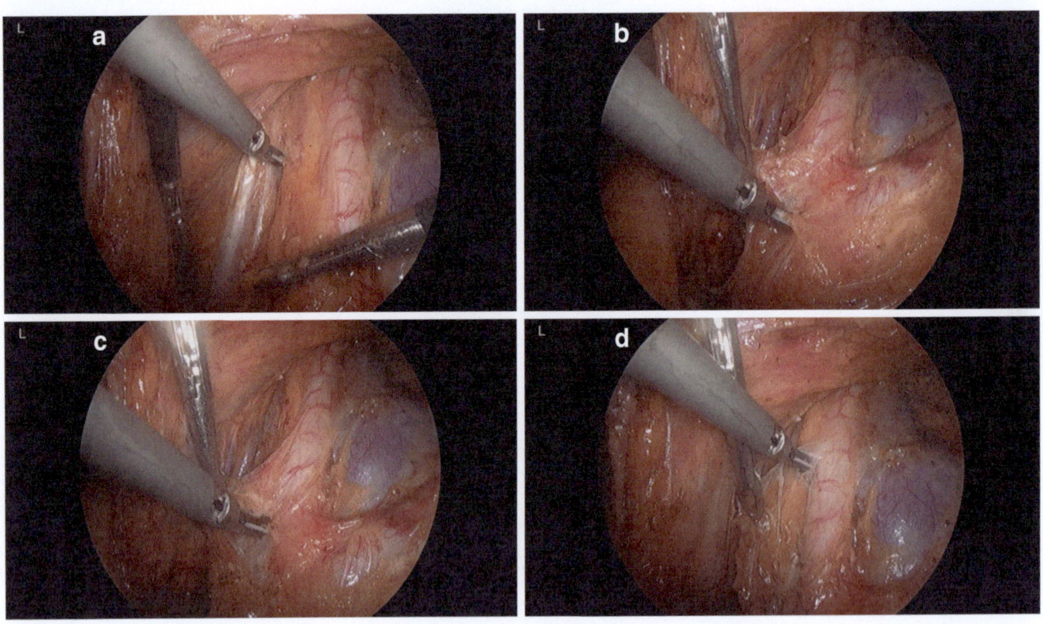

Fig. 14.19 (**a**–**d**) Separate inner boundary of lymph node of left common iliac artery

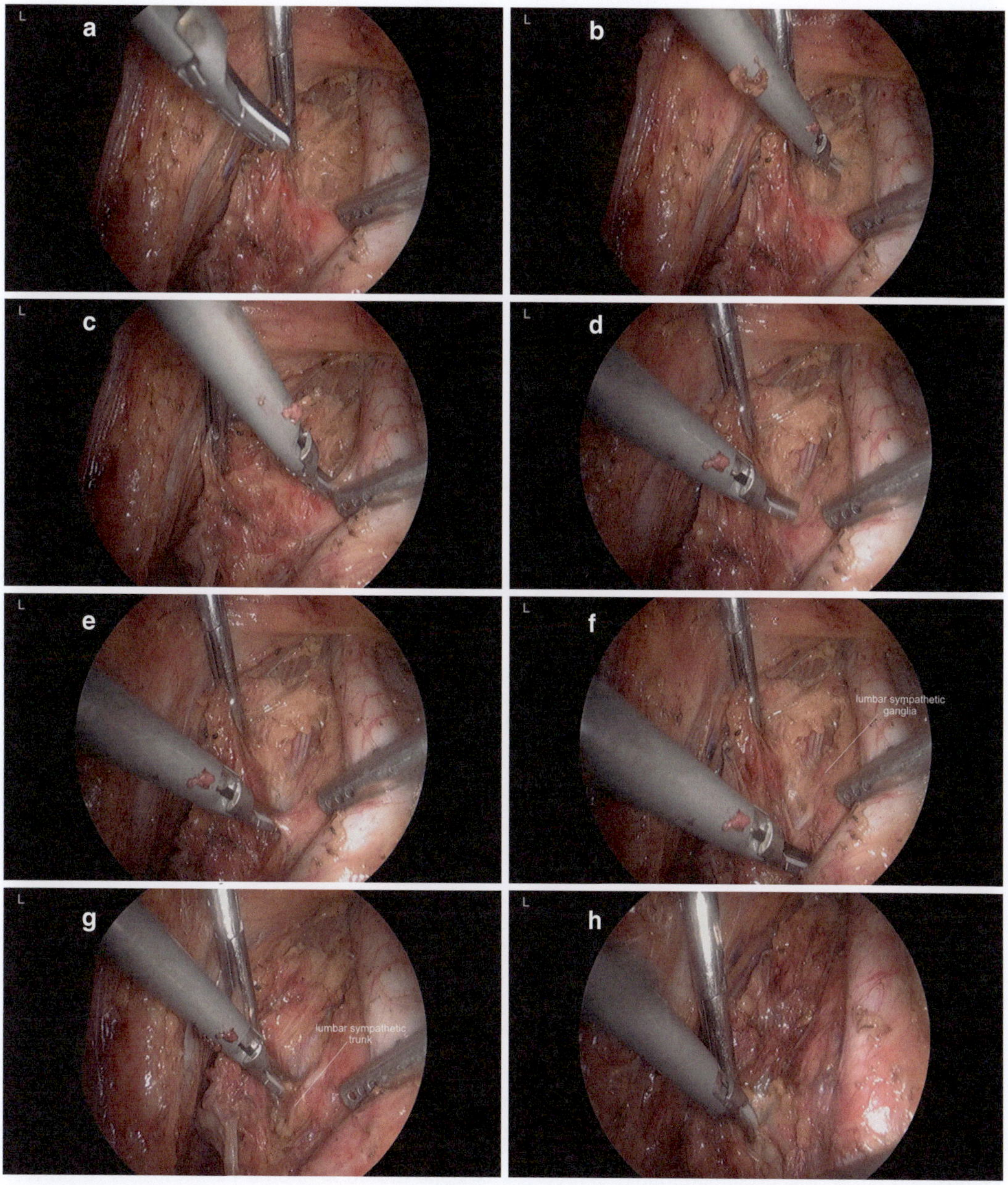

Fig. 14.20 (**a**–**h**) Dissect the left common iliac lymph node, note the lumbar sympathetic trunk and the lumbar sympathetic ganglion

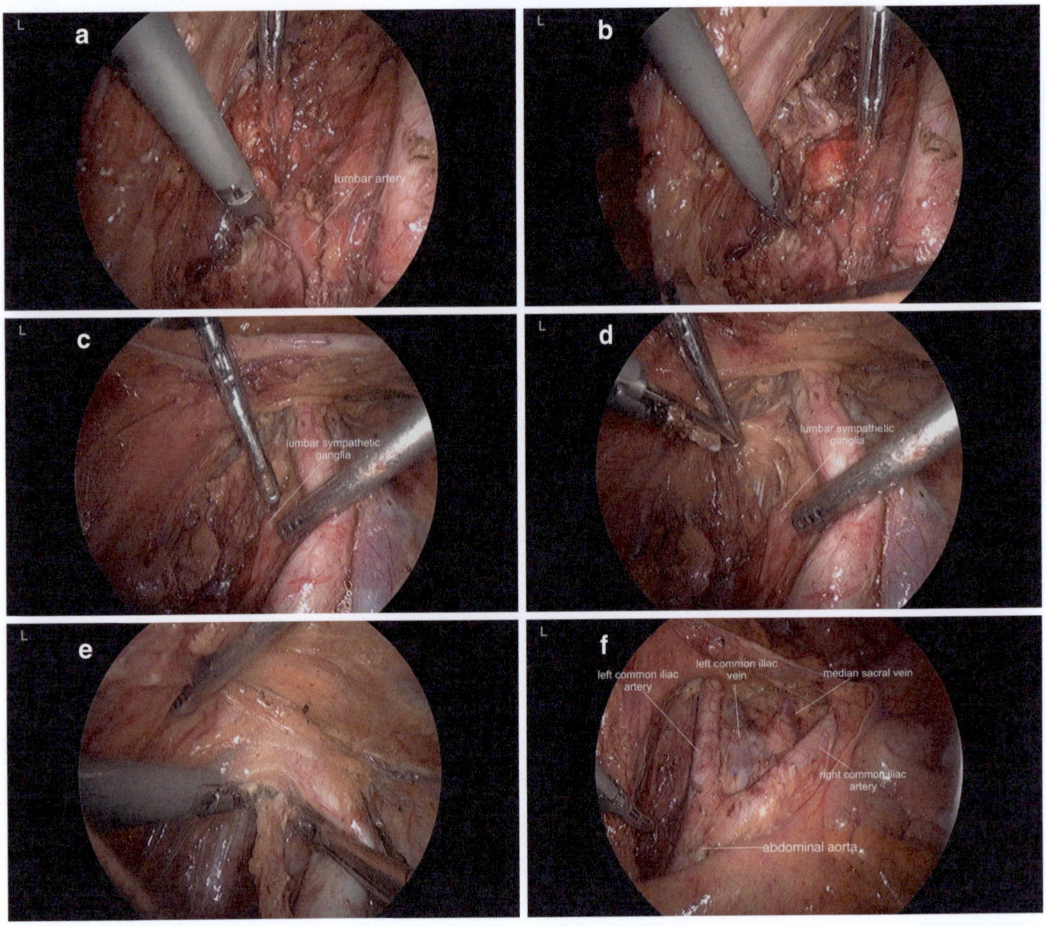

Fig. 14.21 (**a–f**) Remove the lymph nodes on the outer side of the left common iliac artery

14.2 Lymph Node Dissection Along the Surfaces of External Iliac Vessels and Psoas

Gently retracting the ureter cranially, a precise incision is made in its caudal mesentery. The completely excised iliac nodes are then positioned beneath the ureter, adjacent to the surfaces of the external iliac vessels. Careful adherence to the external iliac surface and the surface of the psoas muscle allows for the meticulous separation of lymph nodes situated between these two surfaces, proceeding from the cranial to the caudal direction. Gradually revealing the most inferior segment of the deep circumflex iliac vein, special attention should be dedicated to protecting the genitofemoral nerve and the deep circumflex iliac vein, noting that in certain patients, the deep circumflex vein may traverse along the posterior aspect of the external iliac artery (Figs. 14.22, 14.23, 14.24, and 14.25).

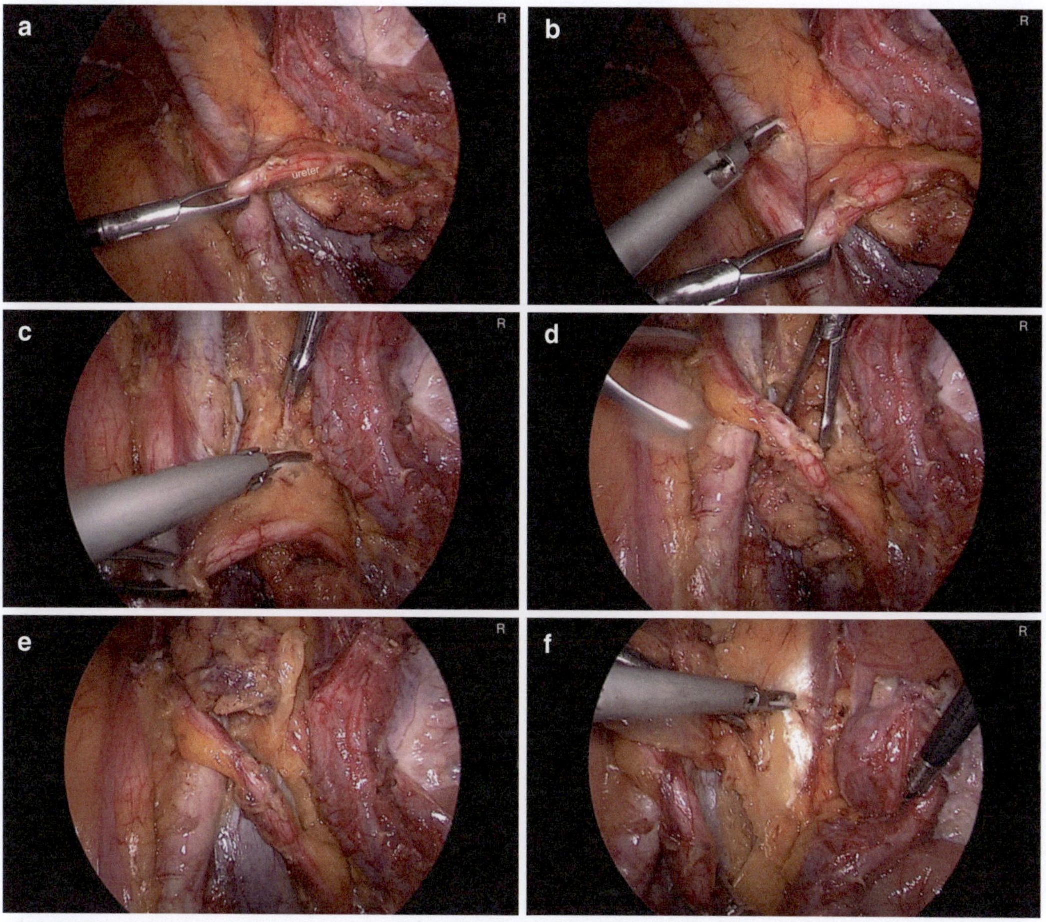

Fig. 14.22 (**a**–**f**) Transfer the common iliac lymph nodes from cranial to caudal direction of ureter

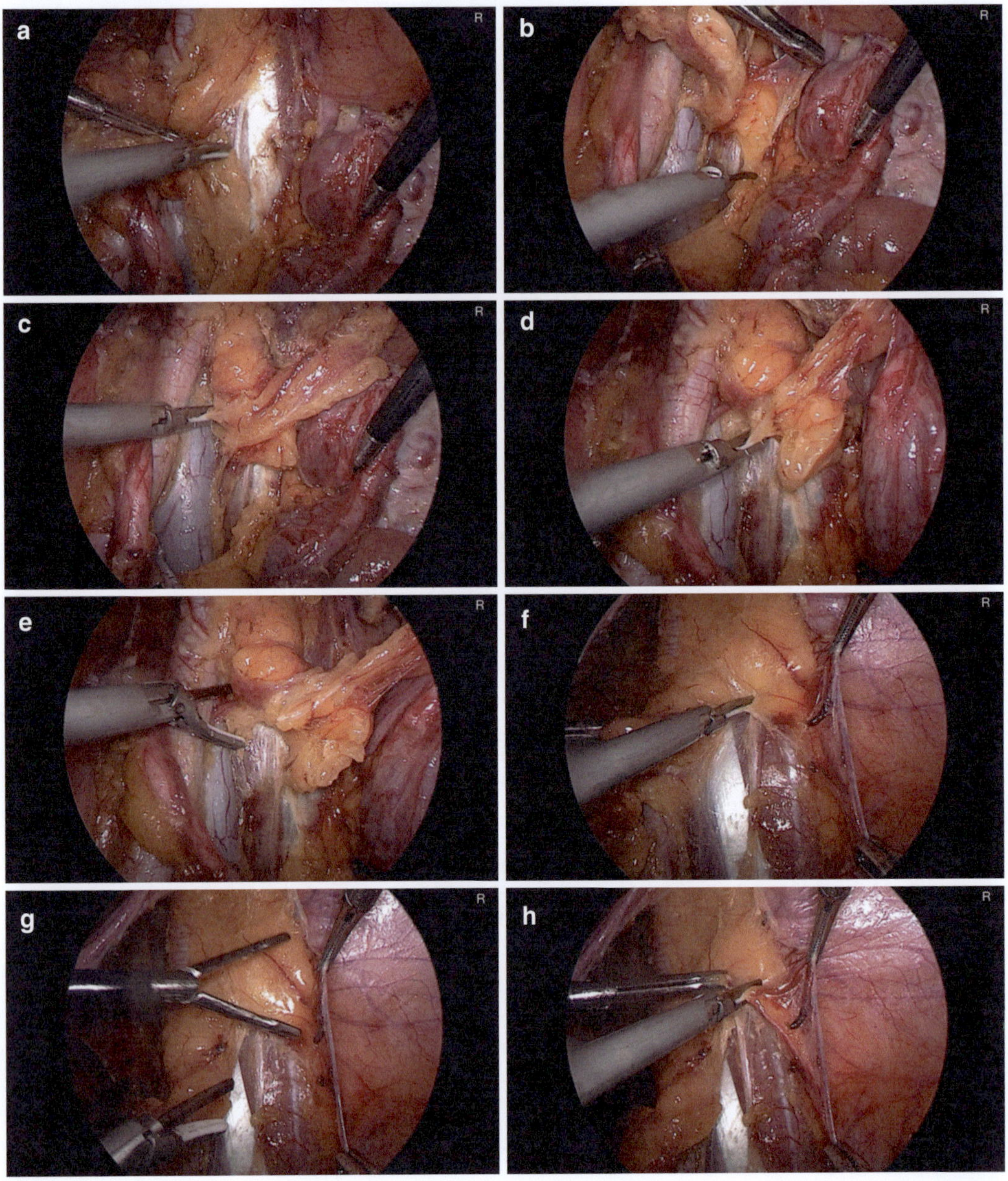

Fig. 14.23 (**a**–**h**) Dissect lymphatic adipose tissue on the surface of external iliac artery from the cranial to the caudal direction

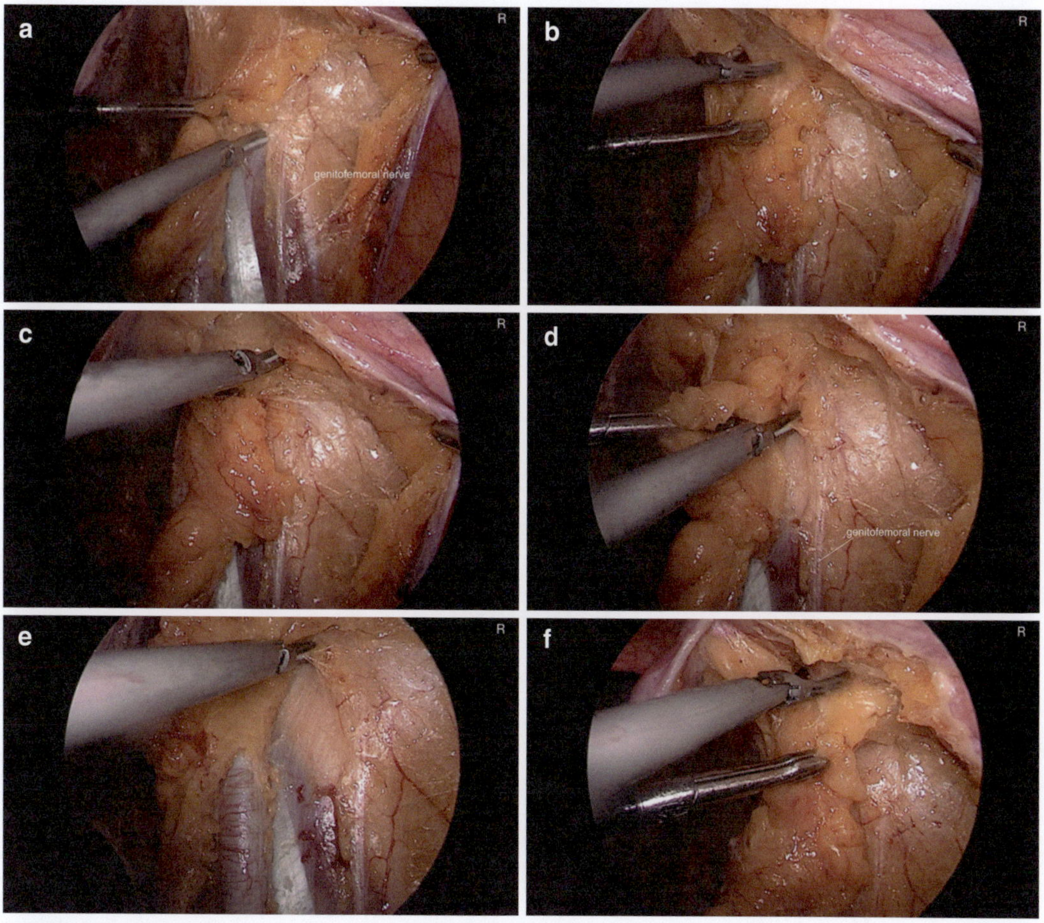

Fig. 14.24 (**a**–**f**) Separate and protect genitocrural nerve

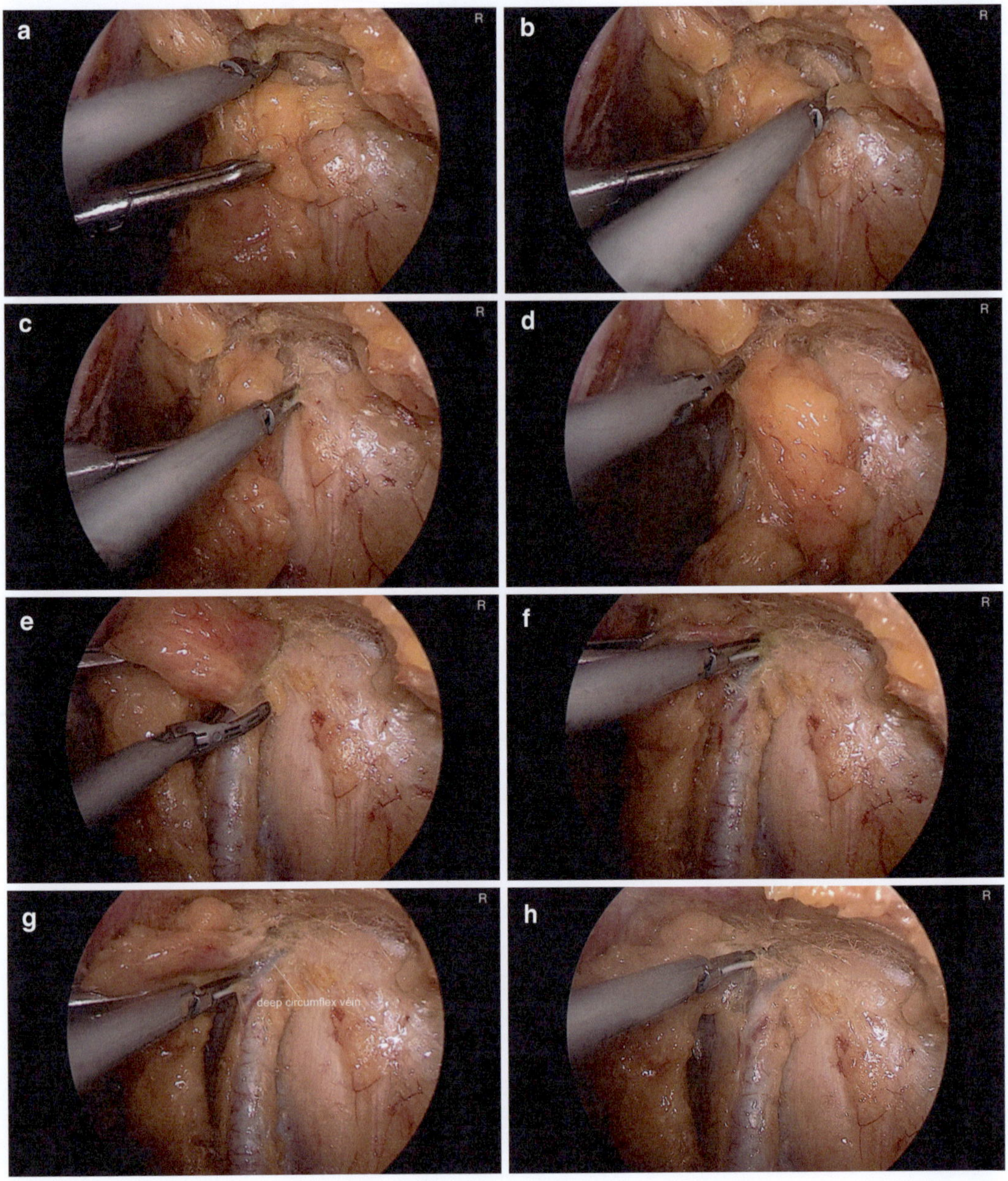

Fig. 14.25 (**a**–**h**) Expose deep circumflex iliac vein

14.3 Complete Dissection of the Obturator Space, Exposing the Pelvic Floor Fascia, and Defining the Medial and Dorsal Boundaries of Lymph Node Dissection

Simultaneously with the handling of the adnexa, our team often conducts partial dissection of the obturator space. Currently, our approach typically involves a staged procedure, with an initial radical hysterectomy followed by pelvic lymph node dissection. In the first step of the radical hysterectomy, lateral parametrial exposure is achieved. Dissection of the obturator space can aid in providing adequate tension for lateral parametrial exposure. Commencing from the origin of the internal iliac artery and closely following its lateral edge, dissection proceeds caudally and dorsally toward the obturator space and the pelvic floor fascia. During this process, the obturator artery and obturator nerve become visible. (Fig. 14.26a–k).

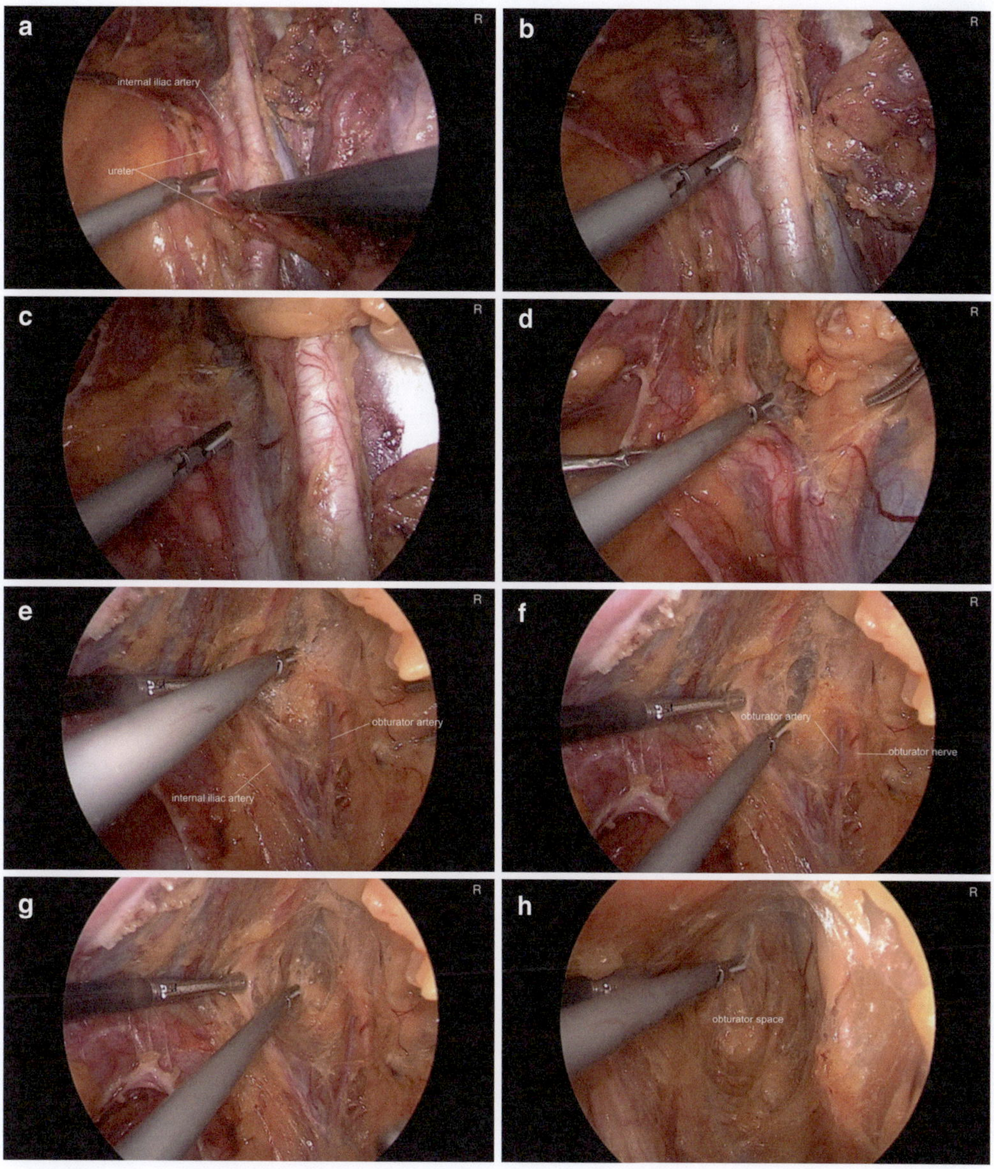

Fig. 14.26 (**a**–**k**) Dissect the obturator space

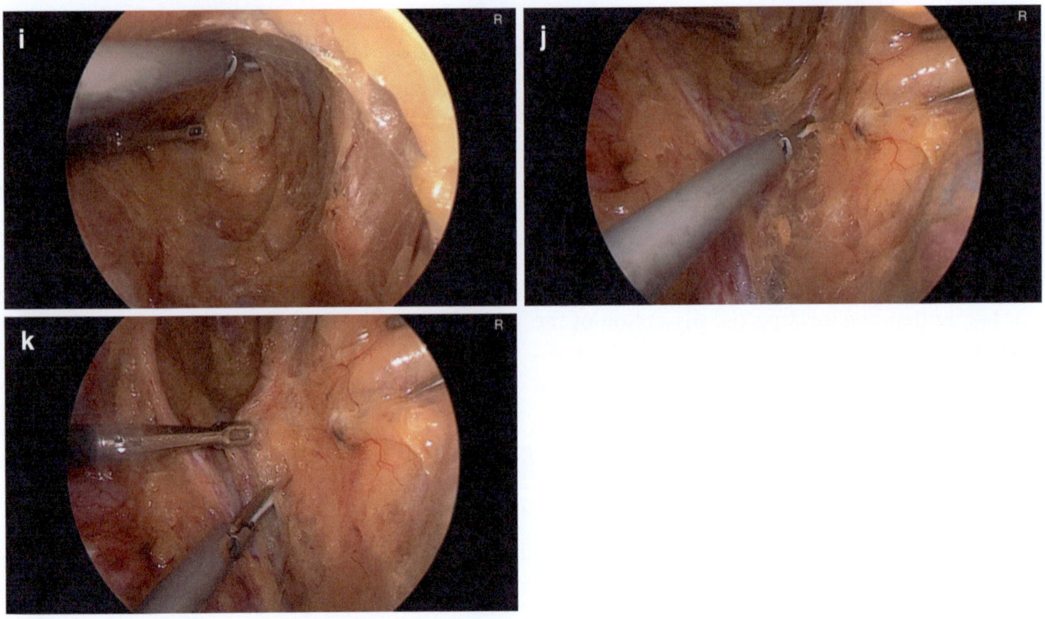

Fig. 14.26 (continued)

14.4 Excision of the Medial Lymph Nodes of the External Iliac Artery and Vein

Starting from the origin of the external iliac artery, the medial lymph nodes of the external iliac artery and vein are dissected in a caudal direction. The lymph nodes that are detached from the surface of the external iliac artery and the psoas muscle converge toward the posterior aspect of the external iliac vein. During this procedure, careful attention is paid to the accessory obturator veins located posteriorly and medially to the external iliac vein, to prevent inadvertent injury (Fig. 14.27a–h).

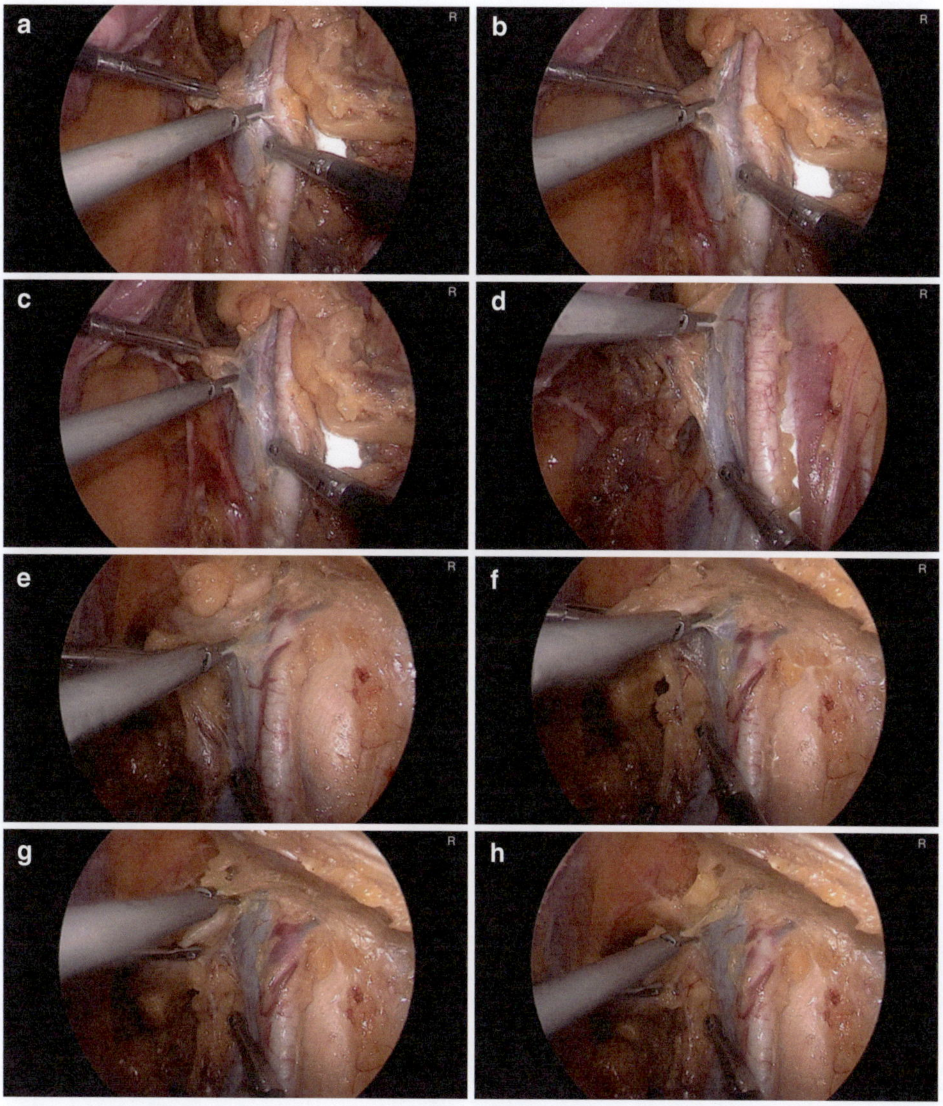

Fig. 14.27 (**a–h**) Starting from the origin of the external iliac artery, the medial lymph nodes of the external iliac artery and vein are dissected in a caudal direction

14.5 Dissect and Remove the Lymph Nodes Between the External Iliac Vessels and the Psoas Muscle, Specifically Exposing the Space Between the External Iliac Vessels and the Psoas Muscle

With a gentle pull, medially retract the external iliac artery and vein, and laterally move the psoas muscle. As a standard procedure, our team initiates dissection within the interval between the external iliac vessels and the lymph nodes (Fig. 14.28a–h). This practice ensures optimal tension and aids in the dissection process. Progressively continue the separation in a caudal direction until the convergence point of the iliac vessels and the psoas muscle is reached (Fig. 14.29a–j). Subsequently, extend the dissection dorsally to the lateral and dorsal aspects of the iliac vessels.

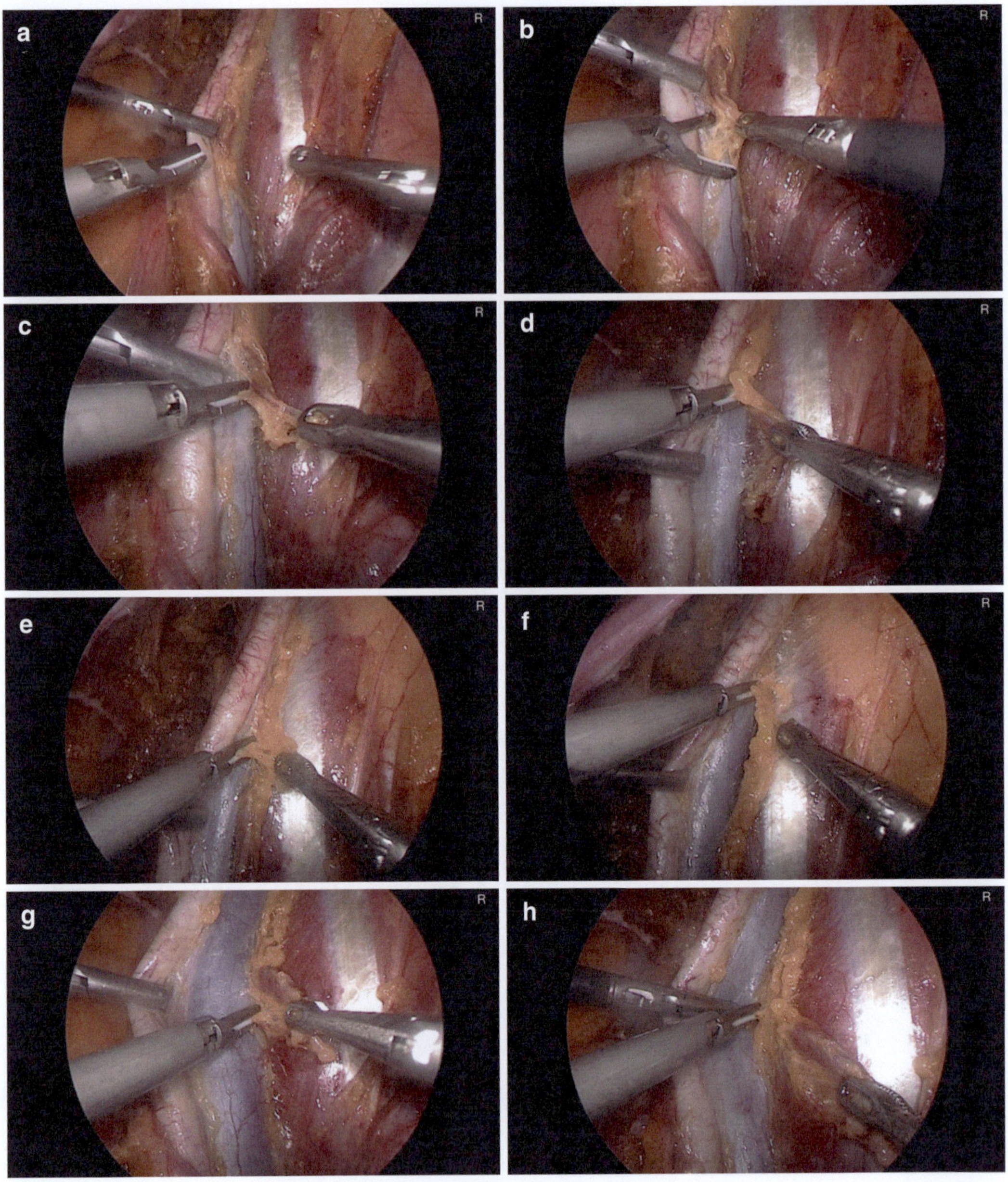

Fig. 14.28 (**a**–**h**) Separate the space between external iliac arteriovenous and lymph nodes

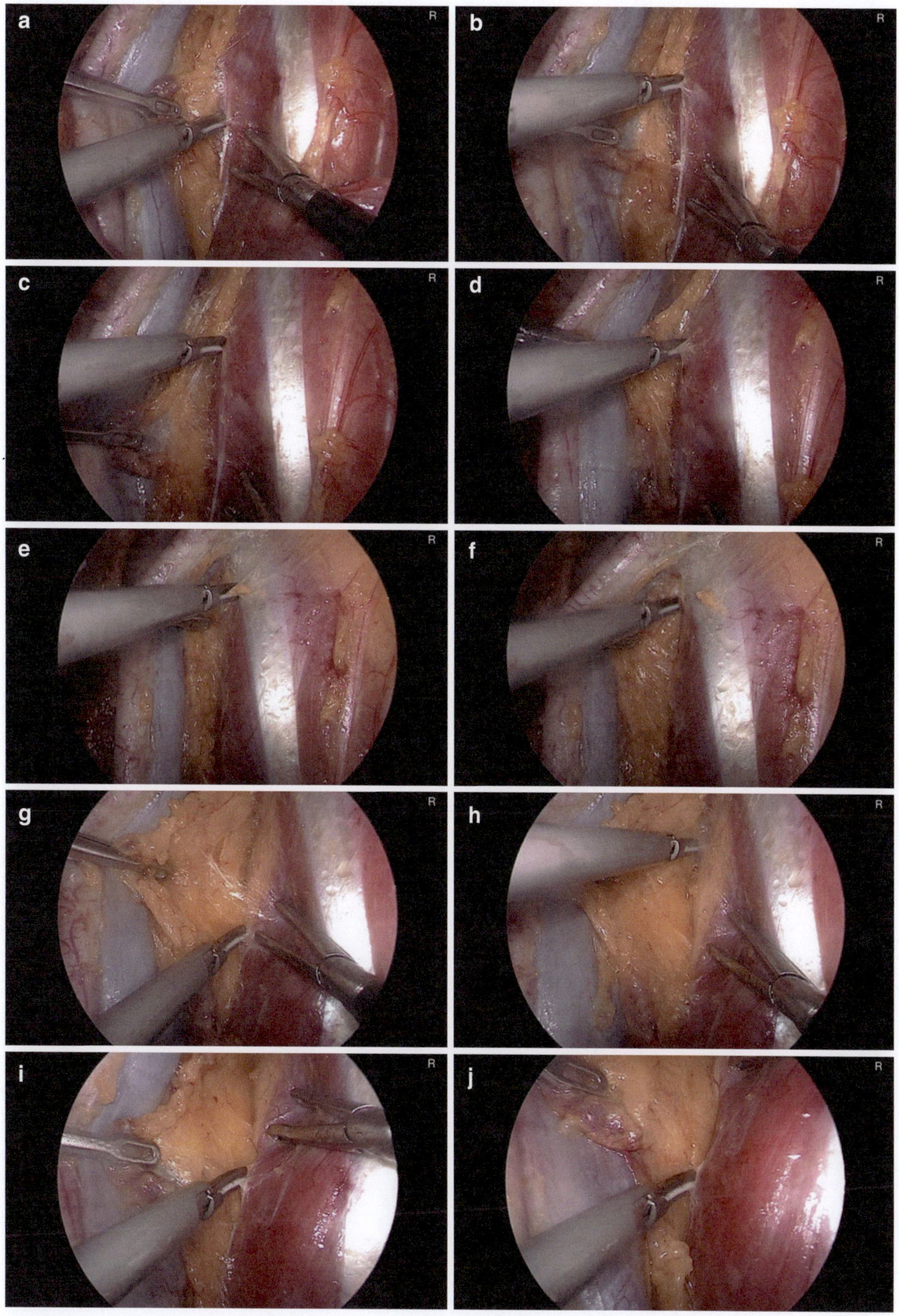

Fig. 14.29 (**a–j**) Separate the space between the psoas muscle and lymph nodes

14.6 Management of Deep Region Lymph Nodes of the Common Iliac Vessels and Exposure of the Upper Segment of the Obturator Nerve

Thoroughly lateralized the psoas major muscle while medially retracting the common iliac vein, facilitating the mobilization of lymph nodes in this region. Initiate the procedure by sharply separating closely along the common iliac vein, progressing from the cranial to the caudal direction, gradually exposing the internal iliac vein (Fig. 14.30a–k). The lumbosacral trunk is situated cranially to the internal iliac vein and posterior to the iliolumbar vein. Proceed sequentially with the removal of lymph nodes from the deep common iliac vessels, moving caudally from the

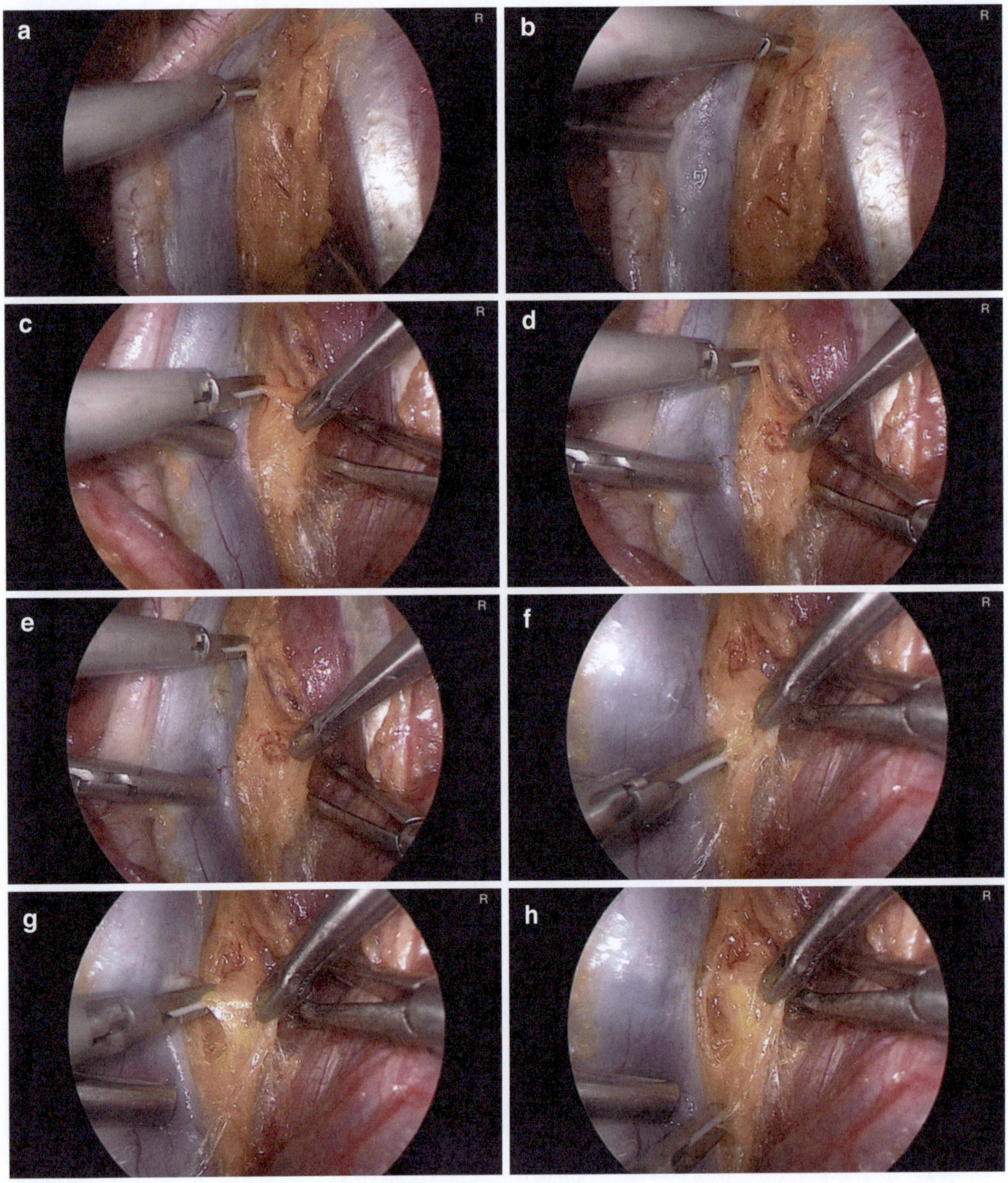

Fig. 14.30 (**a**–**k**) Expose internal iliac vein

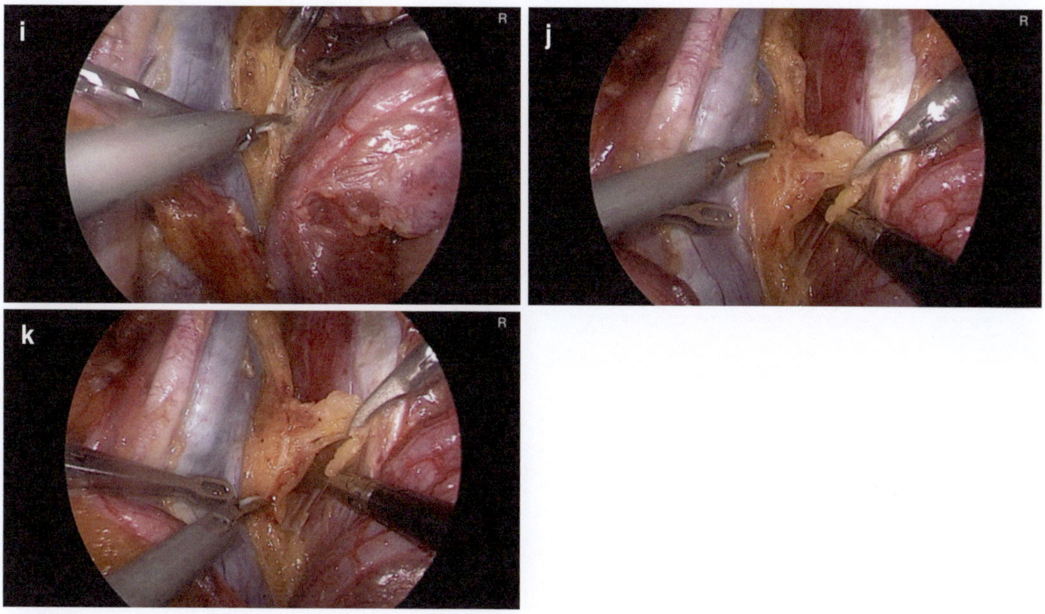

Fig. 14.30 (continued)

cranial direction (Fig. 14.31a–i). During the excision, ensure a significant lateral displacement of the psoas major muscle to facilitate adequate tension for the superior exposure of the proximal obturator nerve (initial segment of the obturator nerve within the pelvic cavity) (Fig. 14.32a–h). Subsequently, continue the excision of lymph nodes in this region until reaching the caudal aspect of the junction between the internal and external iliac veins (Fig. 14.33a–h).

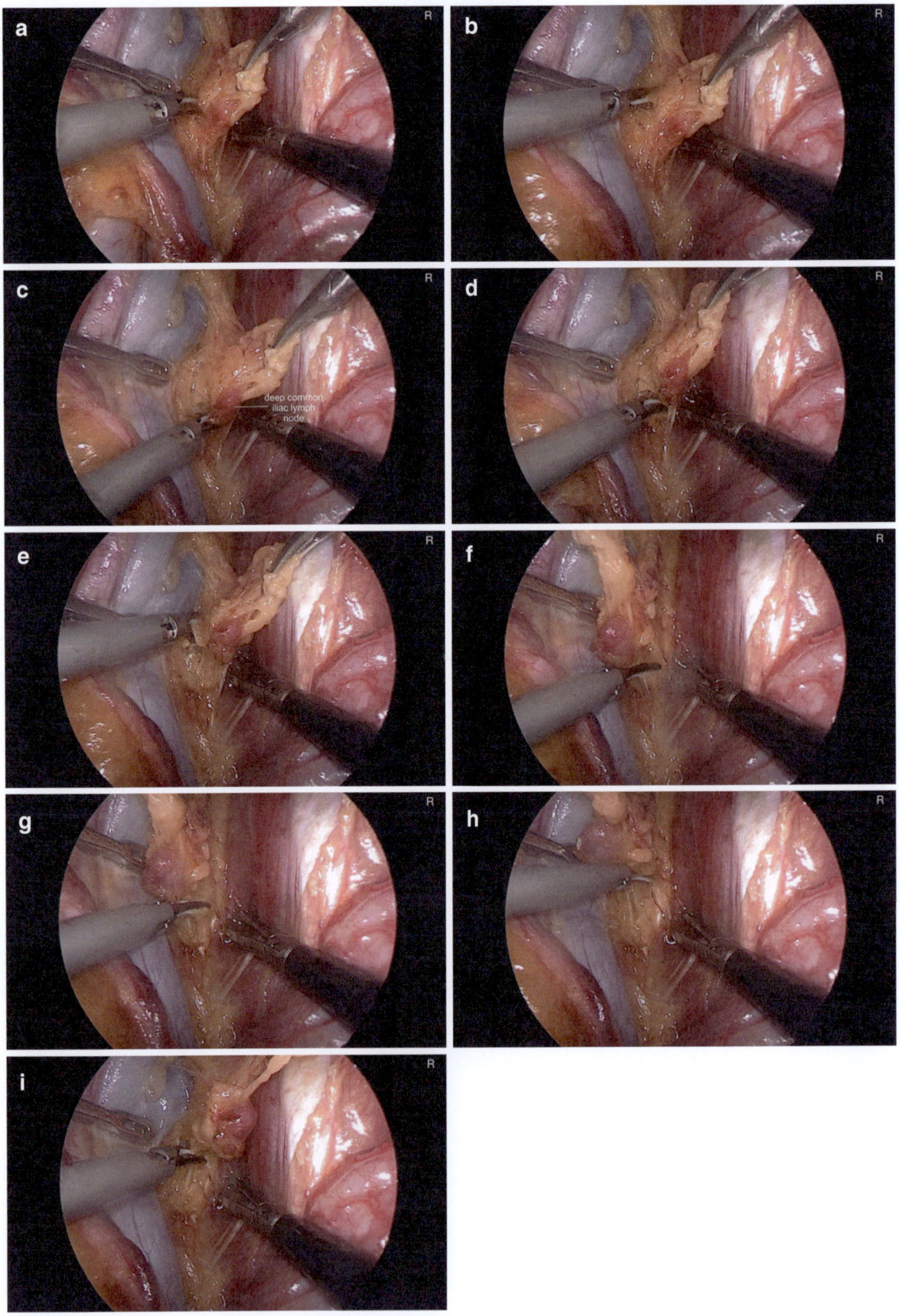

Fig. 14.31 (**a**–**i**) Resect deep region lymph nodes of the common iliac vessels from the cranial to the caudal direction

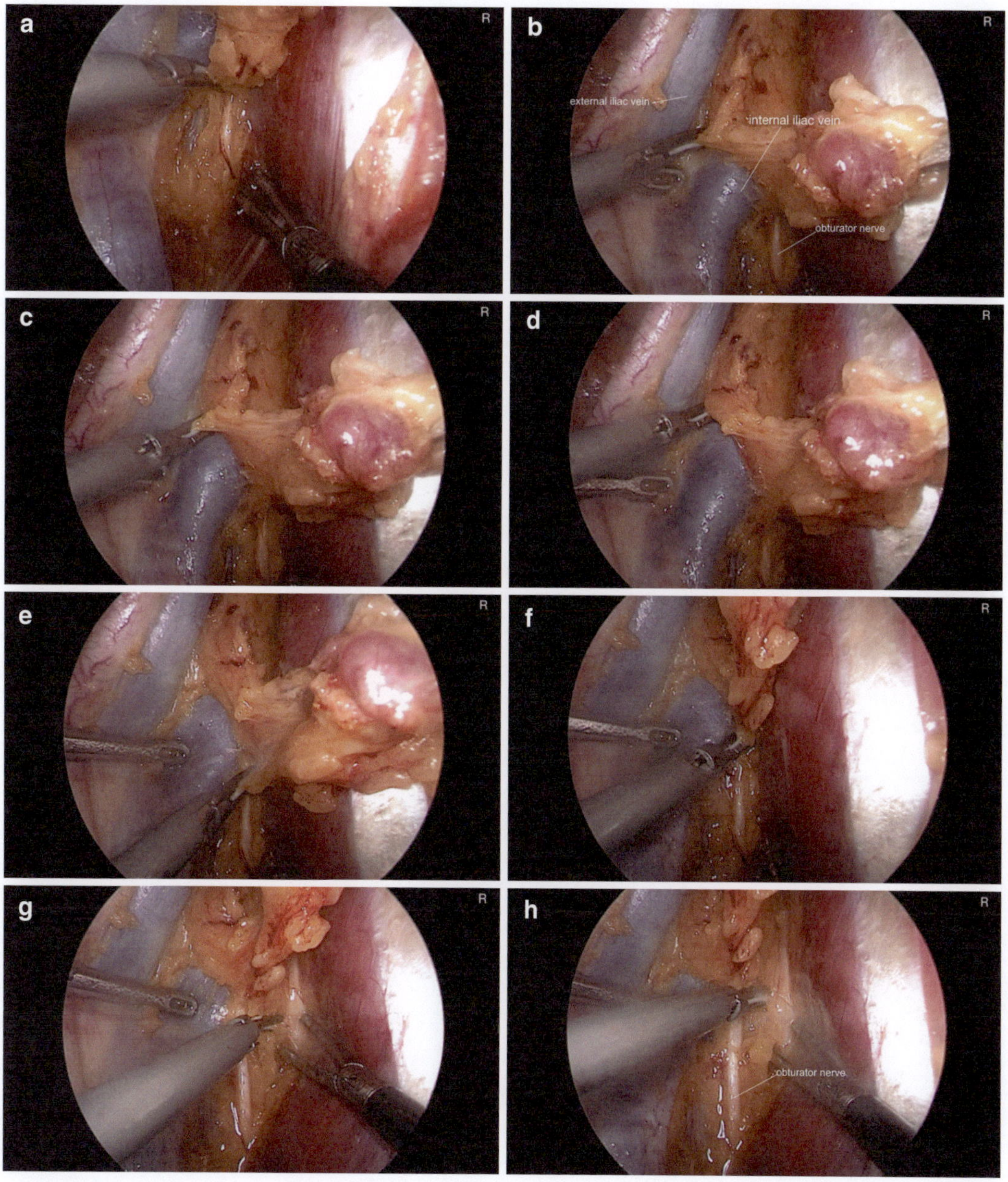

Fig. 14.32 (**a**–**h**) Expose the proximal obturator nerve

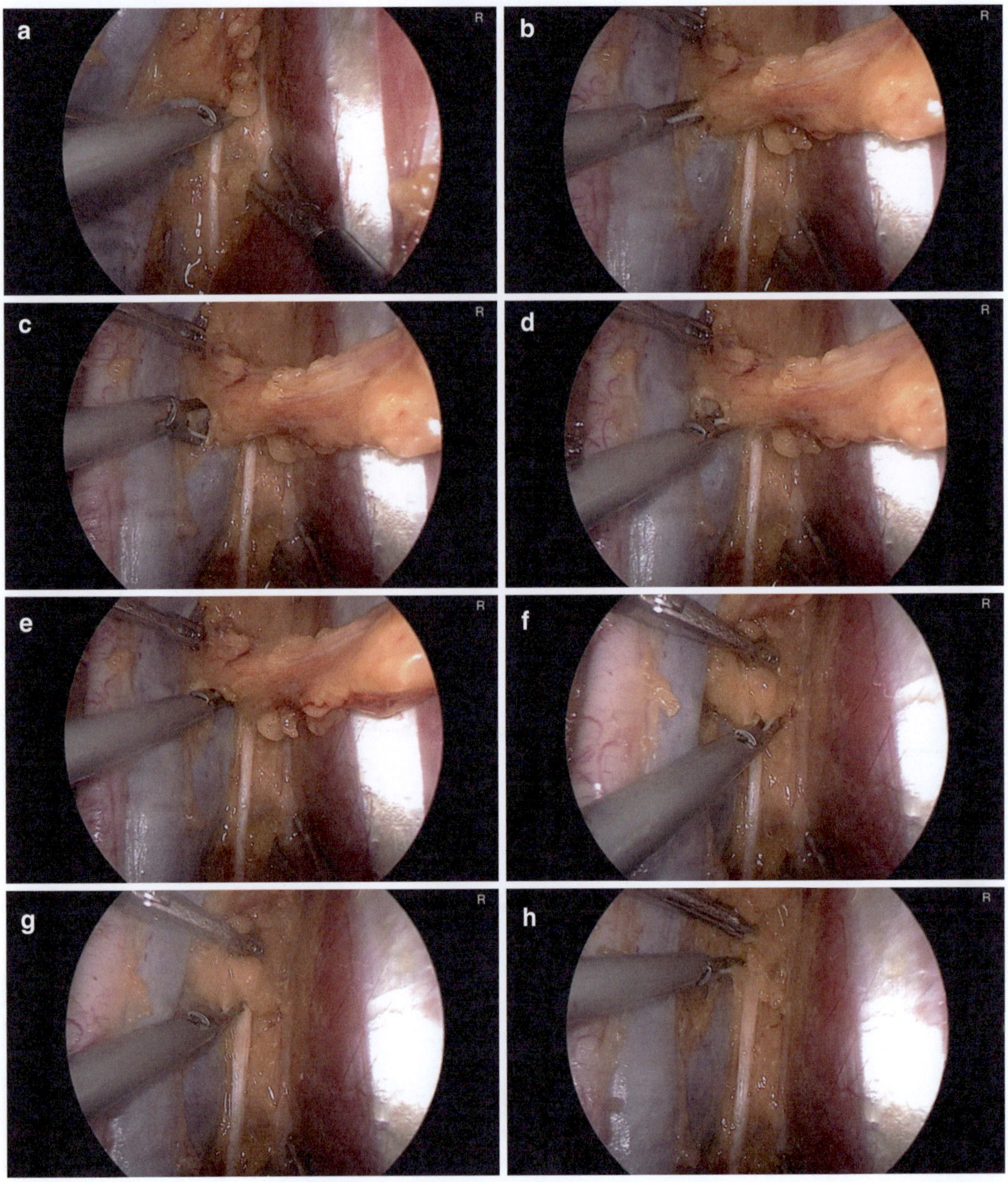

Fig. 14.33 (**a**–**h**) Excise deep region lymph nodes of the common iliac vessels until reaching the caudal aspect of the junction between the internal and external iliac veins

14.7 Management of Lumbosacral Trunk Surface Lymph Nodes and Lymph Nodes Around the Obturator Nerve

Continuing the comprehensive exposure of lymph nodes in the deep area of the common iliac vessels, gently retract the obturator nerve laterally. Employing a combination of blunt and sharp techniques, unveil the lumbosacral trunk, followed by the sequential removal of superficial lymphatic adipose tissue from its surface, progressing caudally. Concurrently, following the isolation of lymphatic adipose tissue encircling the obturator nerve, excise it caudally. Throughout this process, a progressive visualization of the iliolumbar vein, lumbosacral trunk, and obturator nerve can be achieved, potentially accompanied by the presence of an accessory obturator nerve in certain patients (Fig. 14.34a–k).

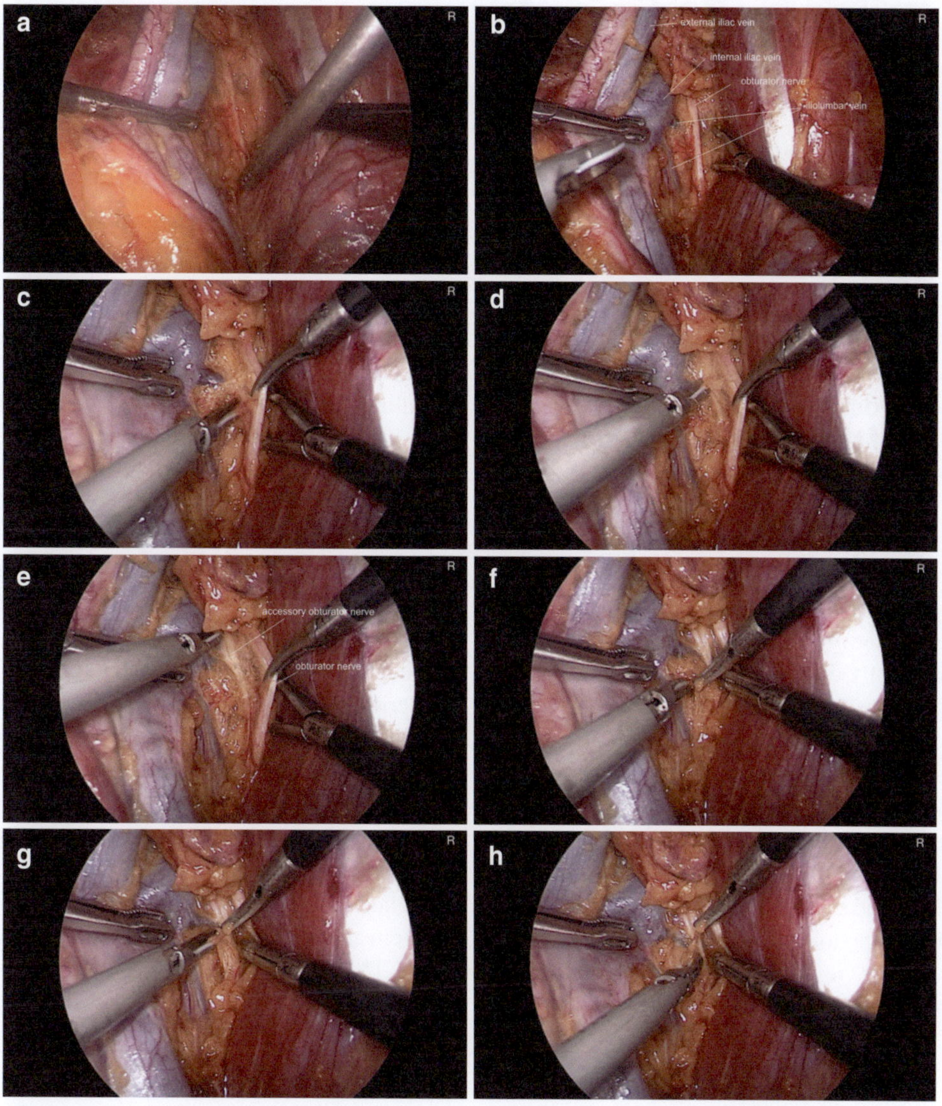

Fig. 14.34 (**a–k**) Expose iliolumbar vein, lumbosacral trunk, obturator nerve, and accessory obturator nerve

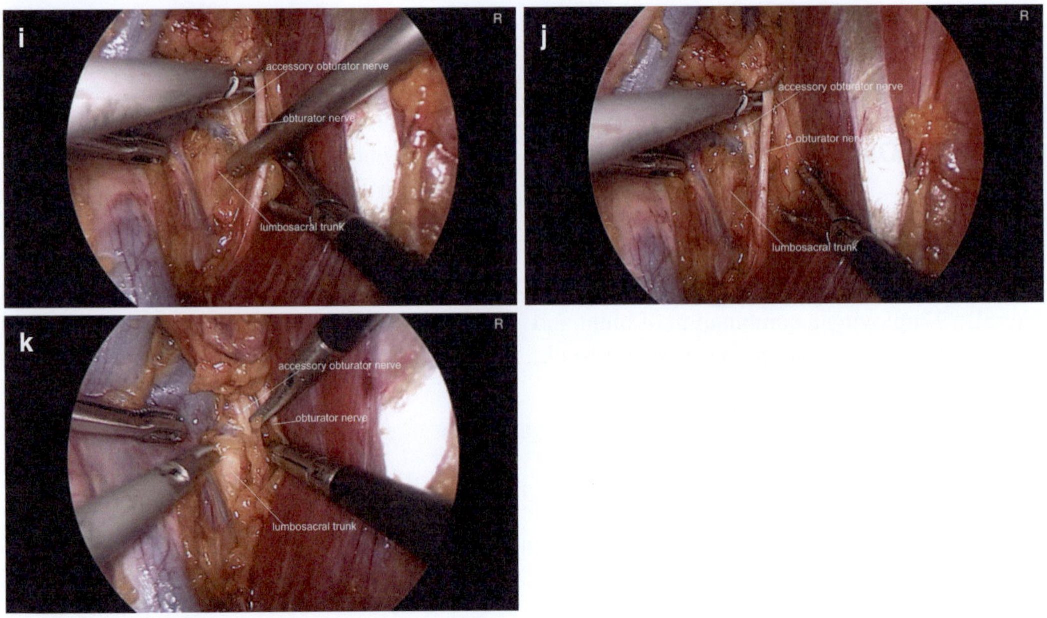

Fig. 14.34 (continued)

14.8 Management of the Bifurcation of the Common Iliac Vessels, Posterior Medial Aspect of the External Iliac Vein, and Accessory Obturator Vein Region

Our team's practice involves initiating the procedure with the mobilization and removal of lymph nodes in the deep common iliac vessels area. Subsequently, we proceed to expose and excise lymph nodes in the caudal region of the common iliac vessels' bifurcation. This sequencing is driven by the anatomical presence of the obturator nerve, which is embedded within and passes through lymphatic tissue in the caudal region of the common iliac vessels' bifurcation. Direct handling and dissection of lymphatic adipose tissue in this region could potentially lead to unintended injury to the obturator nerve.

The internal iliac vein is also covered by lymphatic adipose tissue in this region, making direct manipulation risky. Following the prior handling of lymph nodes in the deep common iliac vessels area, the obturator nerve and internal iliac vein can be exposed adequately beforehand. This approach enhances precision during the procedure. The mobilized lymph nodes from the deep common iliac vessels area are carefully brought out from the surgical field and repositioned medially and anteriorly. They are positioned closely to the external iliac vein, with its posterior aspect serving as a guide for dissection. Gradually progressing caudally, the lymph nodes are freed and removed until reaching the vicinity of the accessory obturator vein. Subsequently, once the lymph nodes adjoining the accessory obturator vein are adequately detached, they are mobilized posteriorly along the vein and then further toward its cranial aspect (Figs. 14.35, 14.36, 14.37, and 14.38).

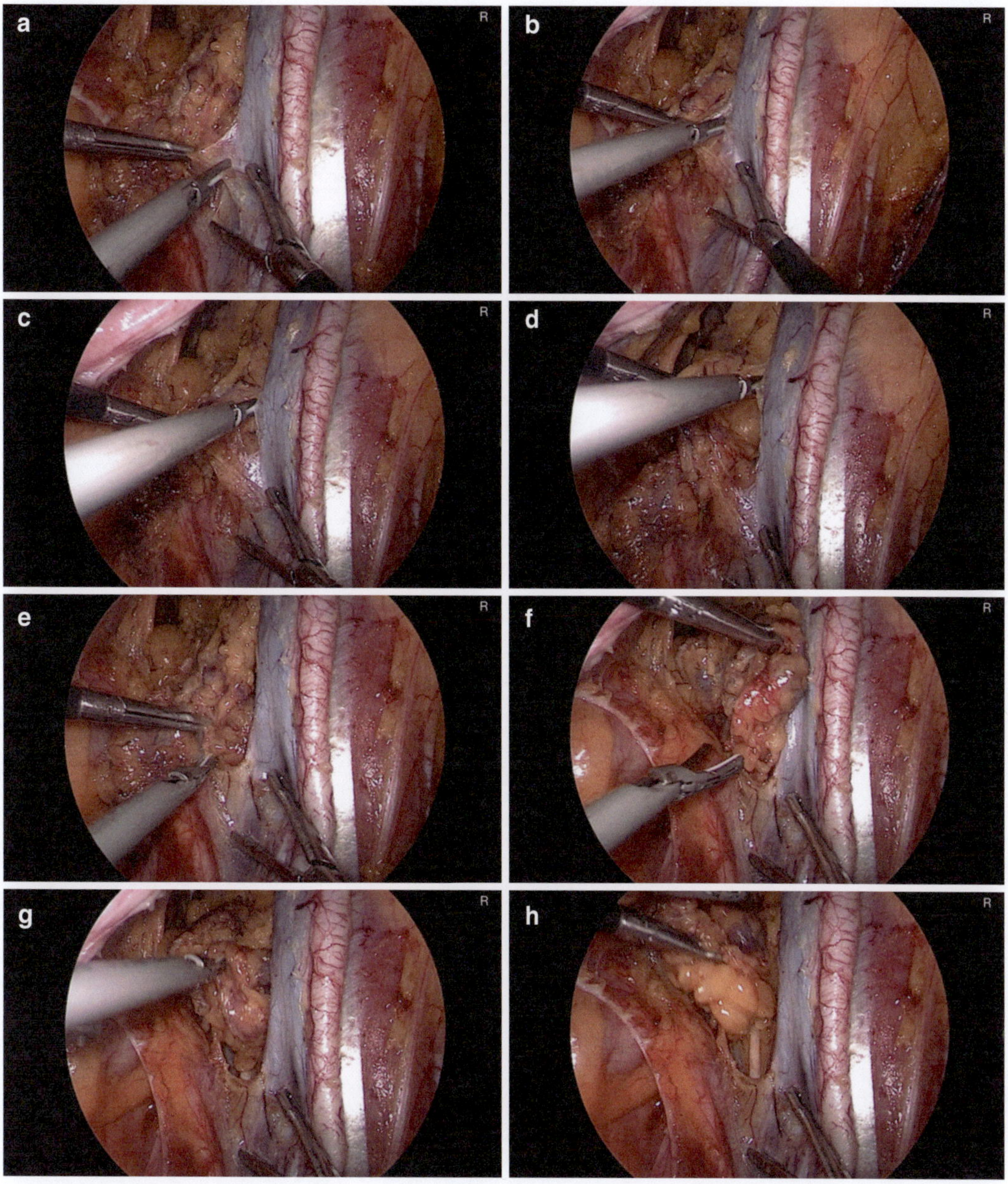

Fig. 14.35 (**a–h**) Move the common deep iliac lymph nodes to the medial side of the external iliac vein

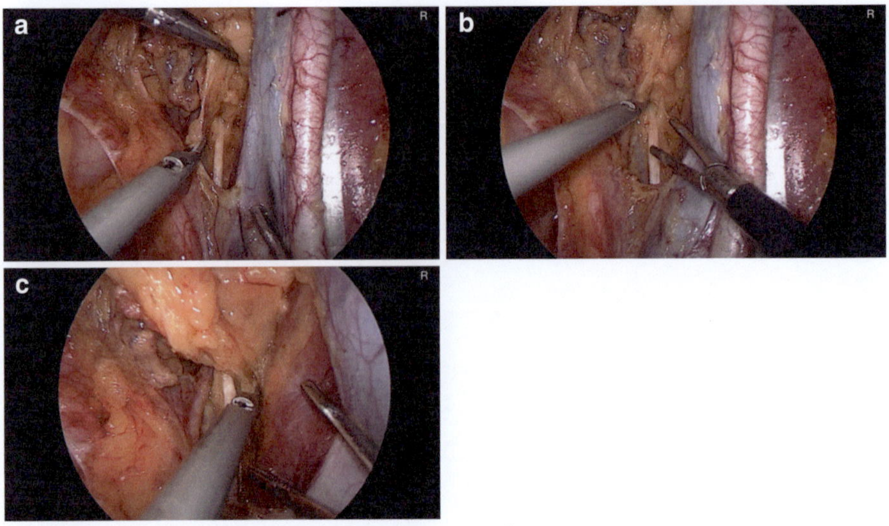

Fig. 14.36 (**a**–**c**) Expose obturator nerve shape

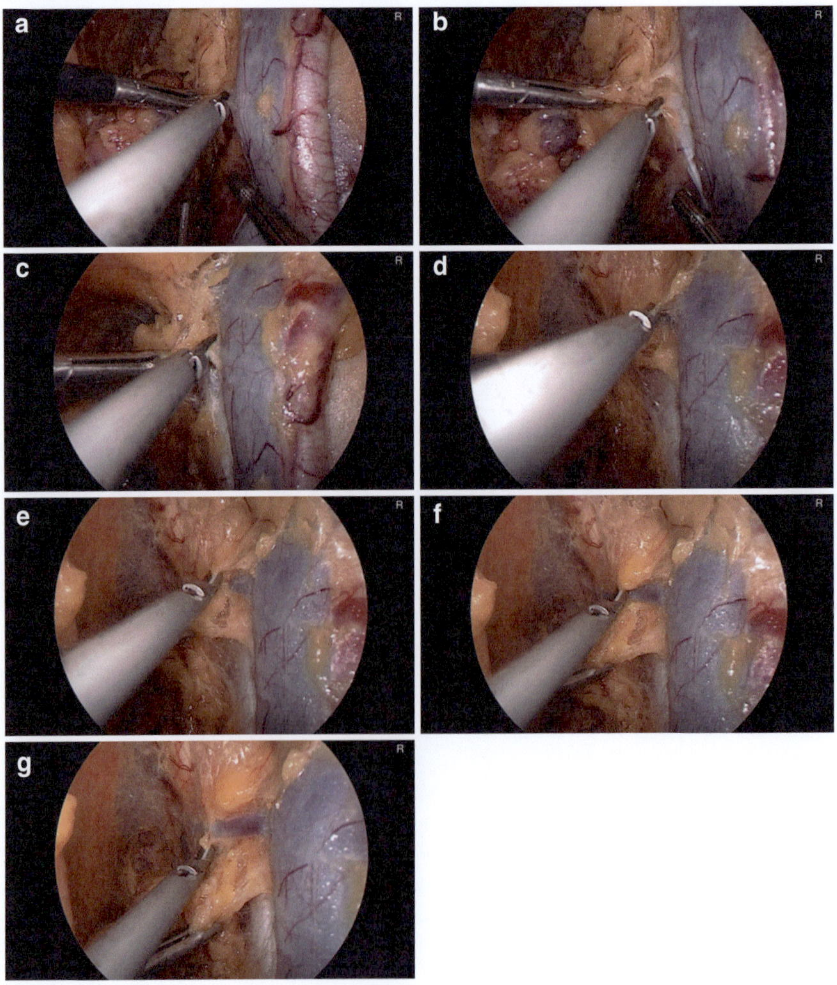

Fig. 14.37 (**a**–**g**) Dissect lymph nodes attached to external iliac vein (note accessory obturator vein)

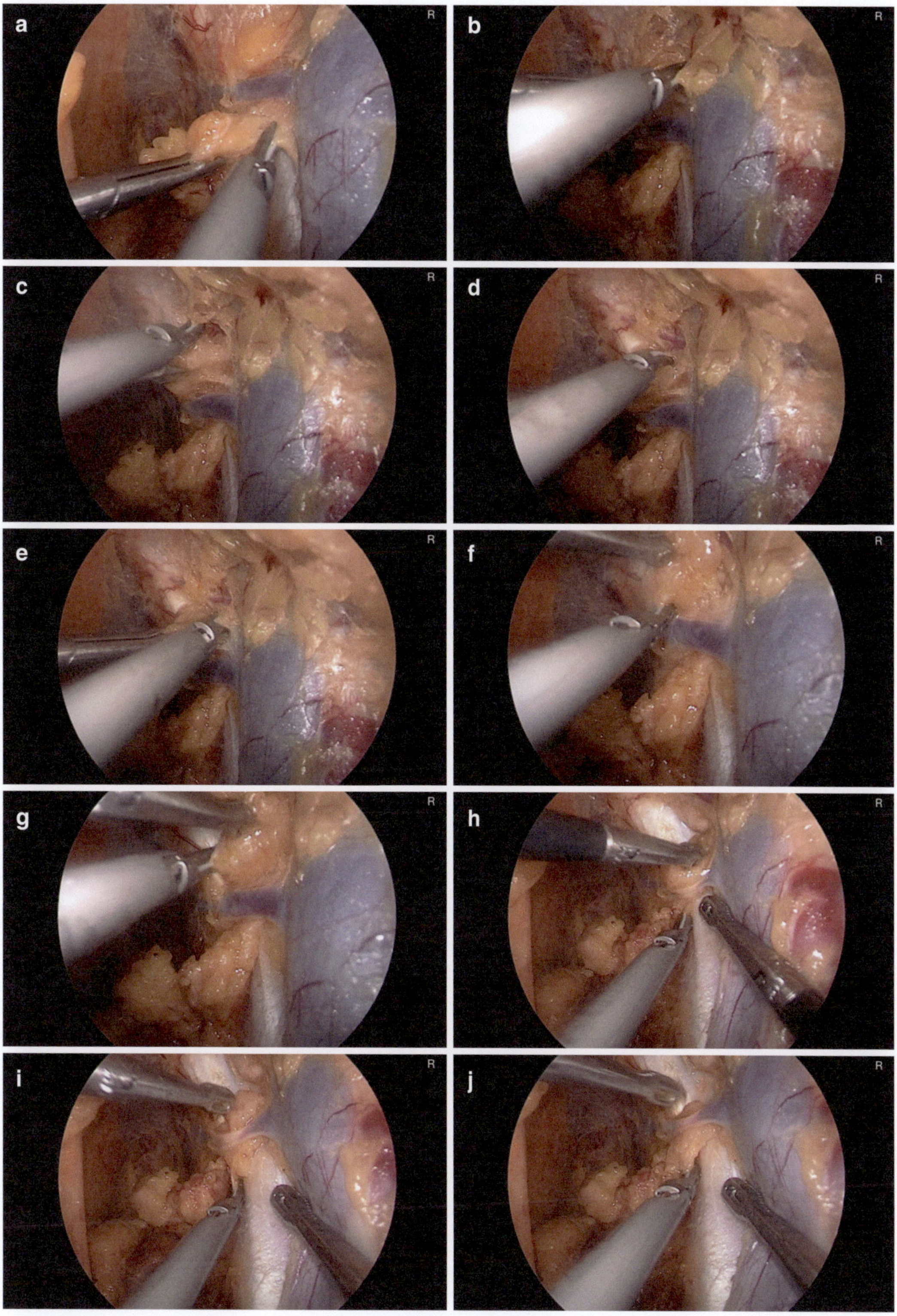

Fig. 14.38 (**a**–**l**) Dissect periaccessory-obturator-vein lymph nodes

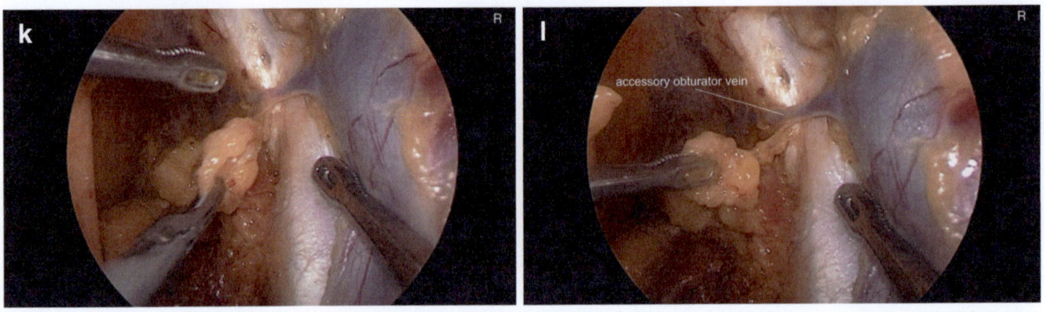

Fig. 14.38 (continued)

14.9 Dissection of the Space Between Lymph Nodes and the Medial Aspect of the Psoas Major Muscle

Gently dissect the interstitial space between the lymph nodes and the medial aspect of the psoas major muscle until the pelvic floor fascia becomes visible (Fig. 14.39a–m). Exercise caution during this dissection. Firstly, ensure that enlarged lymph nodes are not inadvertently missed. Secondly, be attentive to the pelvic floor venous plexus and nerves (such as the sciatic nerve).

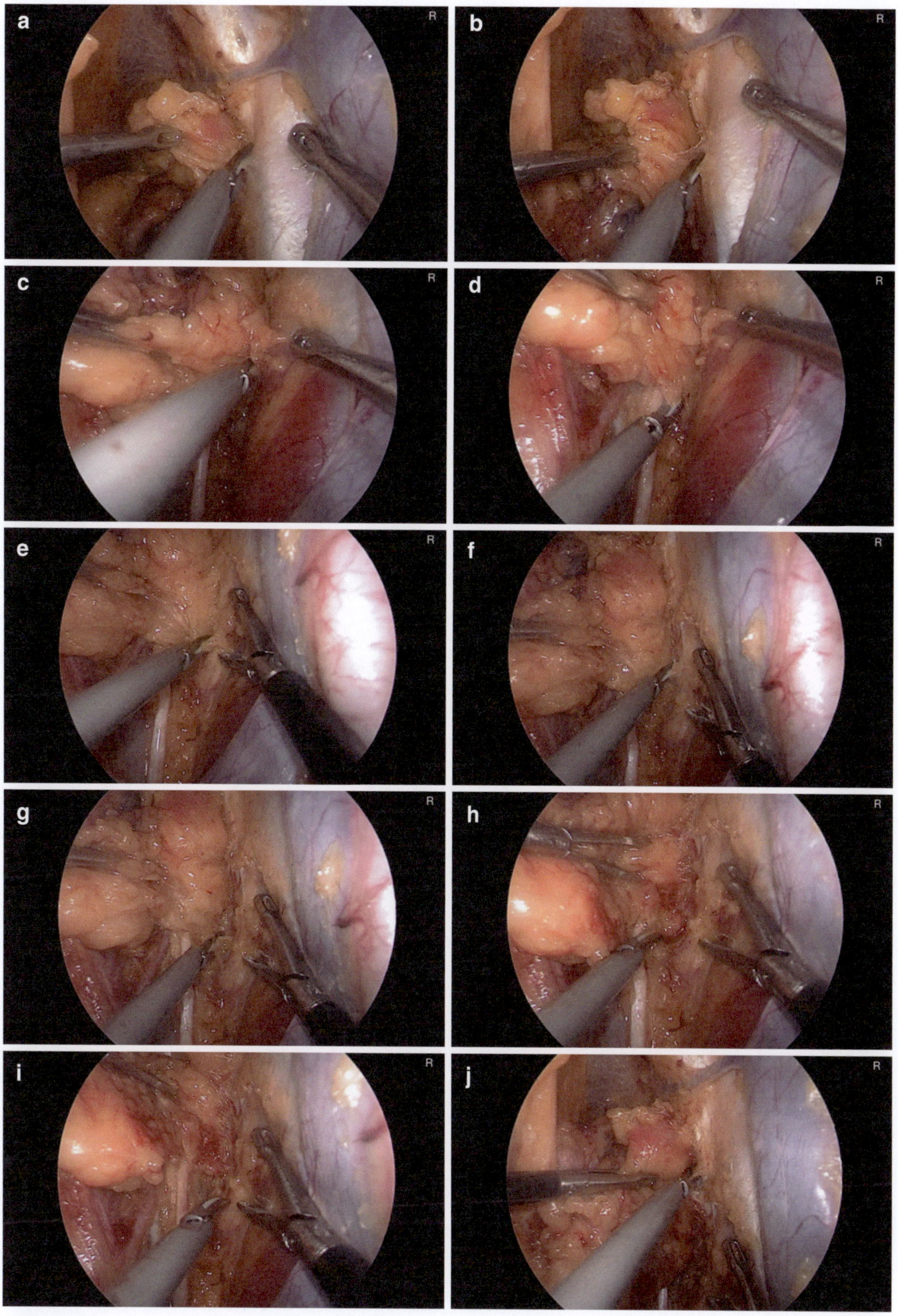

Fig. 14.39 (**a–l**) Dissect the interstitial space between the lymph nodes and the medial aspect of the psoas major muscle

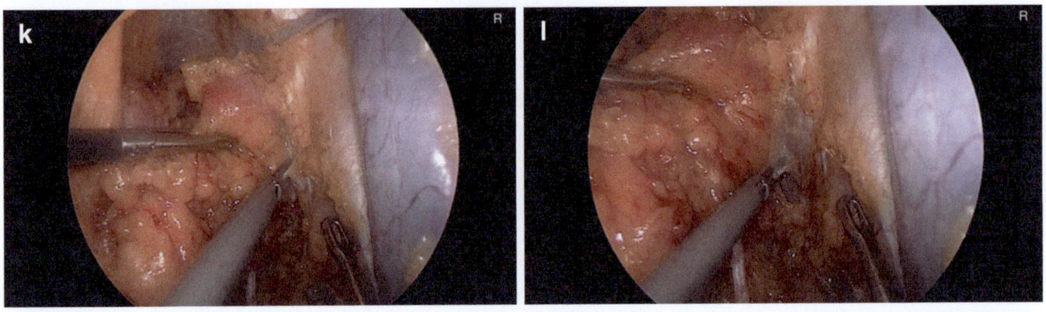

Fig. 14.39 (continued)

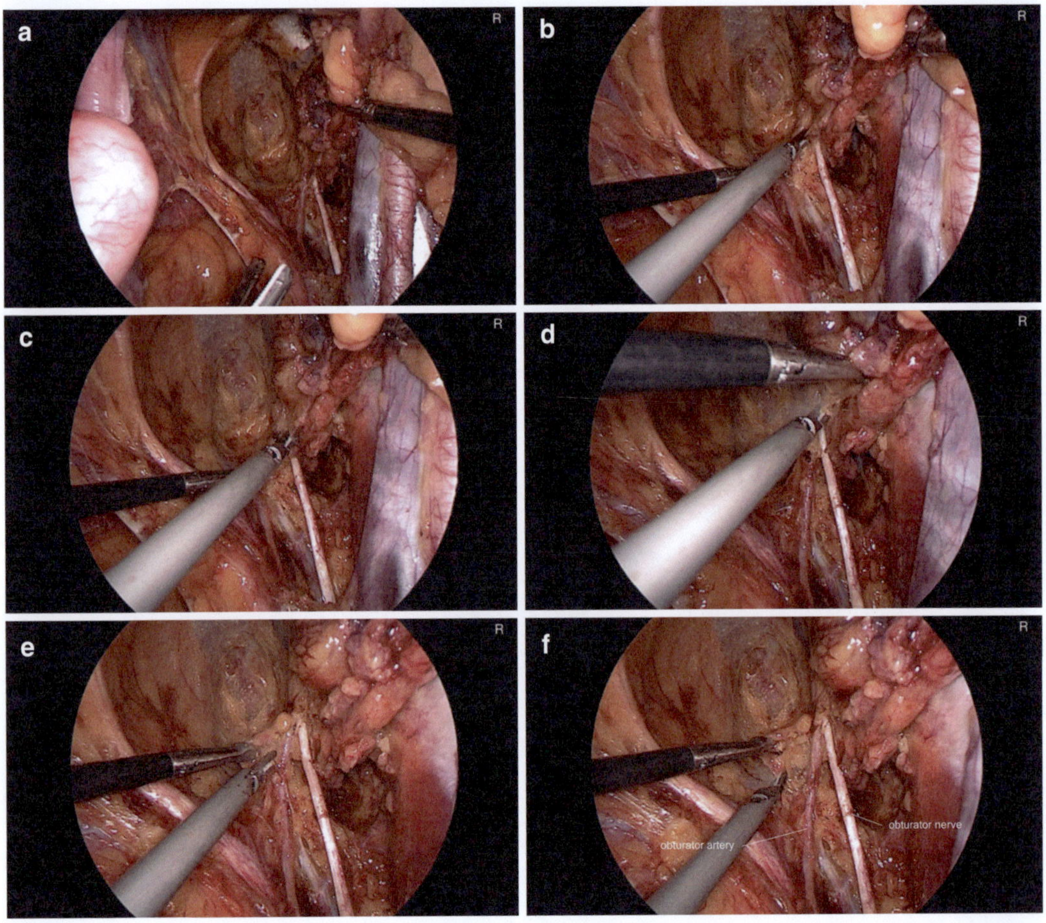

Fig. 14.40 (**a**–**f**) Dissect obturator nerves and blood vessels in the lymphatic adipose tissue gathered in the obturator space

14.10 Excision of Pelvic Lymph Nodes

At this point, all lymphatic adipose tissue converges around the obturator nerve and vasculature. Gently pull the lymphatic adipose tissue toward the ventral and lateral aspects, freeing the obturator nerve, arteries, and venous plexus from within. This concludes the excision of pelvic lymph nodes (Figs. 14.40, 14.41, 14.42, and 14.43).

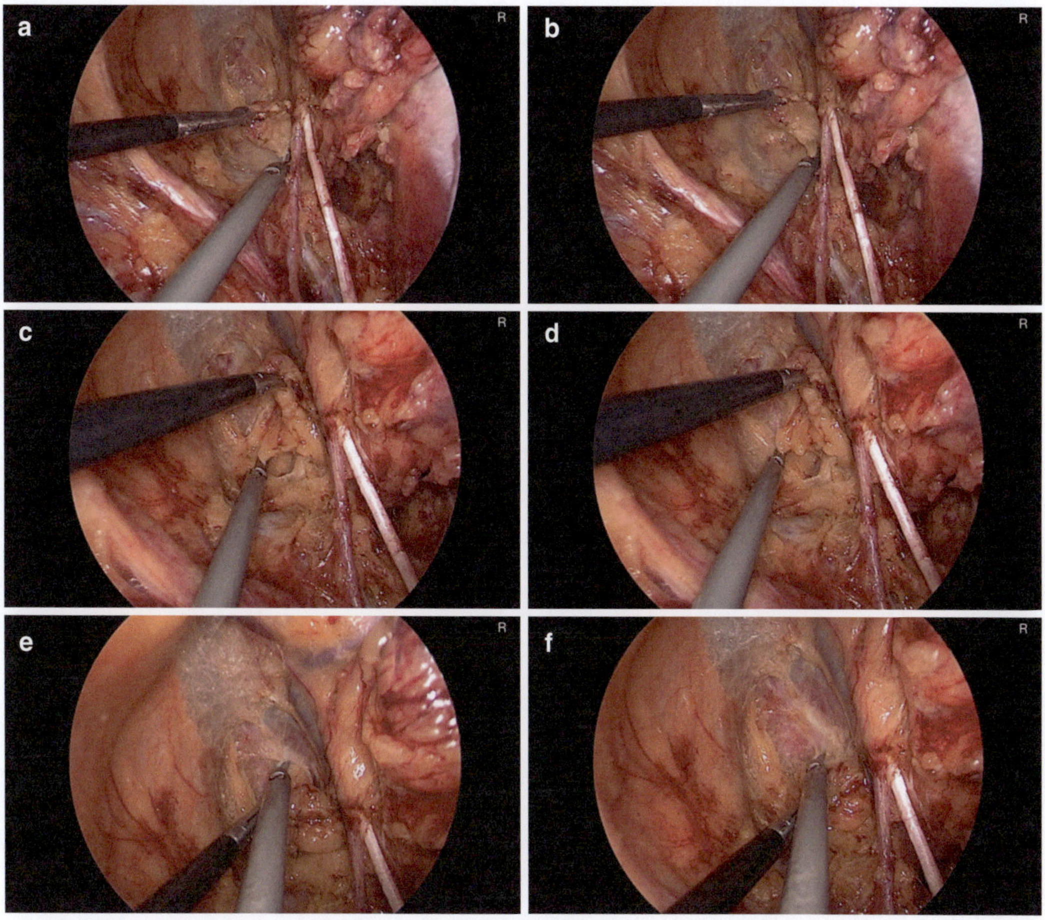

Fig. 14.41 (**a**–**f**) Separate lymphoid adipose tissue to pelvic floor fascia

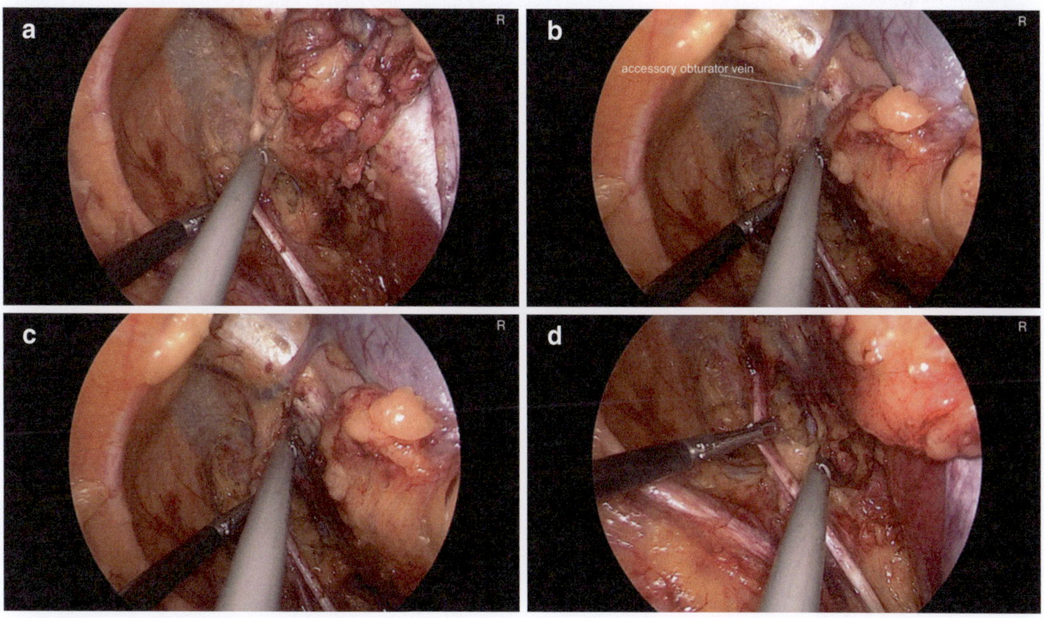

Fig. 14.42 (**a**–**d**) Dissect obturator vein

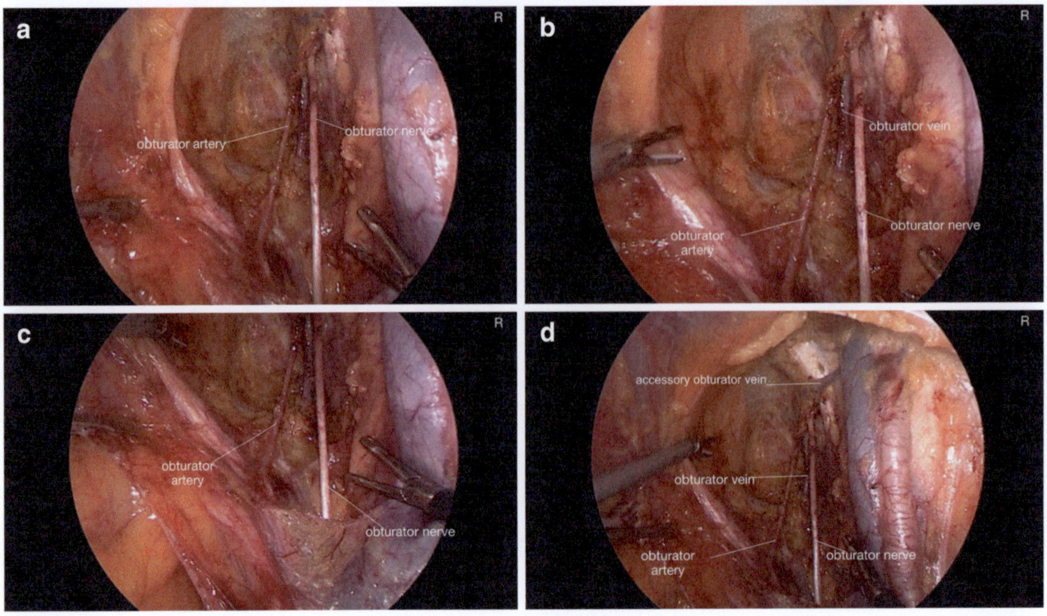

Fig. 14.43 (**a–d**) Presentation after complete resection of pelvic lymph nodes

Pelvic lymphadenectomy procedure can be found in Video 14.1.

References

1. NCCN. NCCN clinical practice guidelines in oncology—cervical cancer. (2022-12-23) [2023-03-15]. https://www.nccn.org/professionals/physician_gls/pdf/cervical.pdf
2. Cibula D, Abu-Rustum NR. Pelvic lymphadenectomy in cervical cancer—surgical anatomy and proposal for a new classification system. Gynecol Oncol. 2010;116:33–7.
3. Ramirez PT, Frumovitz M, Pareja R, et al. Minimally invasive versus abdominal radical hysterectomy for cervical cancer. N Engl J Med. 2018;379:1895–904.
4. Chinese Anti-Cancer Association Gynecological Tumor Professional Committee. 2022 Chinese expert consensus on fertility-sparing treatment of early-stage cervical cancer. Chin J Pract Gynecol Obstet. 2022;38(6):634–41. https://doi.org/10.19538/j.fk2022060114.

15 Parametrial Lymphadenectomy

Shichao Han and Ya Li

The distinction of Type B2 from Type B1 radical hysterectomy lies in the selective excision of parametrial lymph nodes. It is indicated for patients with Stage IA1 cervical cancer accompanied by lymphovascular invasion (+) or Stage IA2 patients. Parametrial lymph nodes mainly refer to the lymphatic adipose tissue within the parametrial region, spanning from the cervix to the pelvic lymph nodes. The lateral boundary of pelvic lymphadenectomy is the outer edge of the internal iliac artery. Consequently, parametrial lymph nodes primarily exist within the lateral aspect of the cervix and the medial aspect of the internal iliac artery, including the pelvic lymph nodes situated around the uterine artery, uterine veins, deep uterine veins, internal iliac artery, and internal iliac veins [1, 2].

15.1 Exposure of Parametrial Lymph Nodes

Parametrial lymph nodes refer to the lymphatic adipose tissue located between the parametrial vessels. This specifically involves the lymphatic adipose tissue situated on the lateral aspects of the cervix. As a result, the initial step involves exposing the lateral parametrial region. By gently retracting the ureter medially and the internal iliac artery laterally, a precise separation is conducted using an ultrasonic scalpel to reveal the space between these structures. Over time, this process gradually exposes the Latzko's pararectal space and the paravesical space (Figs. 15.1 and 15.2).

Supplementary Information The online version contains supplementary material available at https://doi.org/10.1007/978-981-97-7687-0_15.

S. Han (✉) · Y. Li
Department of Gynecology and Obstetrics, Second Affiliated Hospital of Dalian Medical University, Dalian, China

S. Han, J. Wang (eds.), *Open, Laparoscopic, and Robotic Surgery for Cervical Cancer*, https://doi.org/10.1007/978-981-97-7687-0_15

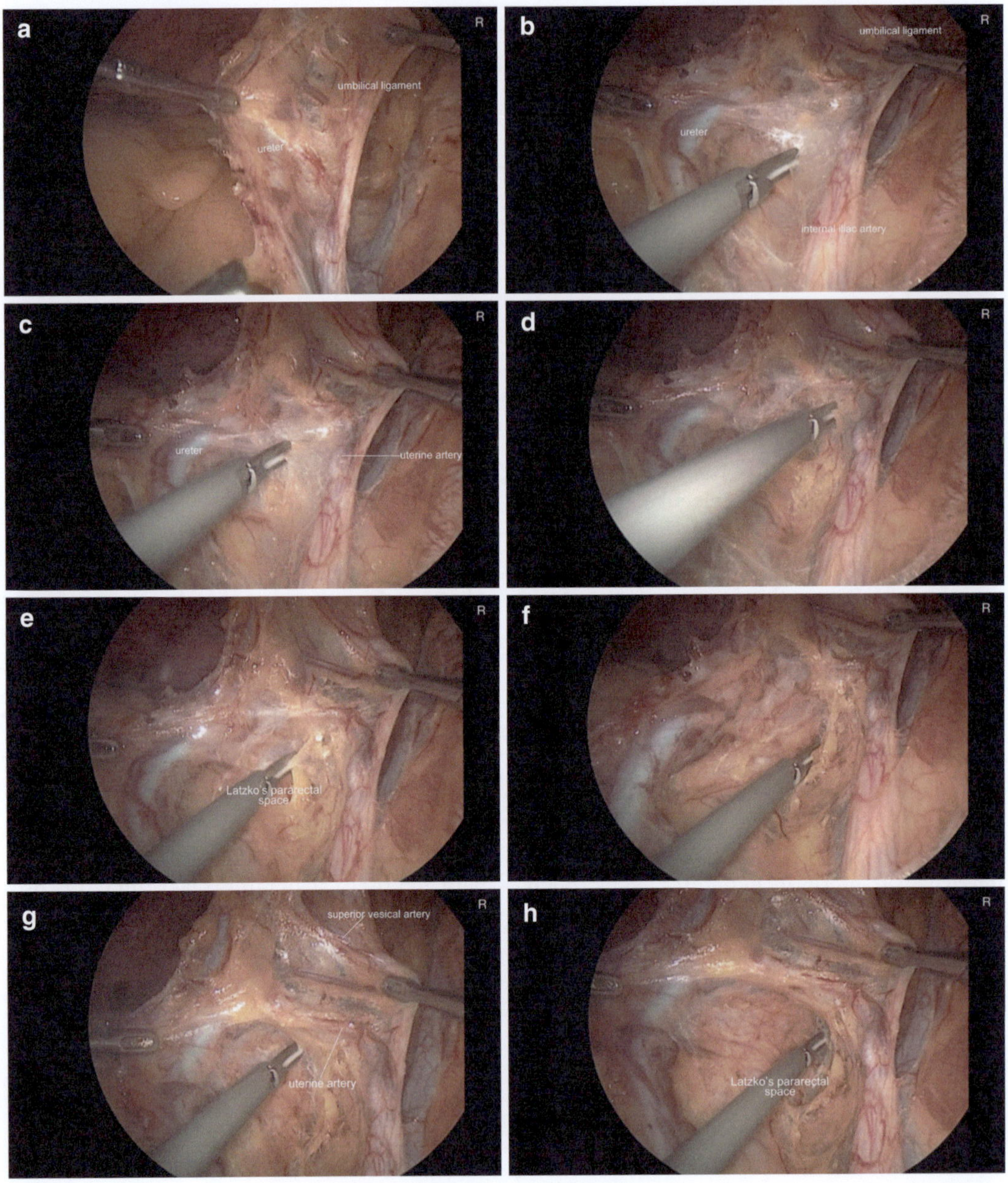

Fig. 15.1 (**a**–**h**) Separate the Latzko's pararectal space

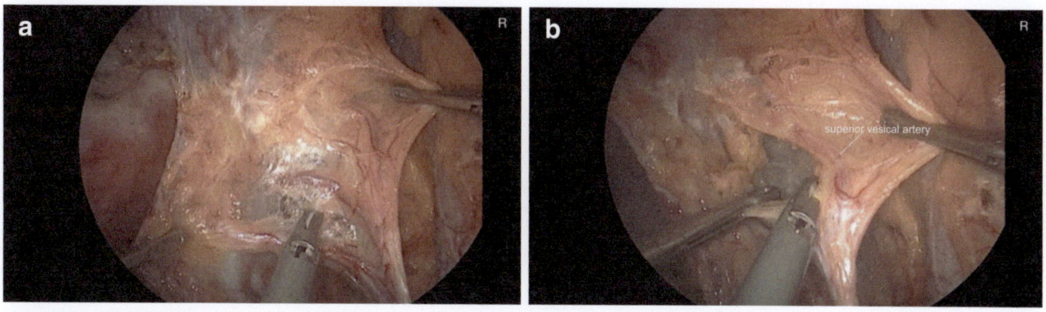

Fig. 15.2 (**a**, **b**) Separate the paravesical space

15.2 Dissecting and Excising Lymph Nodes Within the "Latzko's Pararectal Space" Along the Medial Side of the Internal Iliac Artery and Vein

Starting from the origin of the internal iliac artery and vein, carefully and progressively dissect and excise the lymph nodes on their medial surfaces, moving toward the dorsal and caudal sides. This process requires extreme caution, as rupture and bleeding of the internal iliac vein can lead to catastrophic complications, often necessitating open surgery for vascular repair. In handling the lymphatic adipose tissue in this region, our team practices thorough dissection of the space between the rectal sidewall and the internal iliac vein to adequately expose the internal iliac vein. Simultaneously, an assistant retracts the internal iliac artery laterally to provide sufficient tension (Fig. 15.3a–j).

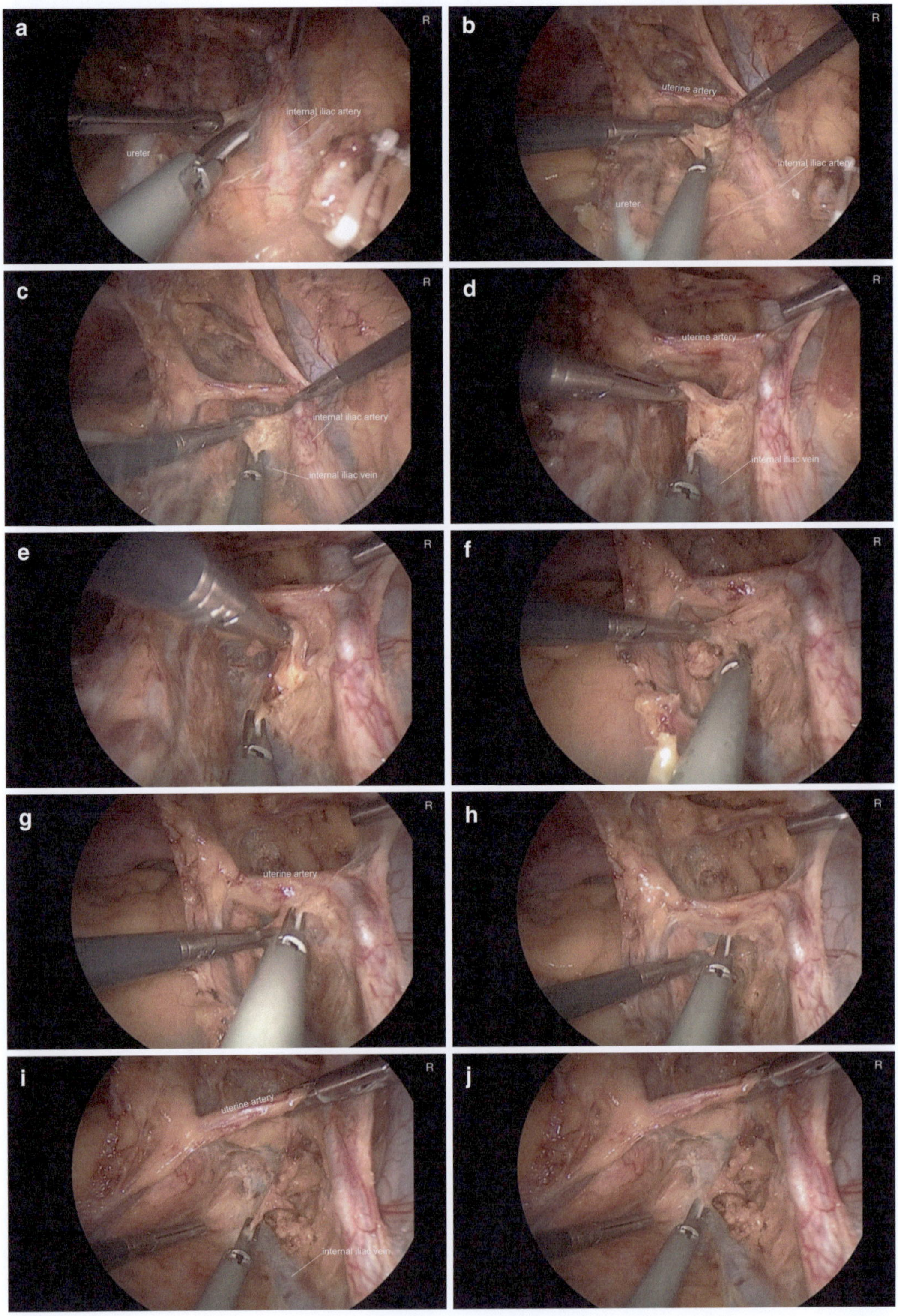

Fig. 15.3 (**a**–**j**) Dissect lymph nodes along the medial surface of the internal iliac artery and vein, from the cranial aspect to the caudal aspect

15.3 Exposure of the Deep Uterine Vein

Gently retract the internal iliac artery laterally, and pull the ureter and lateral peritoneum medially to fully expose the Latzko's pararectal space. Carefully dissect the area adjacent to the internal iliac vein in a caudal direction, gradually revealing the deep uterine vein (Figs. 15.4, 15.5, 15.6, and 15.7).

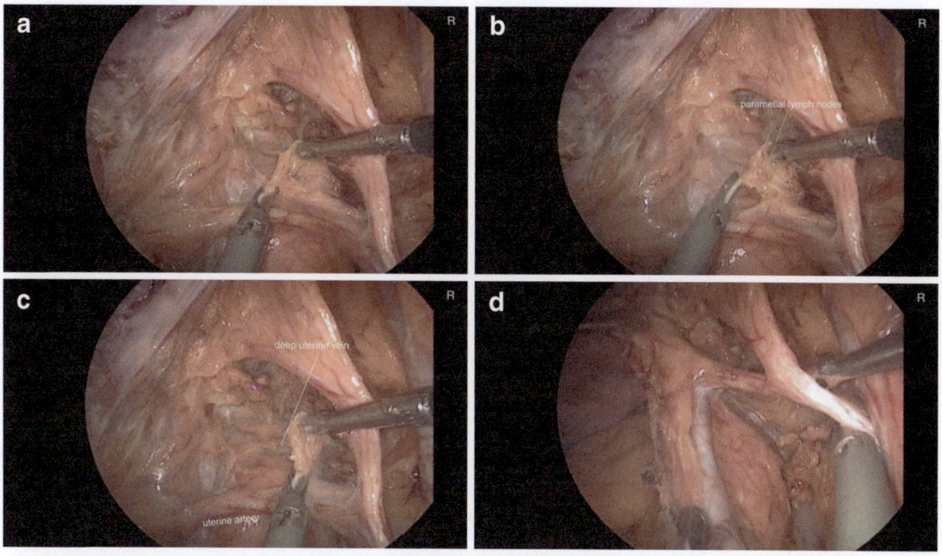

Fig. 15.4 (**a**–**d**) Dissect the uterine artery

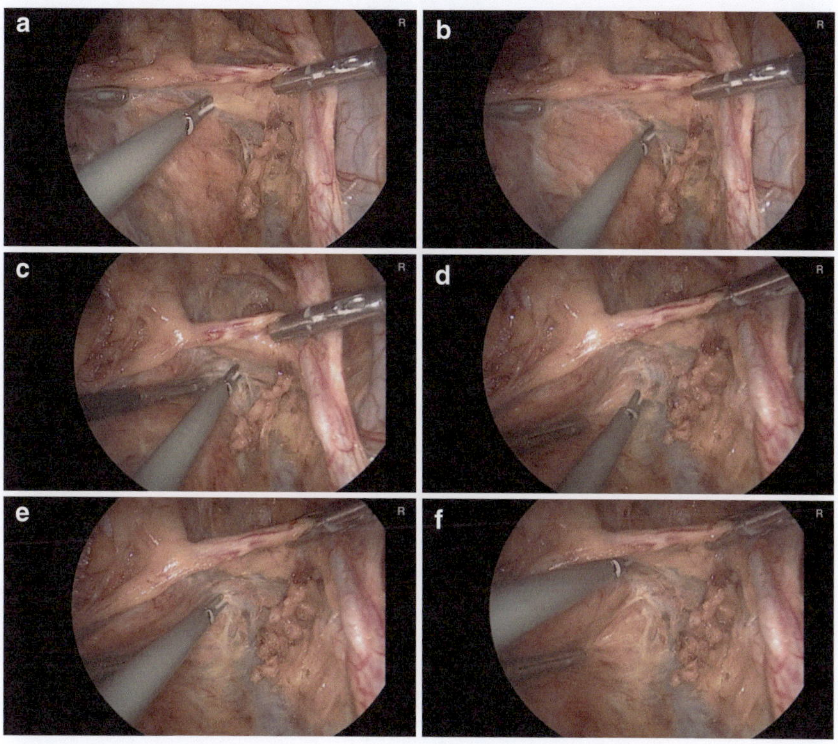

Fig. 15.5 (**a**–**f**) Expose the deep uterine vein

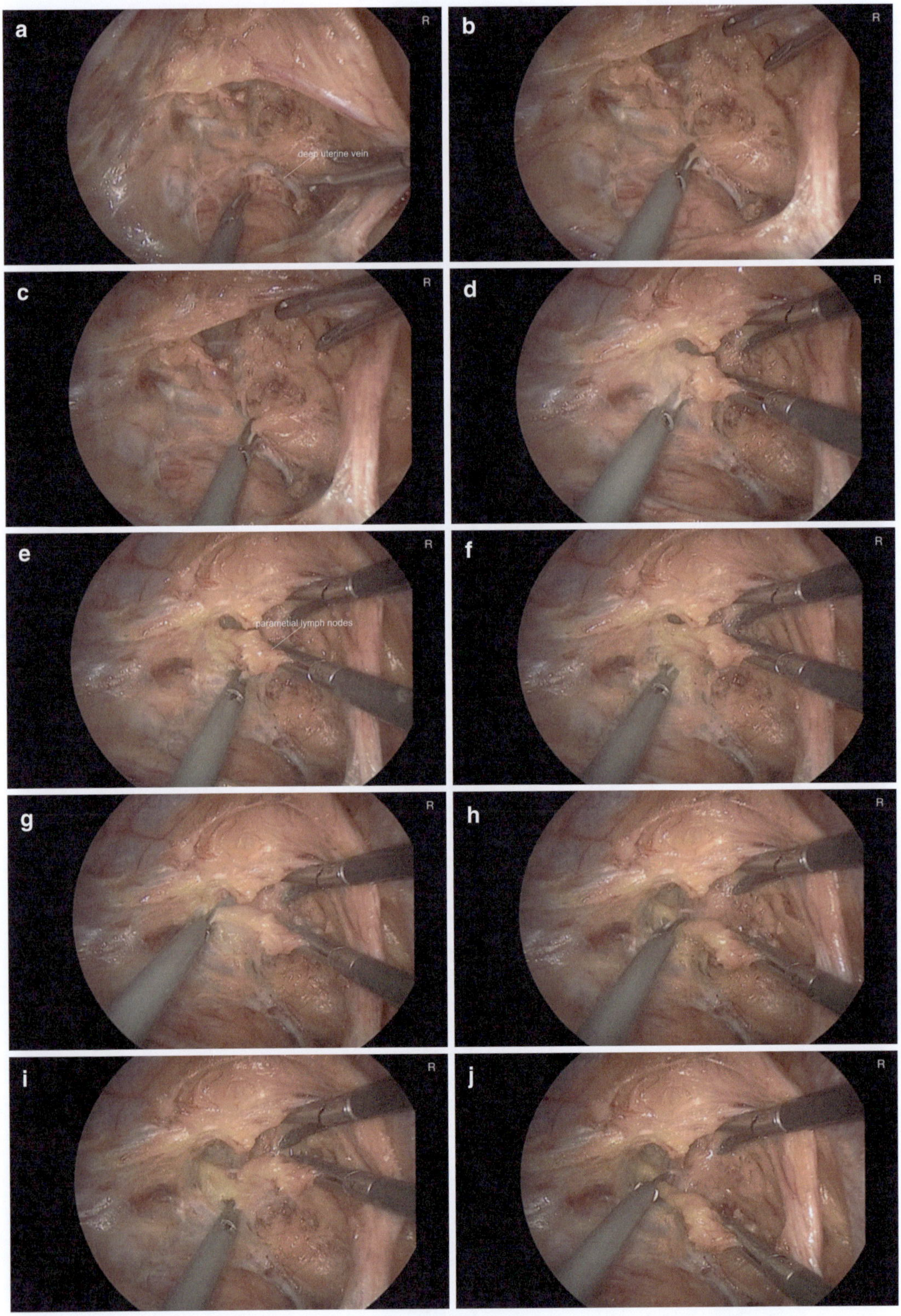

Fig. 15.6 (**a**–**j**) Dissect closely to the deep uterine vein, freeing the space between the lateral peritoneum and the lymphatic adipose tissue

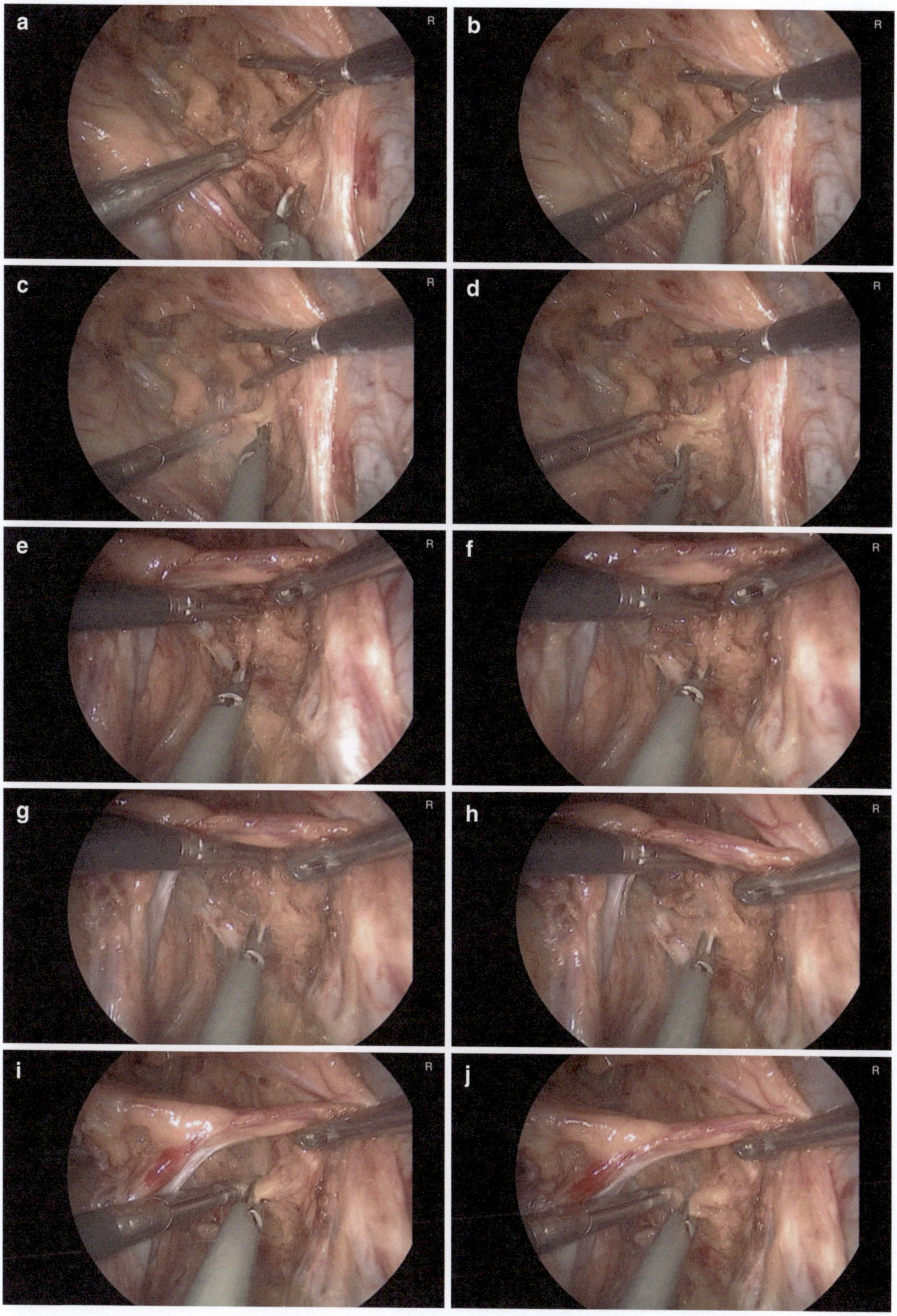

Fig. 15.7 (**a**–**j**) Dissect closely to the deep uterine vein, freeing the lymphatic adipose tissue on the medial side of the internal iliac artery

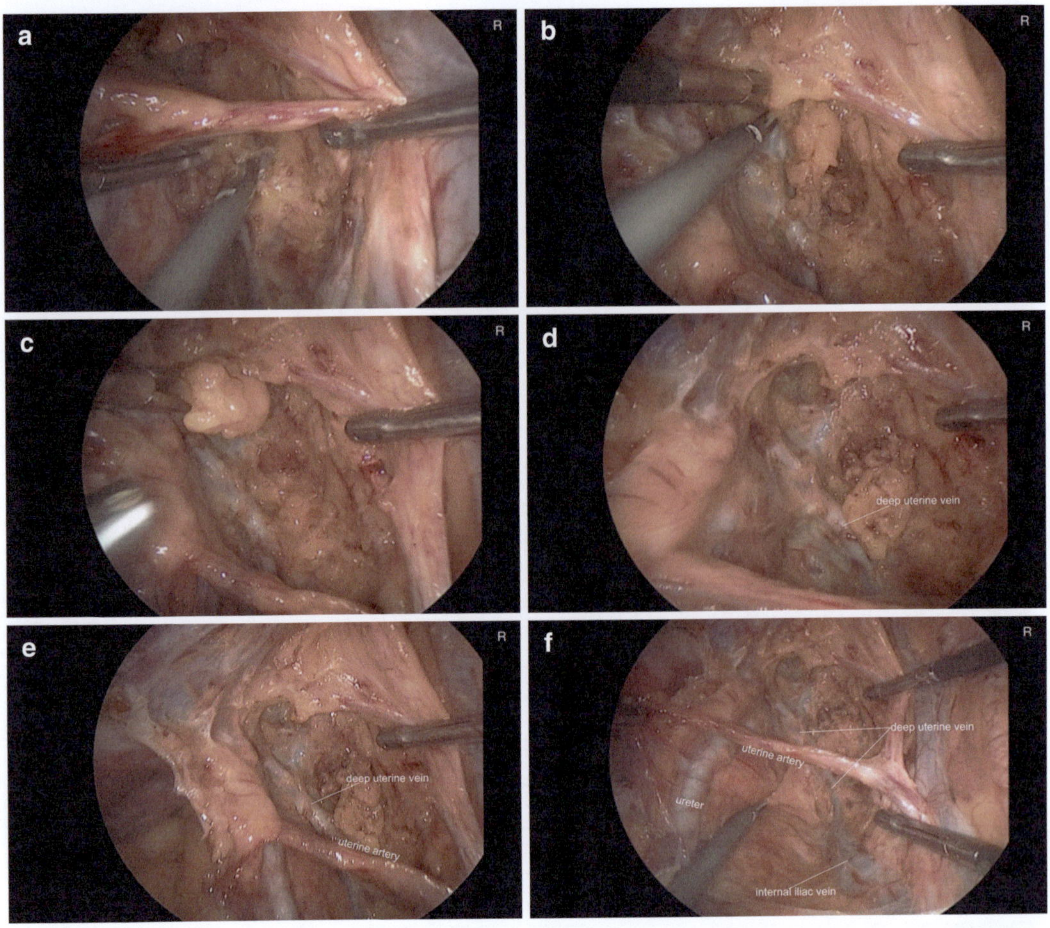

Fig. 15.8 (**a**–**f**) Dissect the deep uterine vein, en bloc resection of parametrial lymph nodes

15.4 En Bloc Resection of Parametrial Lymph Nodes

Carefully follow the inferior edge of the uterine artery to progressively dissect the lymph nodes on its posterior aspect until reaching the surface of the deep uterine vein. Simultaneously, closely adhere to the surface of the deep uterine vein to excise the parametrial lymph nodes as a whole.

In the excision process of B2-type parametrial lymph nodes, the lymphatic adipose tissue is removed after separating the blood vessels and lymphatic adipose tissue of the parametrial region. Our team believes that this procedure deviates from en bloc resection of the tumor. Therefore, in clinical practice, our team typically opts for a simplified C1-type procedure for B2-type surgeries (Fig. 15.8a–f).

Parametrial lymphadenectomy procedure is demonstrated in Video 15.1.

References

1. NCCN. NCCN clinical practice guidelines in oncology—cervical cancer. (2022-12-23) [2023-03-15]. https://www.nccn.org/professionals/physician_gls/pdf/cervical.pdf
2. Cibula D, Abu-Rustum NR. Pelvic lymphadenectomy in cervical cancer—surgical anatomy and proposal for a new classification system. Gynecol Oncol. 2010;116:33–7.

Lymphadenectomy of the Abdominal Aortic Region

16

Shichao Han and Xinyou Wang

Para-aortic lymph node assessment research investigating the frequency and pattern of lymph node metastases in individuals diagnosed with stage IB to IIB cervical cancers indicates a strong correlation between para-aortic lymph node engagement and the presence of metastases in pelvic lymph nodes, as well as larger primary tumor size (>2 cm) and involvement of the common iliac nodes [1, 2].

The methods of lymphadenectomy in this region primarily consist of the antegrade (from cranial to caudal) approach and the retrograde (from caudal to cranial) approach. In our team's experience with the antegrade approach, especially during lymphadenectomy in the upper abdominal aortic region, an important observation is that the ultrasonic scalpel and the blood vessels are oriented perpendicular (given that our team comprises right-handed surgeons, performing left-handed ultrasonic scalpel lymphadenectomy is not feasible). This setup often creates a feeling of vertically cutting the vessels, inducing a significant sense of insecurity. Consequently, our team opts for the retrograde approach when performing lymphadenectomy in the upper abdominal aortic region.

Supplementary Information The online version contains supplementary material available at https://doi.org/10.1007/978-981-97-7687-0_16.

S. Han (✉) · X. Wang
Department of Gynecology and Obstetrics, Second Affiliated Hospital of Dalian Medical University, Dalian, China

16.1 Patient Positioning

The patient is placed in a head-down position, generally at an inclination of 15°–30° (depending on the patient's body mass index). It is not recommended to position the head too low, as excessive head lowering can create a sense of excessive depth of the surgical field during the procedure. This can result in discomfort within the field of vision, necessitating an overly deep insertion of the laparoscope into the abdominal cavity. However, this can also increase the likelihood of instrument and laparoscope collisions.

16.2 Elevation of the Intestine

Arrangement of the intestinal loops to expose the peritoneum of the abdominal aortic region.

16.3 Exposure of the Abdominal Aorta, Inferior Vena Cava, and Duodenum

Gently manipulating the intestinal loops toward the cranial and ventral directions exposes the peritoneum covering the abdominal aorta region (Fig. 16.1). Employing a sharp technique with the ultrasonic scalpel, initiate separation and incision from the caudal-to-cranial direction, ensuring careful identification of the

S. Han, J. Wang (eds.), *Open, Laparoscopic, and Robotic Surgery for Cervical Cancer*,
https://doi.org/10.1007/978-981-97-7687-0_16

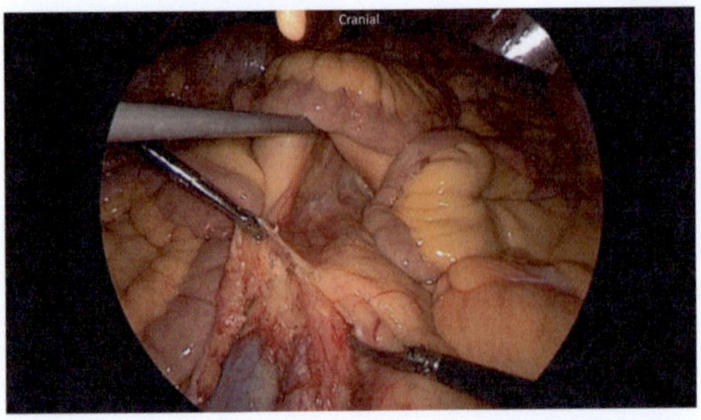

Fig. 16.1 Gently manipulating the intestinal loops toward the cranial and ventral directions exposes the peritoneum covering the abdominal aorta region

duodenum throughout the process. Continue the separation until reaching the vicinity of the duodenum crossing over the abdominal aorta and the inferior vena cava (Figs. 16.2a–j and 16.3a–e). The left renal vein lies cranially at this level. At this point, our team prefers to initially dissect the right peritoneum away from the inferior vena cava (Fig. 16.4a–d), fully exposing the course of the inferior vena cava. This lays the foundation for subsequent suspension of the right peritoneum. During the dissection, meticulous attention should be paid to identifying and locating the right ureter to prevent inadvertent injury.

The left renal vein is located cranially at this level. Our team prefers to initially separate the right side of the peritoneum from the inferior vena cava (see Fig. 16.4a–d), fully exposing the course of the inferior vena cava and establishing a foundation for the subsequent suspension of the right side of the peritoneum. During the dissection, it is important to identify and locate the right ureter to avoid inadvertent injury.

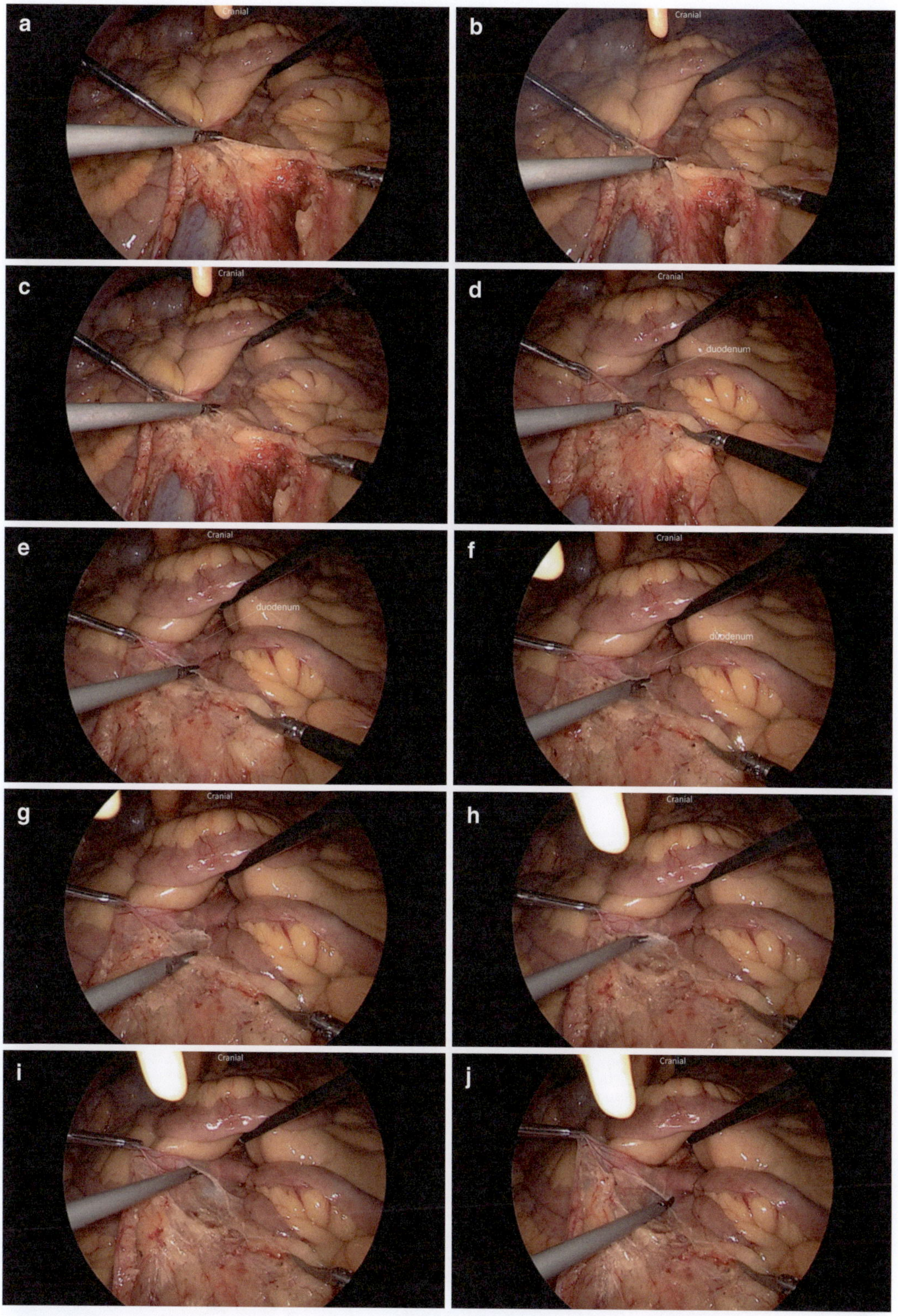

Fig. 16.2 (**a**–**j**) Sharp opening of the main abdominal area peritoneum to the duodenum across the abdominal aorta and adjacent to the inferior vena cava

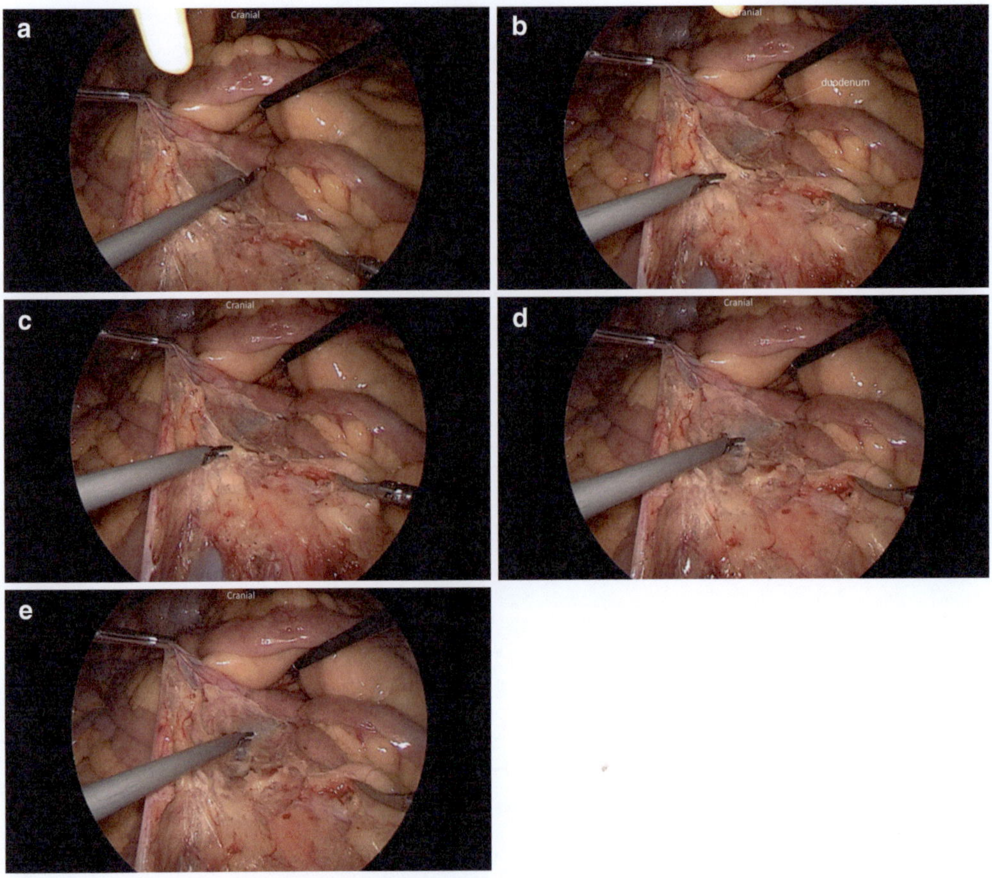

Fig. 16.3 (**a**–**e**) Identify and separate the duodenum

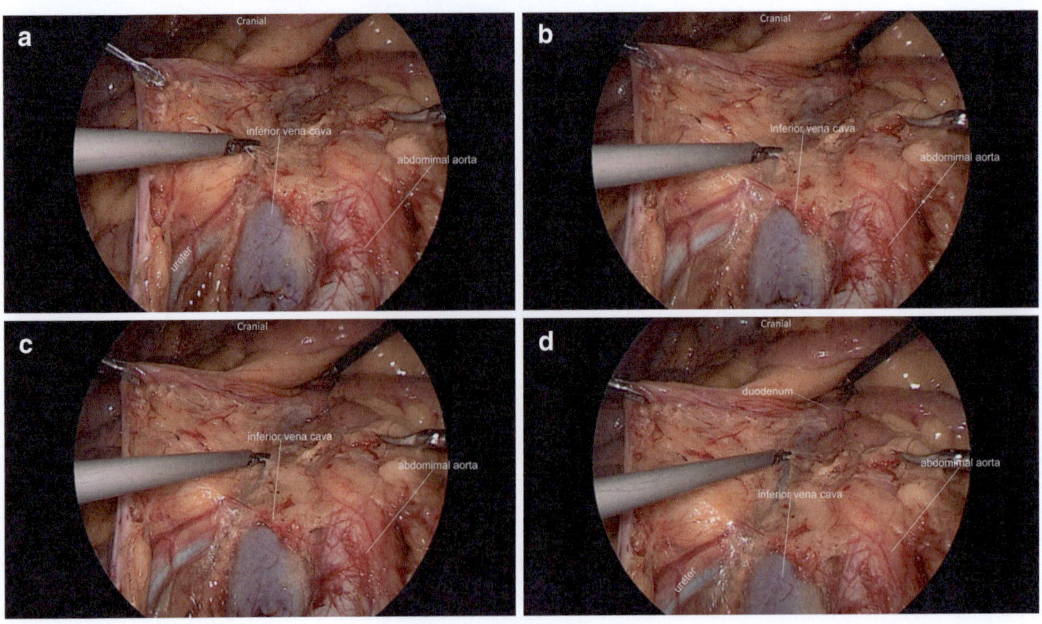

Fig. 16.4 (**a**–**d**) Separate the space between the right peritoneum and inferior vena cava

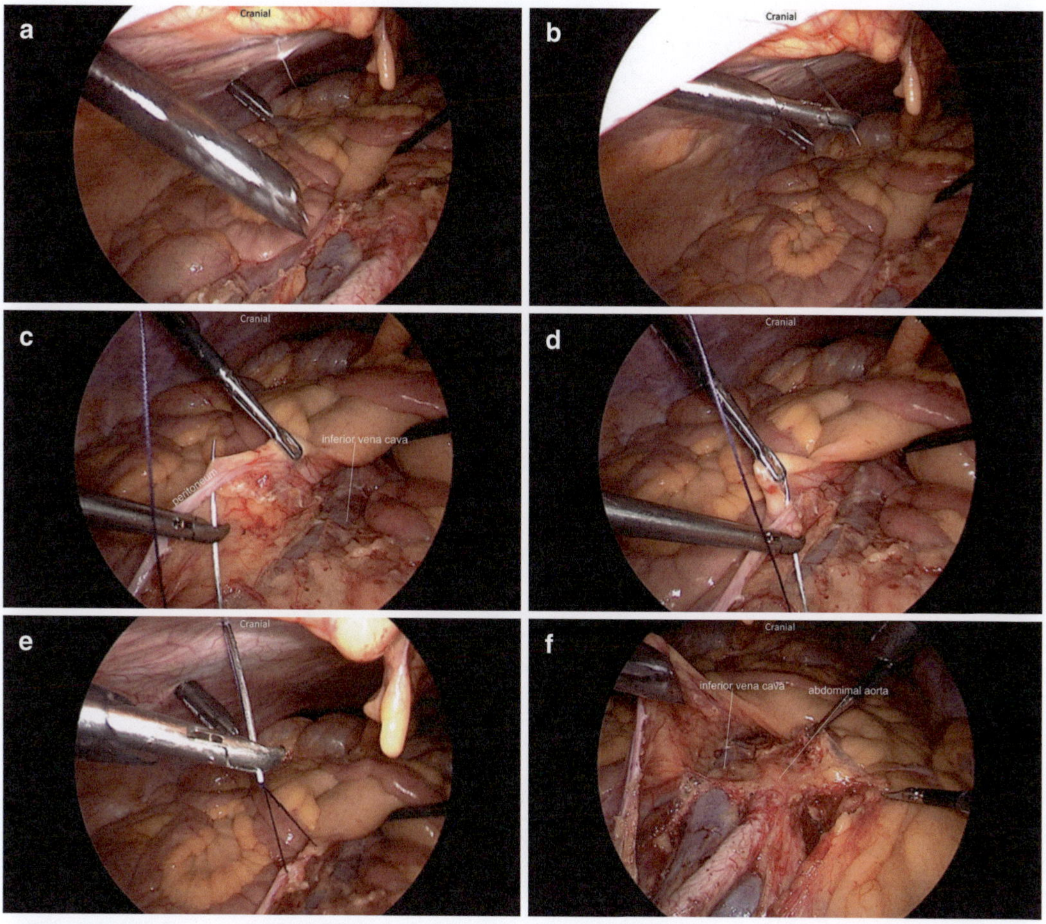

Fig. 16.5 (a–f) Suspend right peritoneum

16.4 Suspension of the Right Peritoneum

Using absorbable 1-0 suture, insert the needle through the abdominal wall, situated between the two puncture holes on the right side, thereby gaining access to the abdominal cavity. After suturing the right peritoneum, guide the needle from within the abdominal cavity back through the abdominal wall, gently applying tension to the peritoneum. Securely anchor the suture to the abdominal wall, ensuring strong fixation, while concurrently maintaining appropriate tension on the peritoneum (Fig. 16.5a–f).

16.5 Exposure of the Right Ovarian Artery, Ovarian Vein, and Left Renal Vein

Gently elevating the intestinal loop ventrally, sharply dissect along the space between the inferior vena cava and the mesentery in a caudal-to-cranial direction (Fig. 16.6a–j). As the dissection progresses, the right ovarian artery may become visible (depending on its size, if the artery is substantial, vascular clamps can be utilized for occlusion; if delicate, an ultrasonic scalpel can be employed for coagulation and division). When the dissection reaches the level

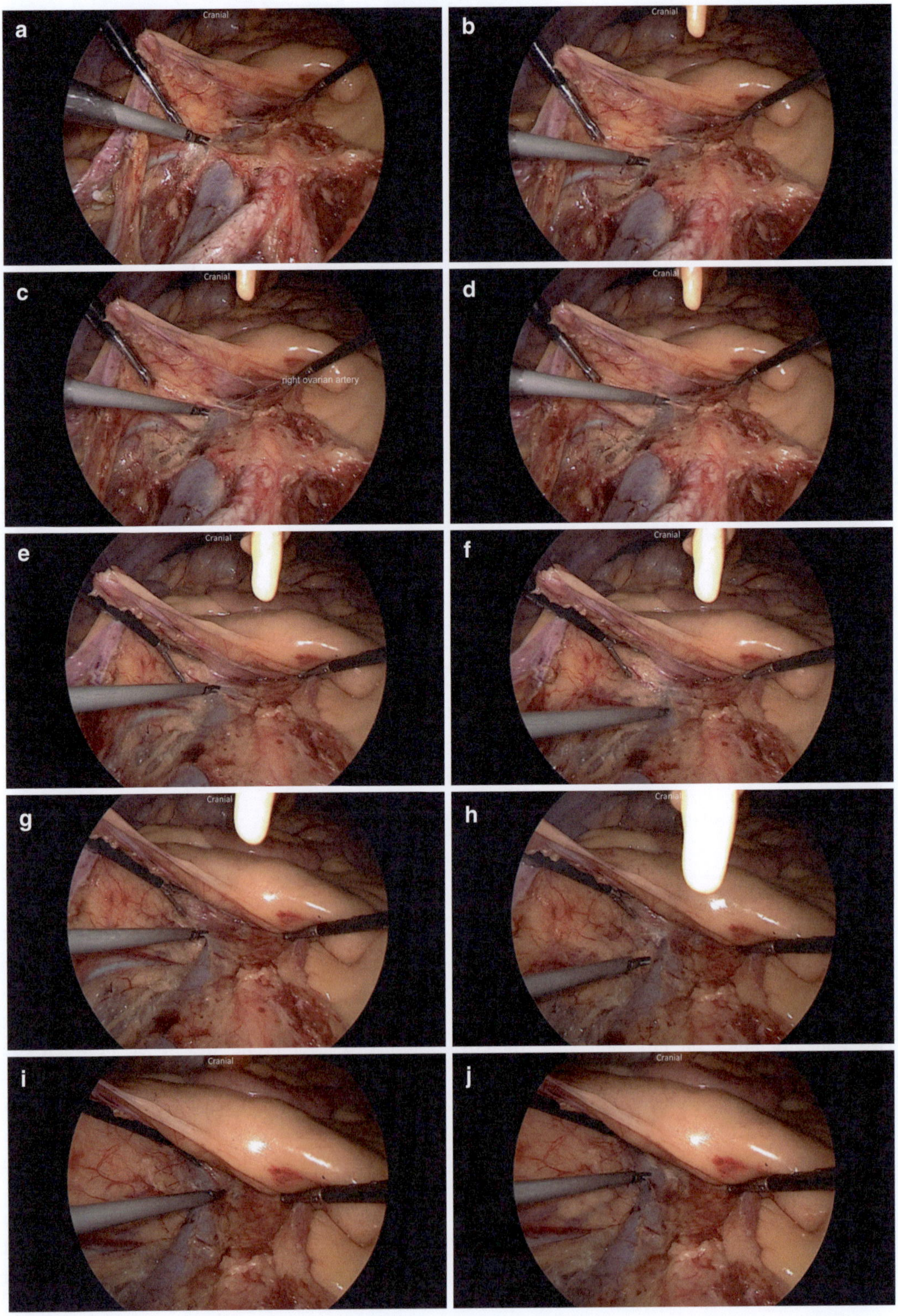

Fig. 16.6 (**a**–**j**) Sharply dissect along the space between the inferior vena cava and the mesentery in a caudal-to-cranial direction

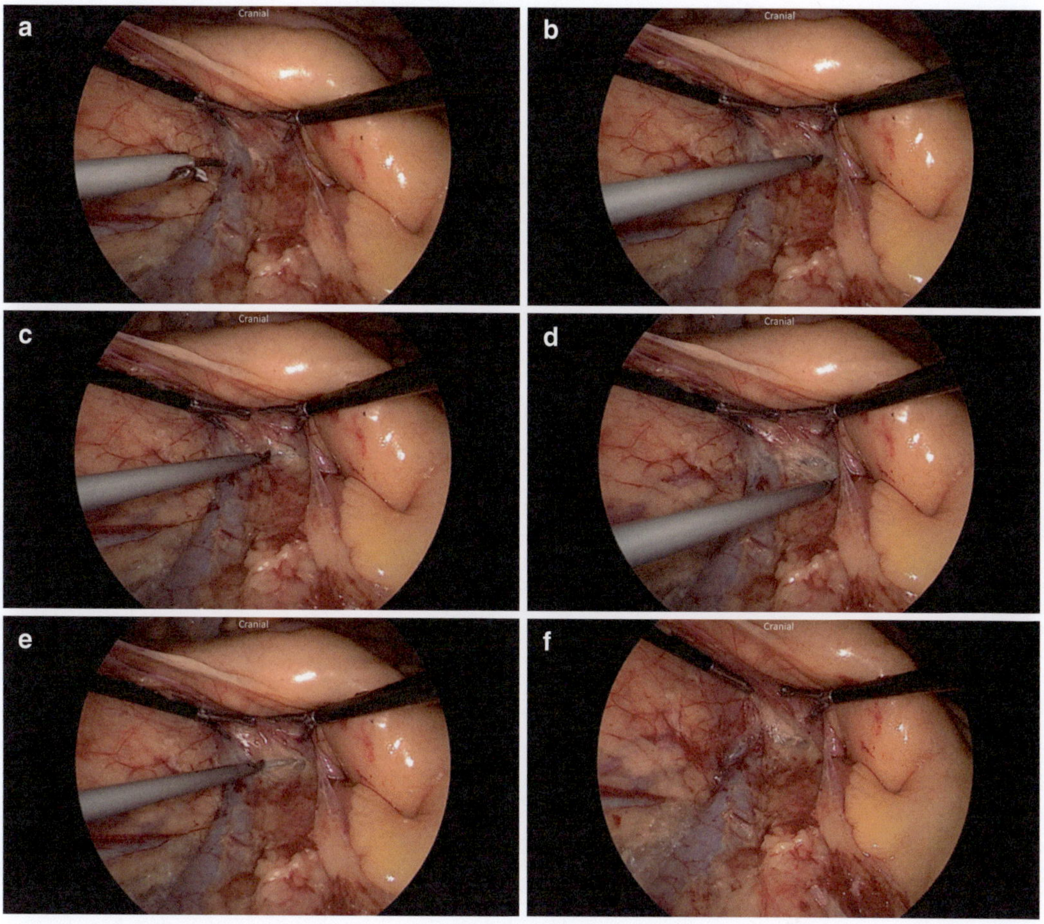

Fig. 16.7 (**a–f**) Separate the inferior vena cava and duodenal space

of the duodenum, it becomes crucial to gently elevate the duodenum ventrally using atraumatic forceps, which exposes the space beneath it situated between the inferior vena cava and the abdominal aorta. Following this, a meticulous separation is executed using the ultrasonic scalpel (Fig. 16.7a–f). As part of this process, our team's approach involves initially dissecting the space between the inferior vena cava and the duodenum. This strategy stems from the observation that lymph nodes are seldom located on the cranial aspect of the right ovarian vessels. Consequently, the dissection of the inferior vena cava in this particular region tends to be comparatively straightforward. Moreover, the left renal vein converges with the inferior vena cava, which simplifies its recognition upon separation from the vessel's surface. After exposing the left renal vein, careful adherence to its surface is performed (Fig. 16.8a–f), guaranteeing a comprehensive outline of its trajectory (Fig. 16.9a–h). This systematic dissection enhances accurate anatomical orientation for the following lymph node excision.

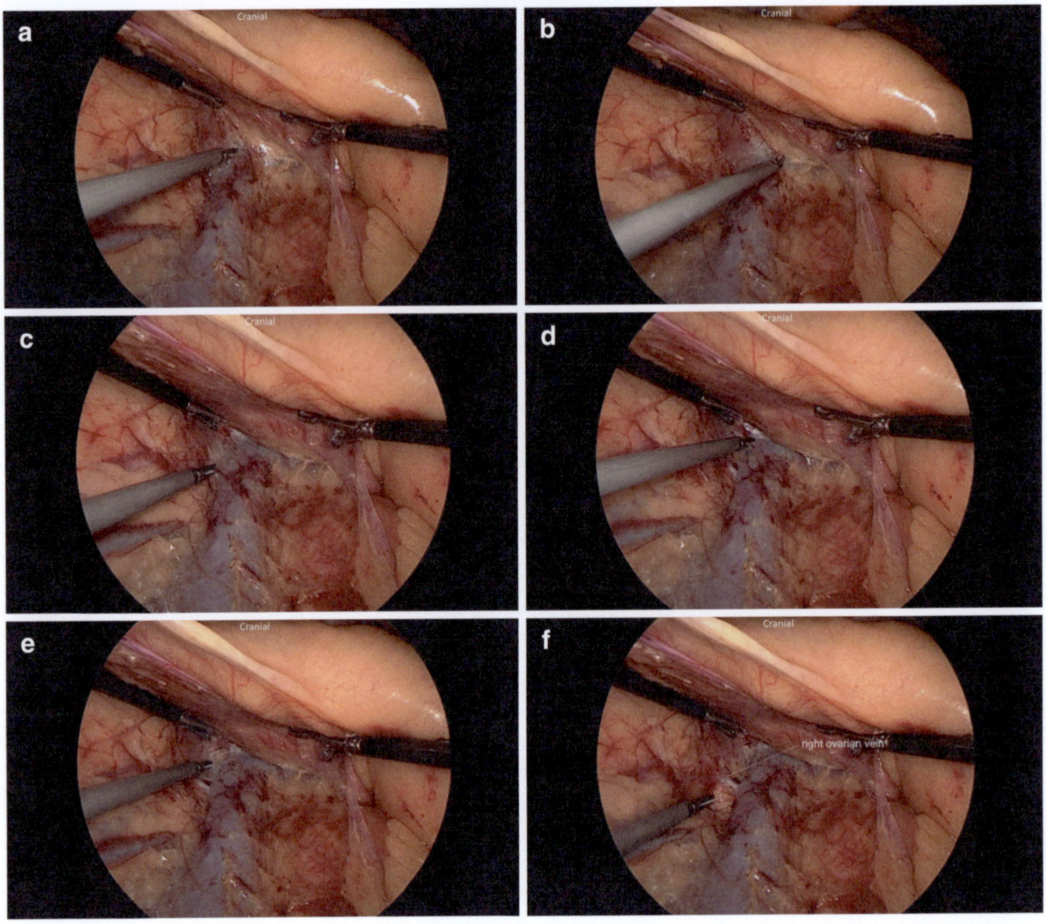

Fig. 16.8 (**a**–**f**) Separate and expose the left renal vein

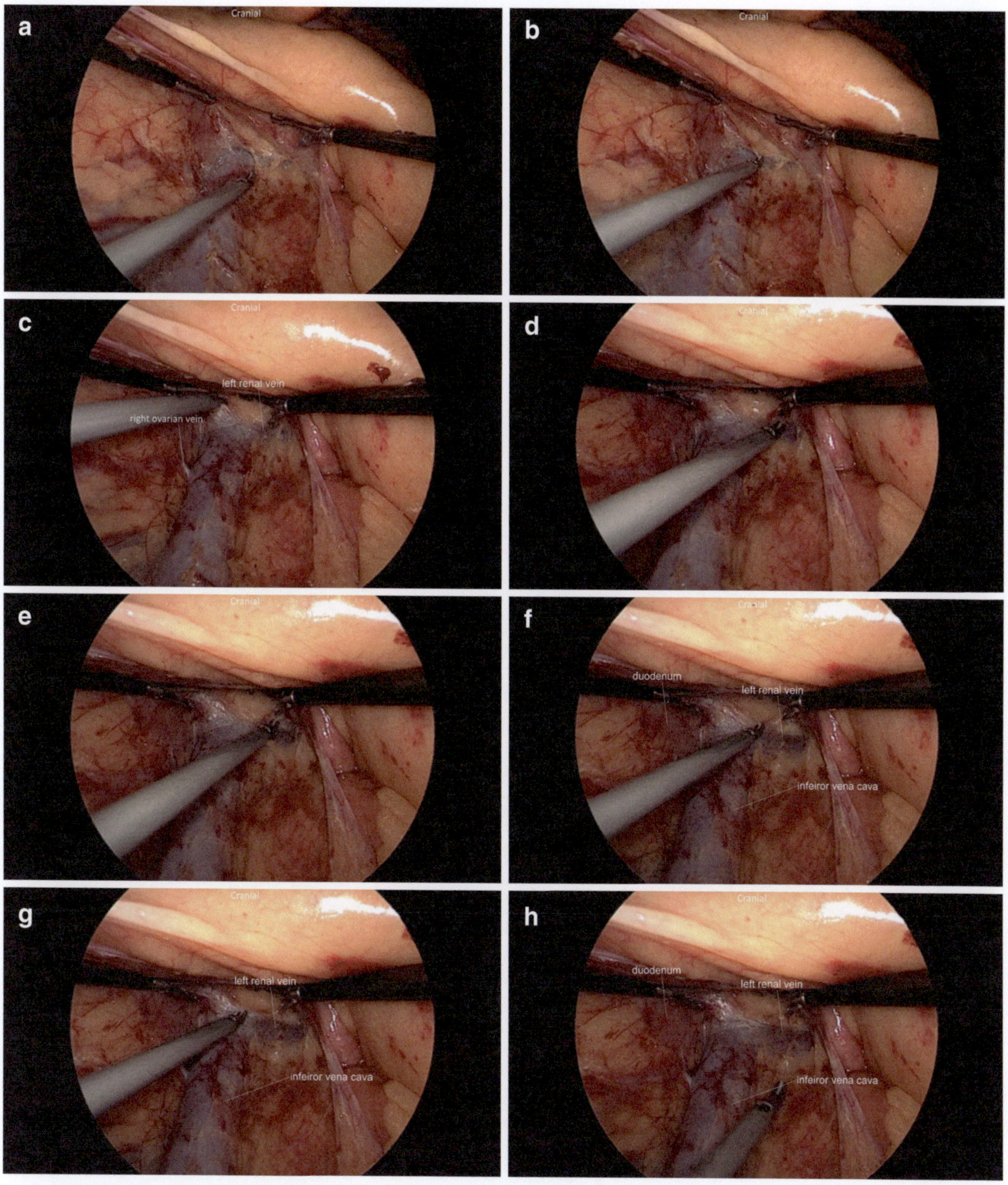

Fig. 16.9 (**a–h**) Expose comprehensive outline of the left renal vein trajectory

16.6 Excision/Detachment of Lymph Nodes from the Surface of the Inferior Vena Cava

Following the principle of en bloc resection, our team performs lymph node excision as a whole. The initial step involves the detachment of lymph nodes from the surface of the inferior vena cava, converging them between the inferior vena cava and the abdominal aorta. During this process, venous tributaries draining from the lymph nodes into the inferior vena cava may be encountered. Handling them with extreme care is crucial to prevent inadvertent tearing and bleeding, as forceful manipulation of the lymph nodes can lead to vascular rupture and bleeding. Hemorrhage management can pose challenges, often necessitating vascular suturing to repair the inferior vena cava in case of bleeding. Typically, these venous tributaries can be safely coagulated and divided using the ultrasonic scalpel after careful separation. If a substantial tributary is encountered, vascular clamps can be contemplated for permanent occlusion (Fig. 16.10a–i).

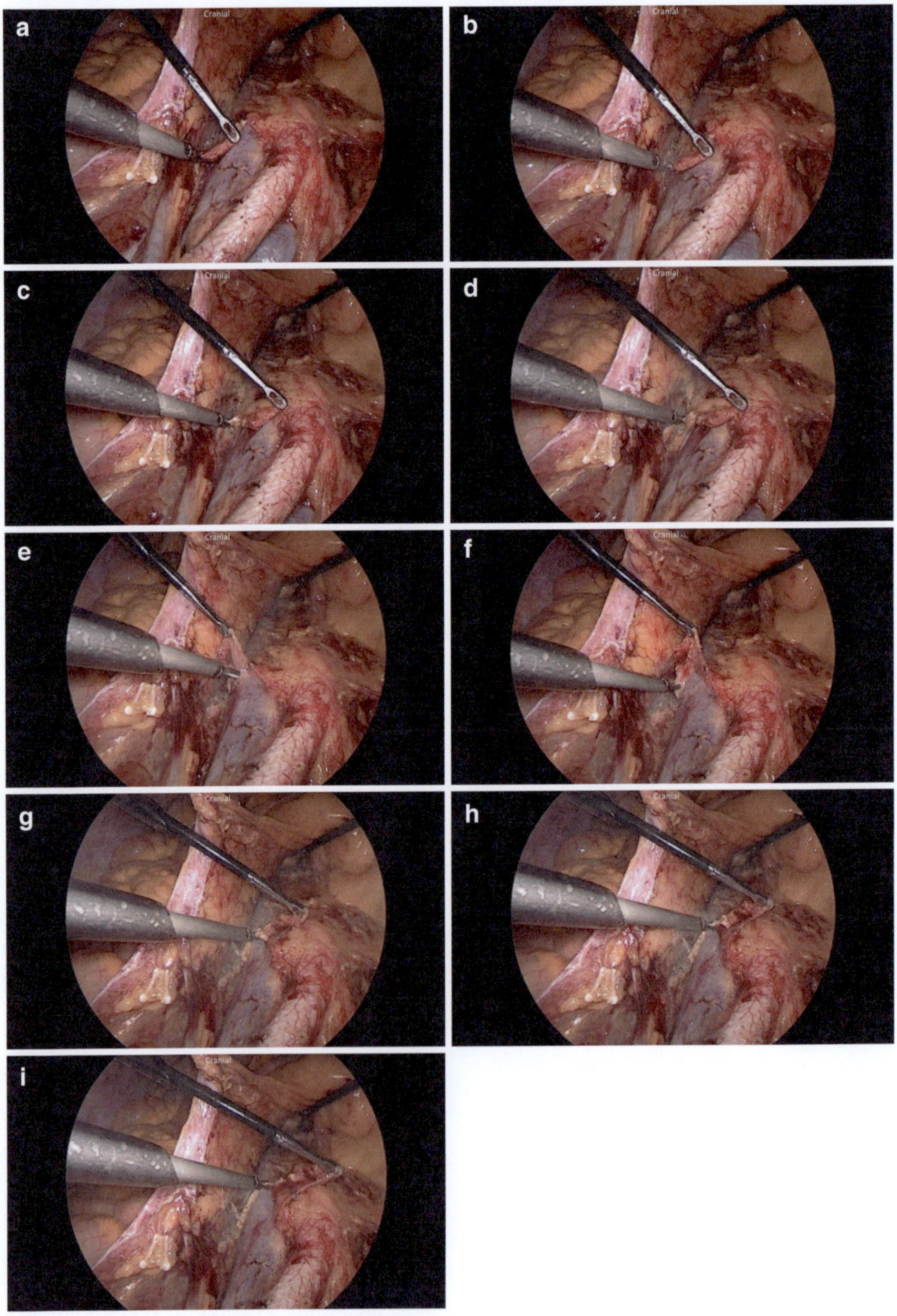

Fig. 16.10 (**a**–**i**) Excise superficial lymph nodes of inferior vena cava

16.7 Detachment of Lymph Nodes in the Area Between the Inferior Vena Cava and the Abdominal Aorta

Gently elevating the lymph nodes toward the left and ventral side, employ the ultrasonic scalpel for precise separation of the lymph node tissue in this area (Fig. 16.11a–c). Continue the dissection from the caudal-to-cranial direction until reaching the vicinity of the lower edge of the left renal vein (Figs. 16.12a–l and 16.13a–d). If there is inadequate tension during the separation, it is permissible to remove a portion of the lymphatic tissue from the surface of the abdominal aorta concurrently (our team typically employs en bloc resection followed by region-specific pathological examination).

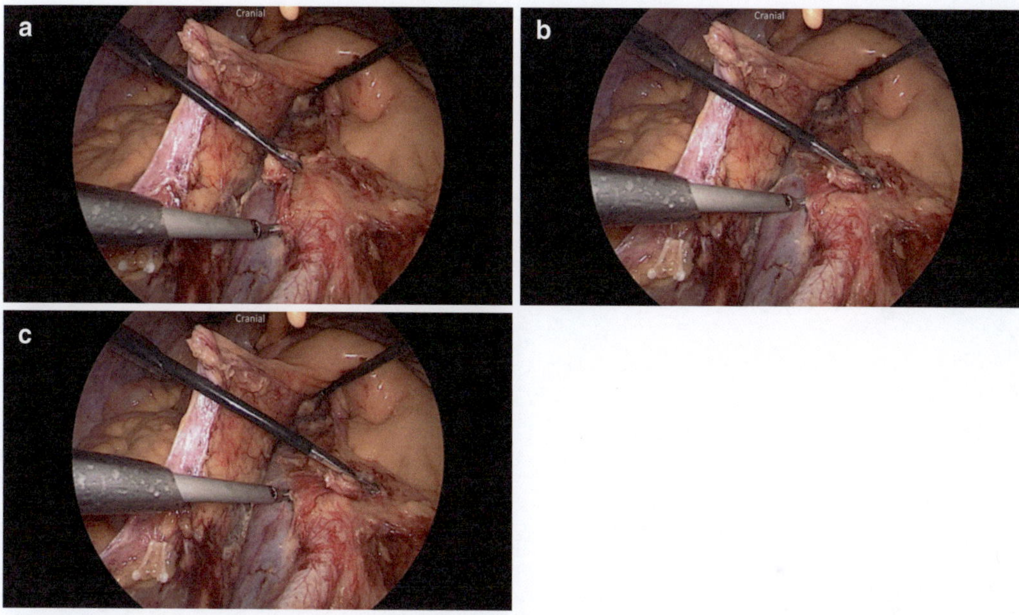

Fig. 16.11 (**a–c**) Dissect lymph nodes from the surface of the inferior vena cava to the area between the inferior vena cava and the abdominal aorta

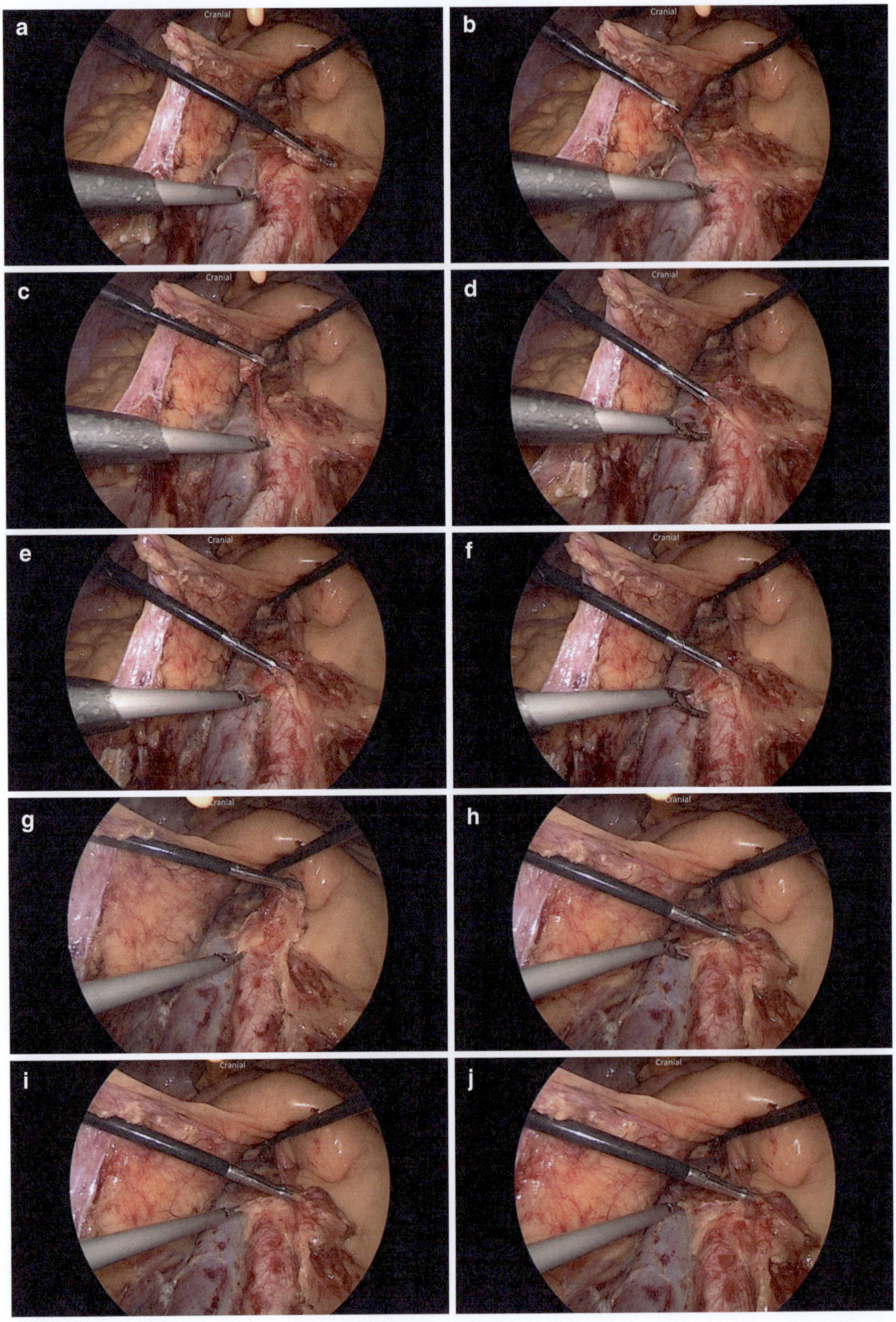

Fig. 16.12 (**a–l**) Dissect lymph nodes in the region between the inferior vena cava and the abdominal aorta, proceeding from the caudal (inferior) to the cranial (superior) direction

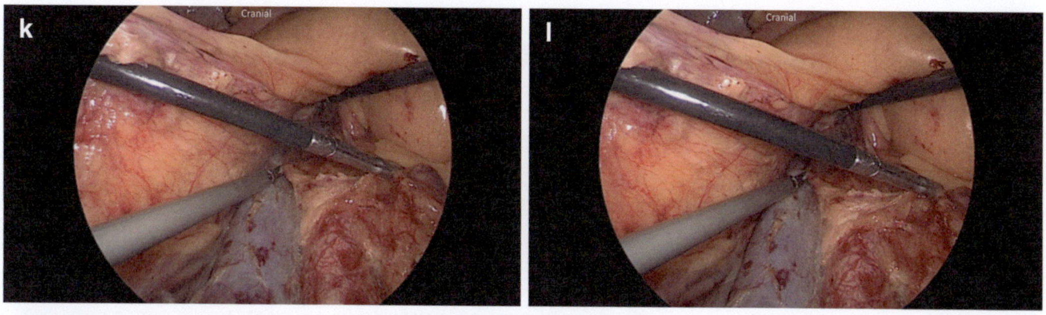

Fig. 16.12 (continued)

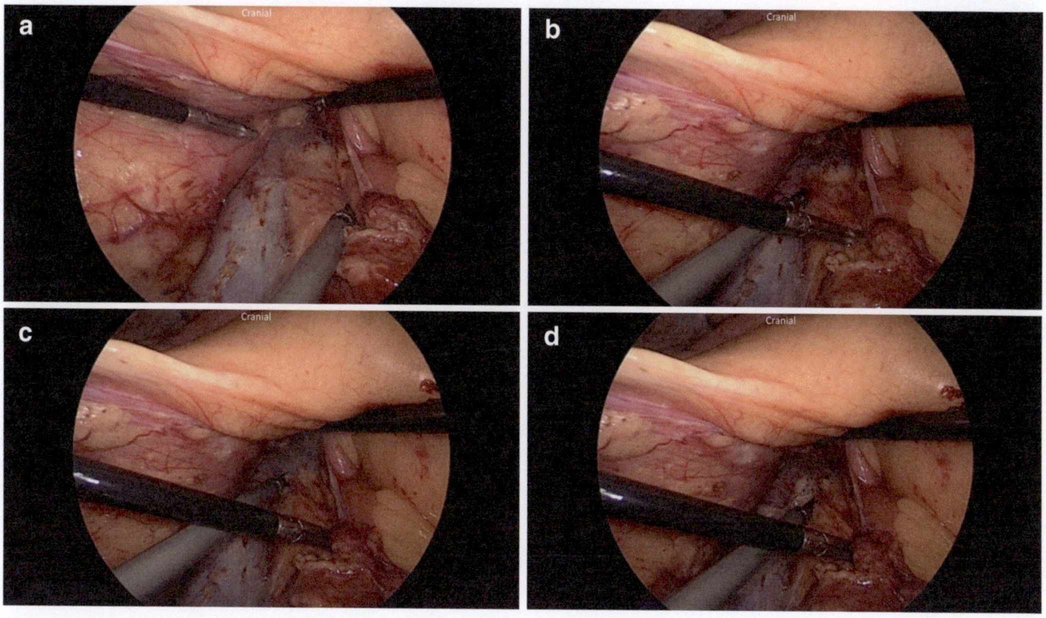

Fig. 16.13 (**a–d**) Dissection extending to the lower margin of the left renal vein

16.8 Exposure of Lymph Nodes in the Caudal Region of the Inferior Mesenteric Artery

Prior to undertaking the retrograde lymph node dissection in the region of the abdominal aorta, our team follows a sequential approach by first performing antegrade excision of bilateral common iliac, presacral, and pelvic lymph nodes. Additionally, we conduct separation and preservation of the superior hypogastric plexus. In this particular region, the lymph nodes and the adipose tissue situate between the inferior mesenteric artery and the superior hypogastric plexus. By excising the common iliac lymph nodes in the antegrade manner, the left ureter is already well exposed, ensuring the safety and reliability of this procedure. The left peritoneum is gently pulled laterally and toward the ventral side (alternatively, it can also be suspended similarly to the right side using sutures). Simultaneously, the abdominal aorta is retracted toward the right side. Employing the ultrasonic scalpel, carefully dissect the lymphatic adipose tissue in this region (Fig. 16.14a–f). During this process, it is crucial to be cautious around the lumbar arteries and veins to prevent inadvertent injury. The lymph nodes in this area are excised from the caudal-to-cranial direction until reaching the posterior aspect of the inferior mesenteric artery (Fig. 16.15a–k).

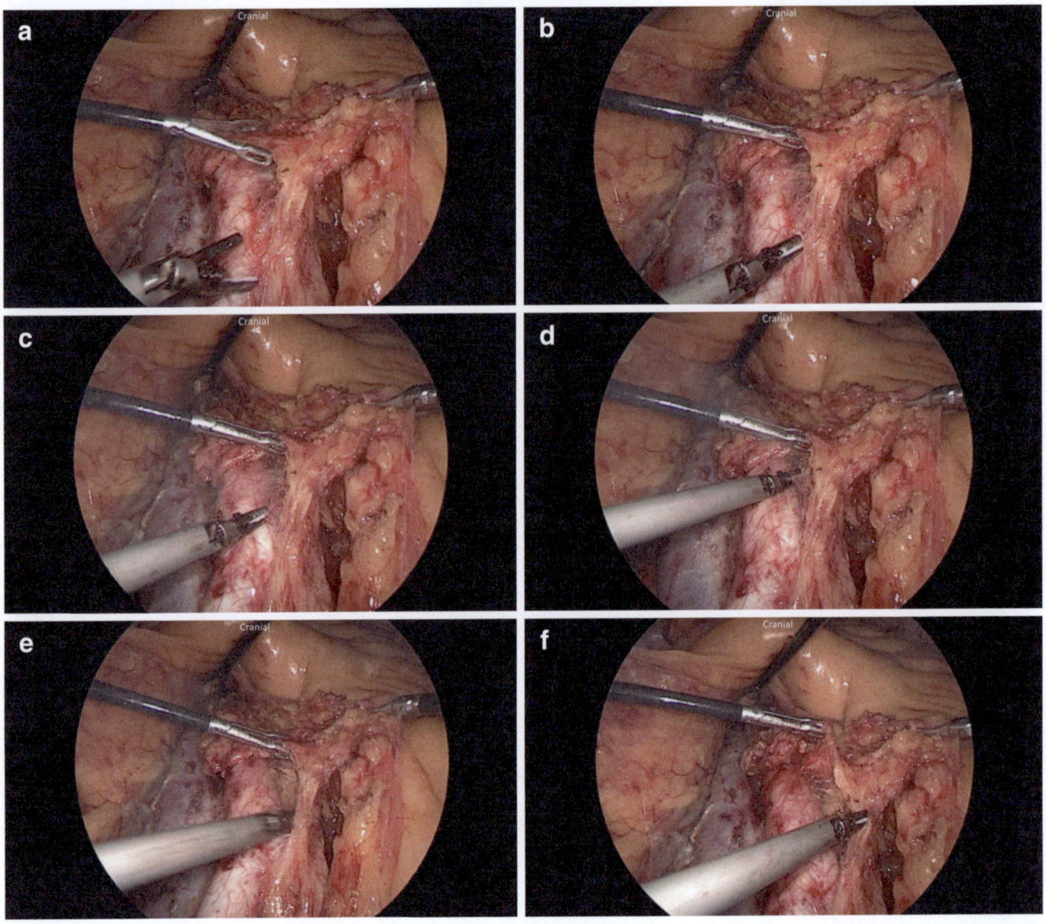

Fig. 16.14 (**a**–**f**) Separate and preserve the abdominal aortic plexus

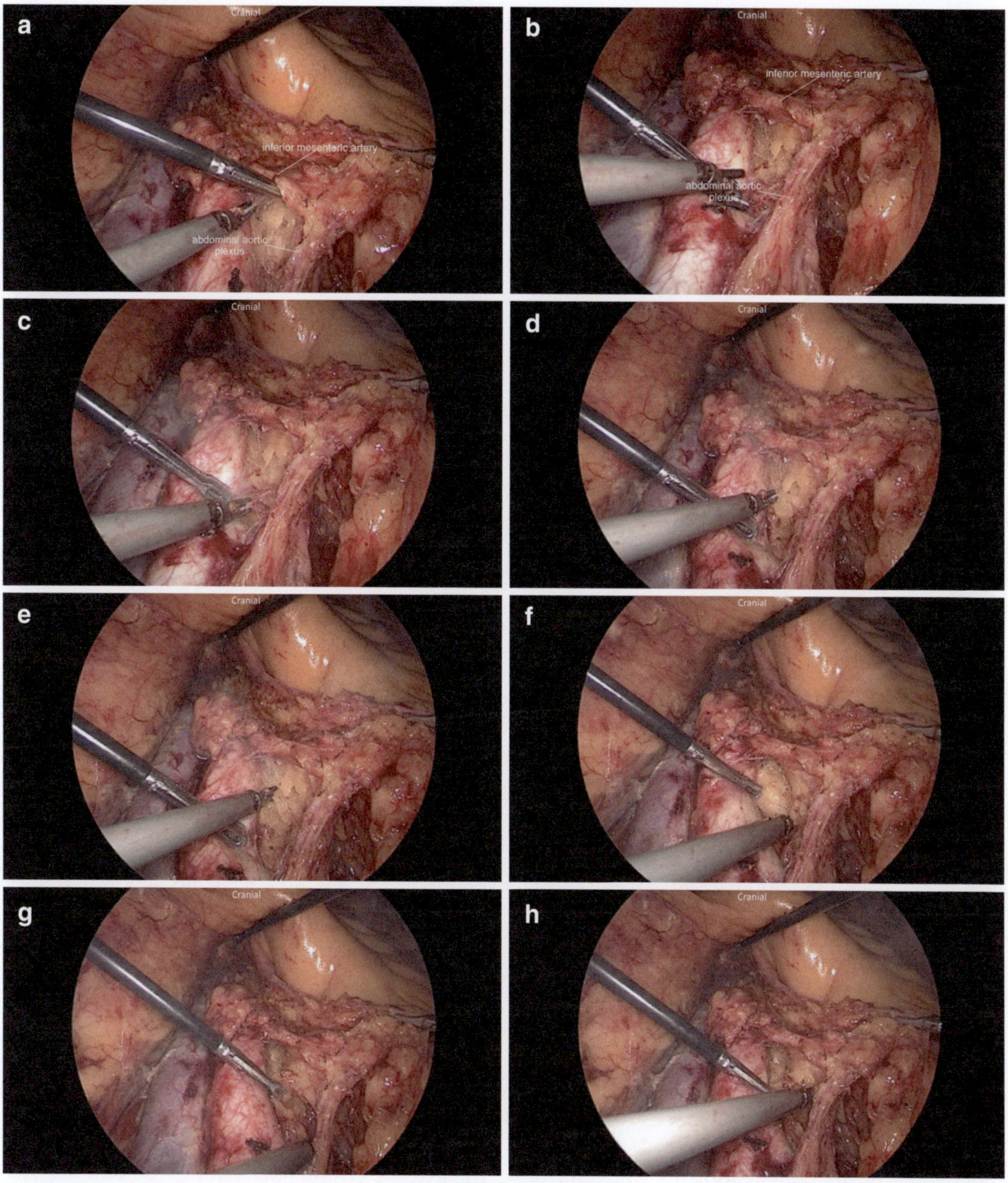

Fig. 16.15 (**a**–**k**) Resect the lymph nodes in the caudal-to-cranial direction in the mesenteric artery's posterior region

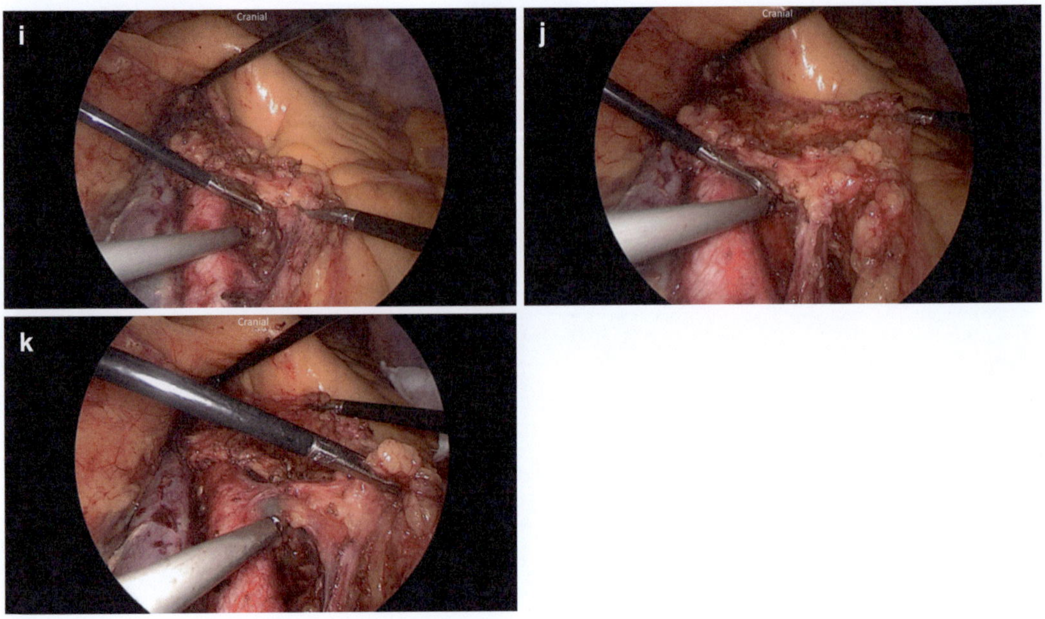

Fig. 16.15 (continued)

16.9 Exposure of Lymph Nodes in the Cranial Region of the Inferior Mesenteric Artery

Our approach involves initially using the ultrasonic scalpel to meticulously dissect the lymph nodes situated on the surface of the abdominal aorta. This dissection takes place in a direction from the caudal to the cranial region, commencing at the point of origin of the inferior mesenteric artery and continuing until reaching the vicinity of the lower border of the left renal vein (Figs. 16.16a–f, 16.17a–h, and 16.18a–e). Following this, the lymph nodes situated in the left area of the abdominal aorta are isolated from the peritoneal space. By gently retracting the left peritoneum both laterally and ventrally, the space between the lymphatic adipose tissue and the peritoneum becomes visible. A precise dissection is performed along this space, proceeding from the caudal-to-cranial and posterior directions, to create separation between the lymphatic adipose tissue and the peritoneum (Figs. 16.19a–l, 16.20a–h, and 16.21a–d). Furthermore, proceeding from the origin of the mesentery, we continue to separate the lymph nodes in the left region of the abdominal aorta toward the cranial direction (Figs. 16.22a–f, 16.23a–d, 16.24a–h, and 16.25a–d). As we move toward the cranial region, it becomes increasingly important to exercise caution regarding the branches of the left ovarian artery to prevent inadvertent injury. Hemorrhage control can be intricate once it occurs; thus, vascular clamps can be employed if necessary (Fig. 16.26a–d). Finally, the lymph nodes in this area are excised at the level of the lower margin of the left renal vein (Fig. 16.27a–e).

Abdominal aortic region lymphadenectomy procedure is demonstrated in Videos 16.1 (Laparoscopic) and 16.2 (Robotic).

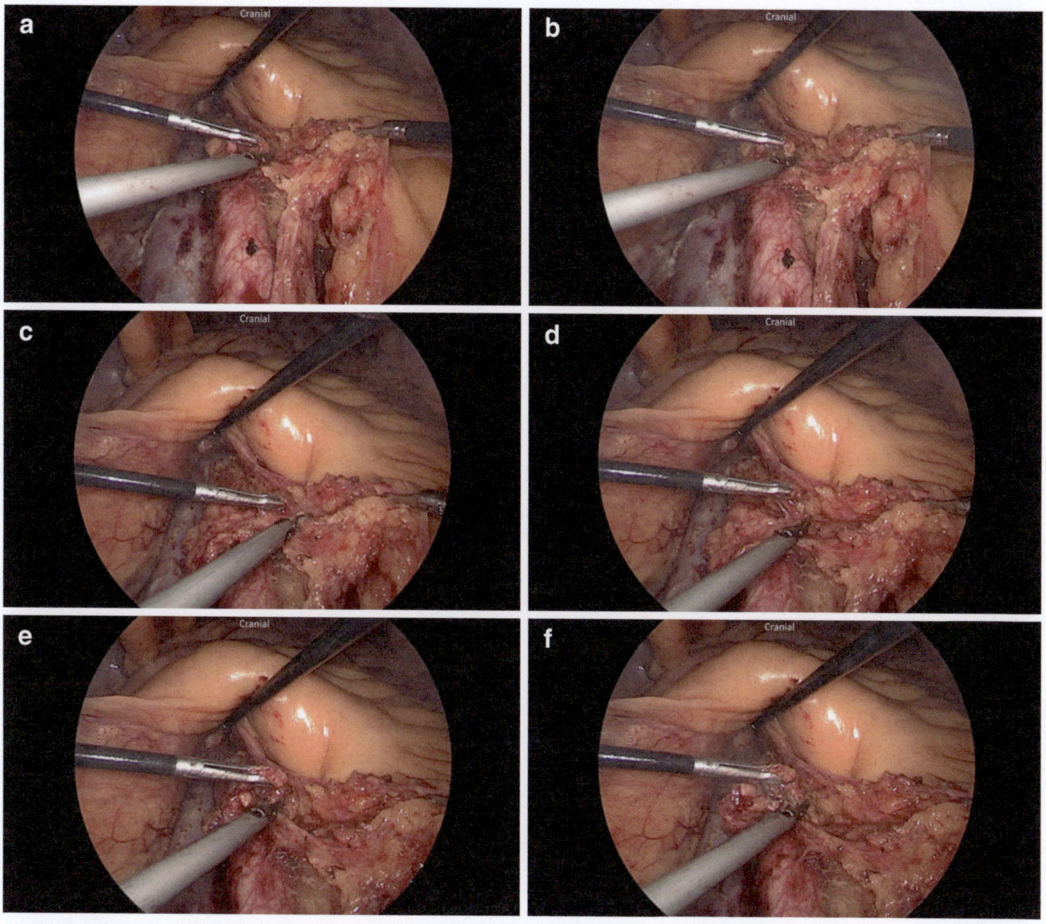

Fig. 16.16 (**a–f**) Separate lymphatic adipose tissue at the origin of the mesenteric artery

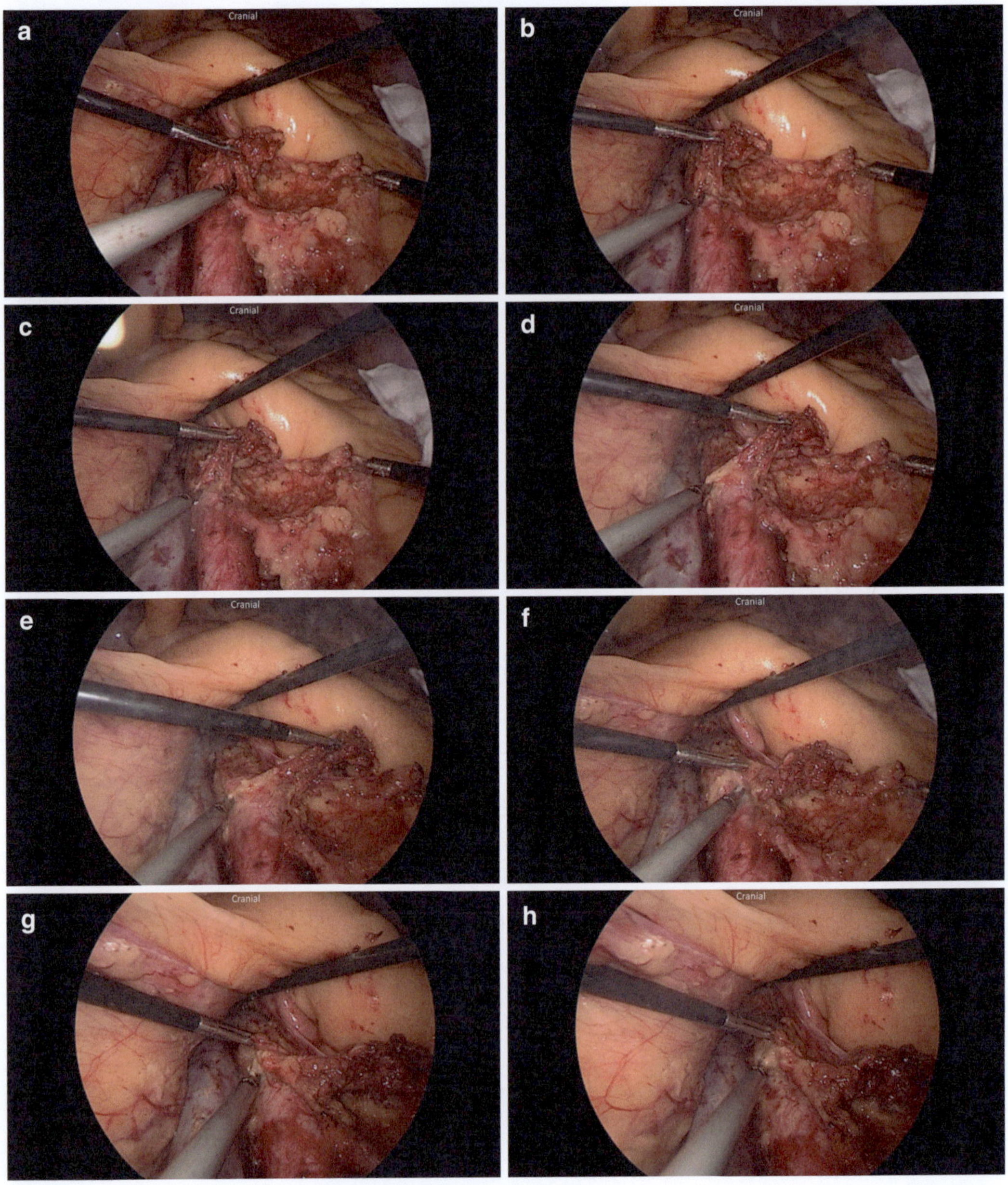

Fig. 16.17 (**a**–**h**) Retrograde separate lymph nodes on the surface of the abdominal aorta

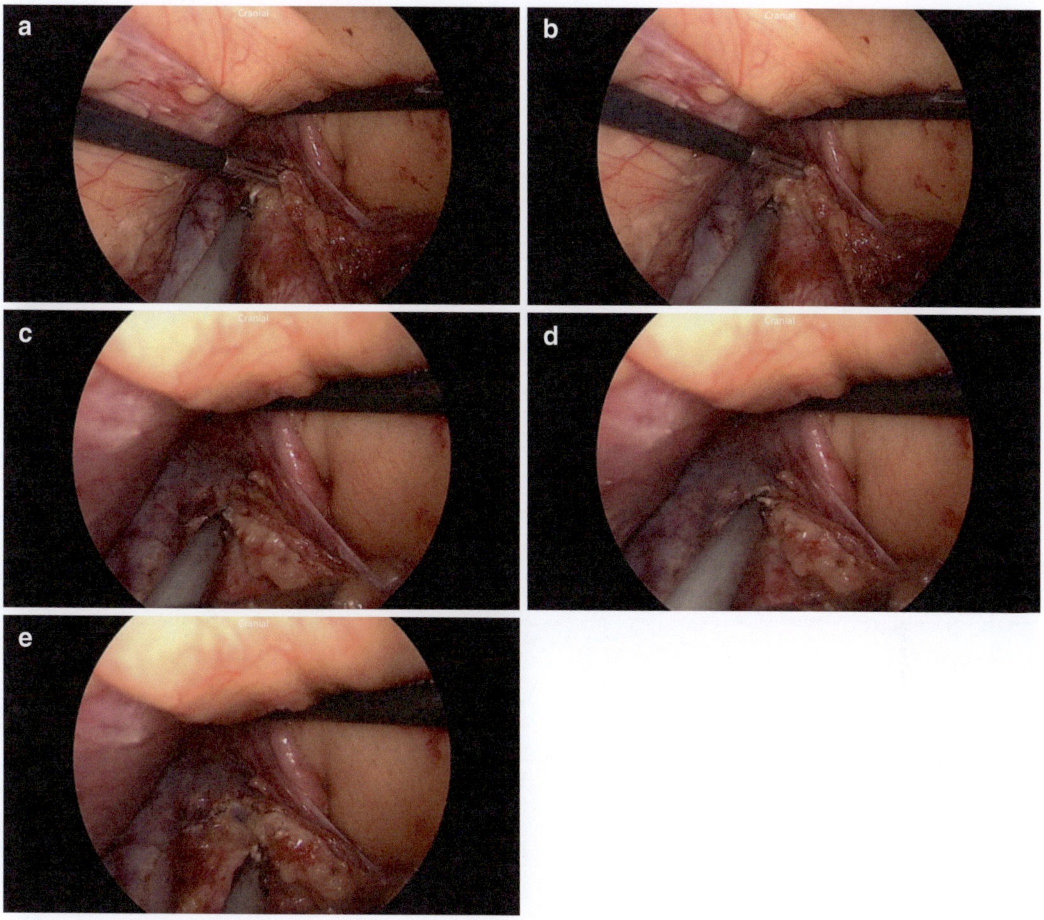

Fig. 16.18 (**a**–**e**) Dissect lymphatic adipose tissue on the surface of the abdominal aorta to the lower margin of the left renal vein

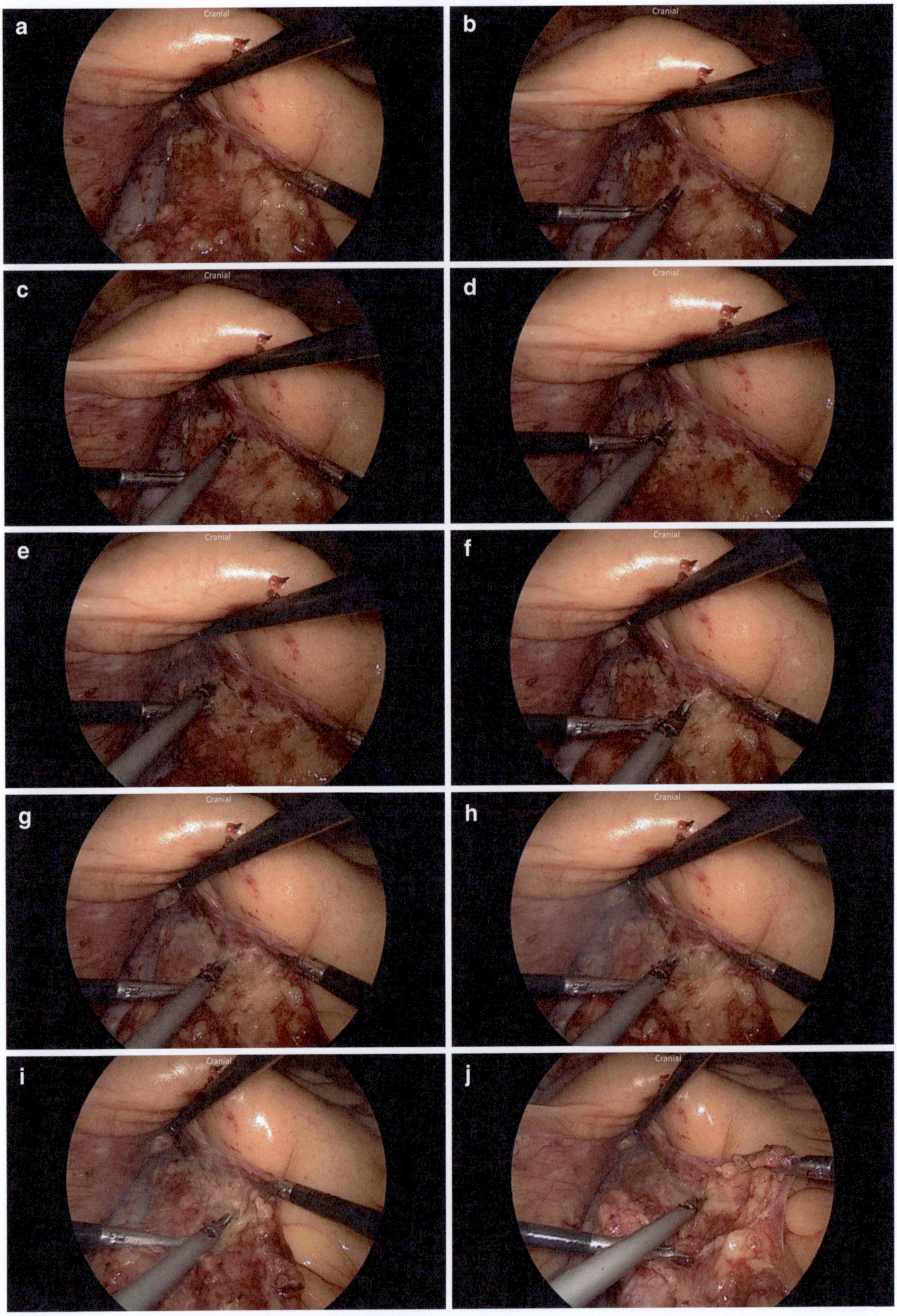

Fig. 16.19 (**a–l**) Dissect lymph nodes in the left region of the abdominal aorta along the peritoneal space

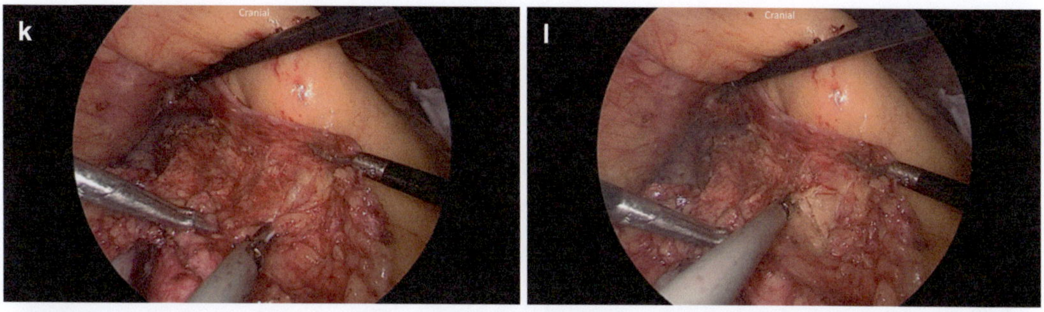

Fig. 16.19 (continued)

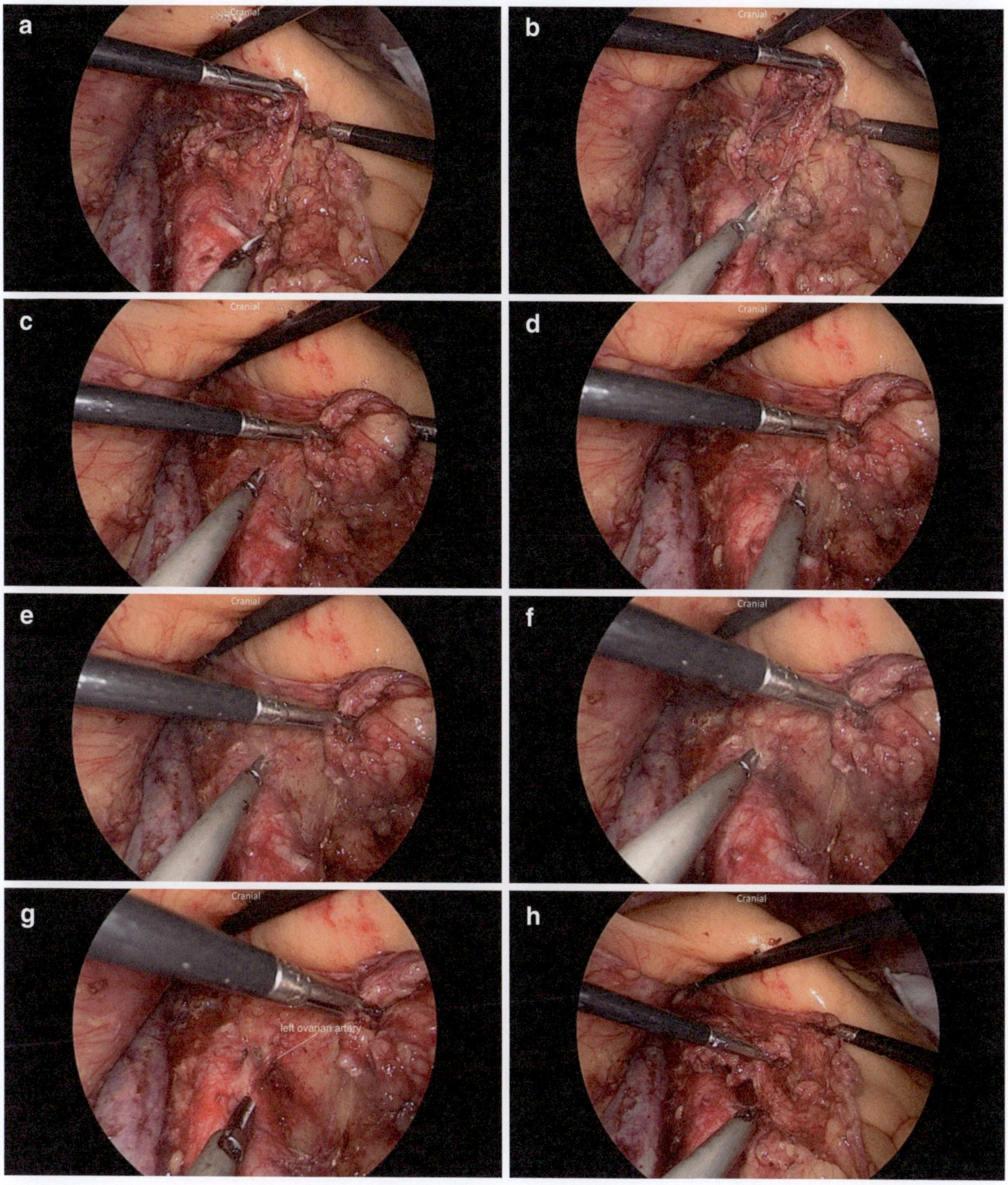

Fig. 16.20 (**a**–**h**) Dissect the gap between the left margin of the abdominal aorta and the lymphatic adipose tissue

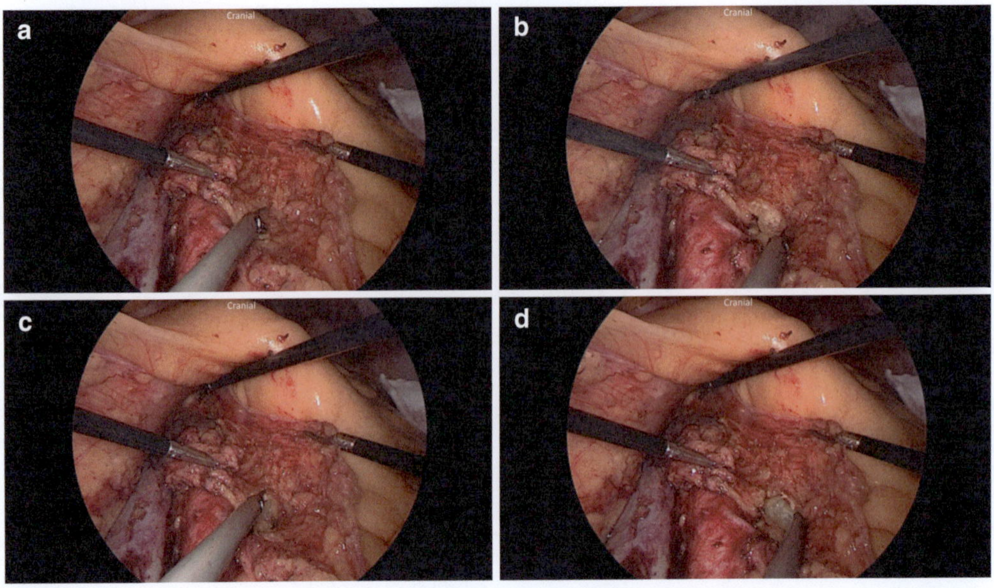

Fig. 16.21 (**a**–**d**) Dissect along the gap toward the cephalad (head) and dorsal (back) directions

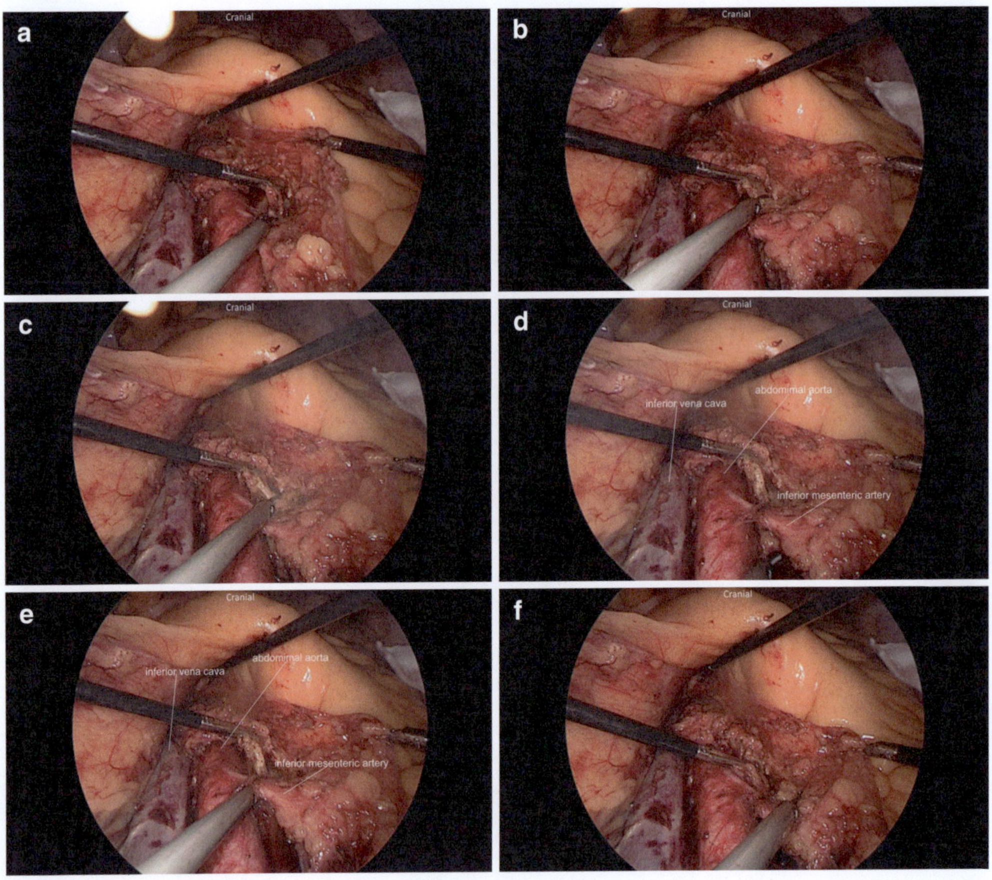

Fig. 16.22 (**a**–**f**) Dissect lymphatic adipose tissue toward the cephalad (head) direction from the origin of the superior mesenteric artery

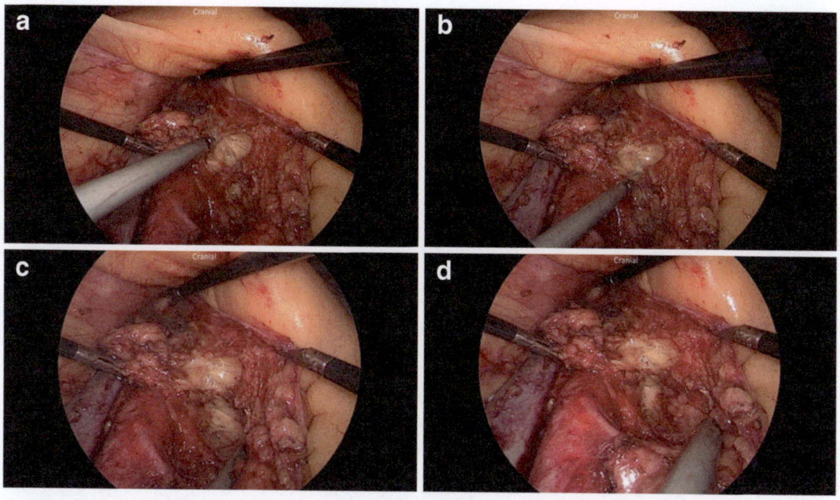

Fig. 16.23 (**a**–**d**) Expose and push out the perirenal fat in the renal hilum region

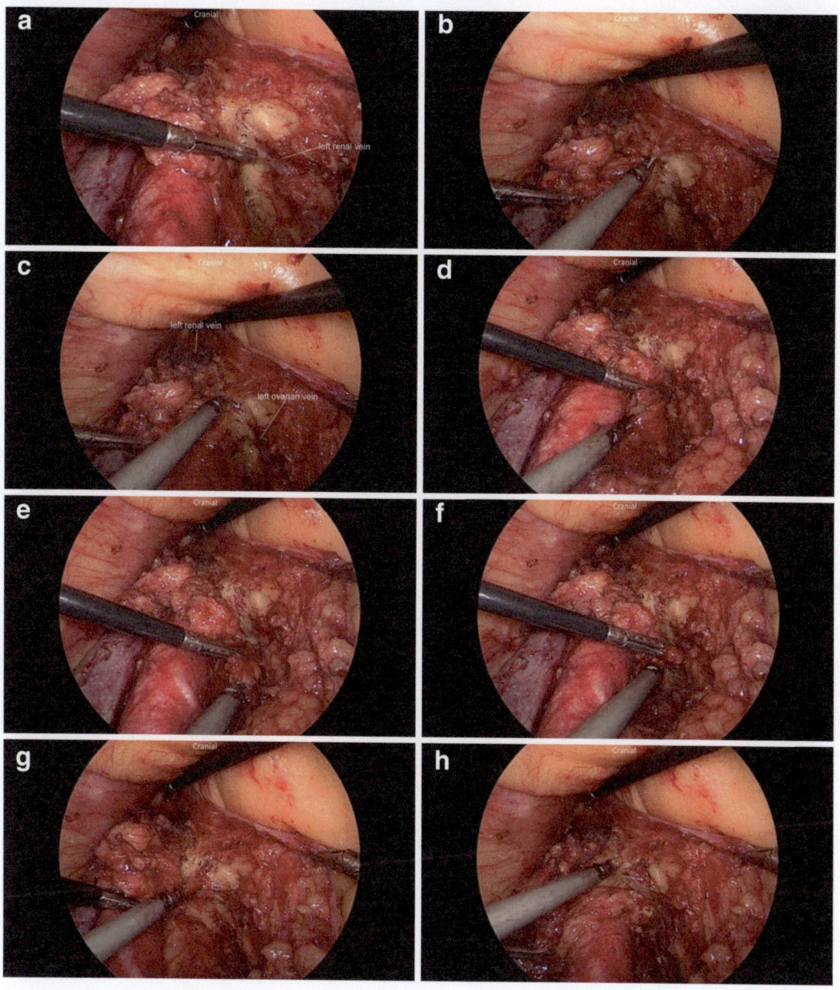

Fig. 16.24 (**a**–**h**) Separate the lymph nodes in the left-sided region of the abdominal aorta by dissecting along the inner side of the renal fat

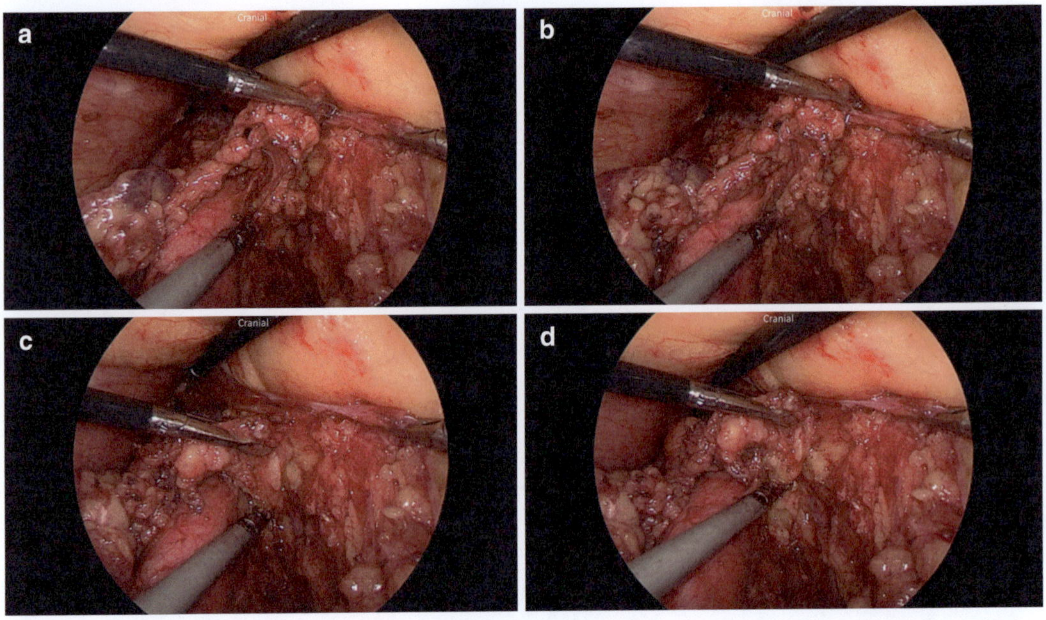

Fig. 16.25 (**a**–**d**) Dissect and separate the left ovarian artery

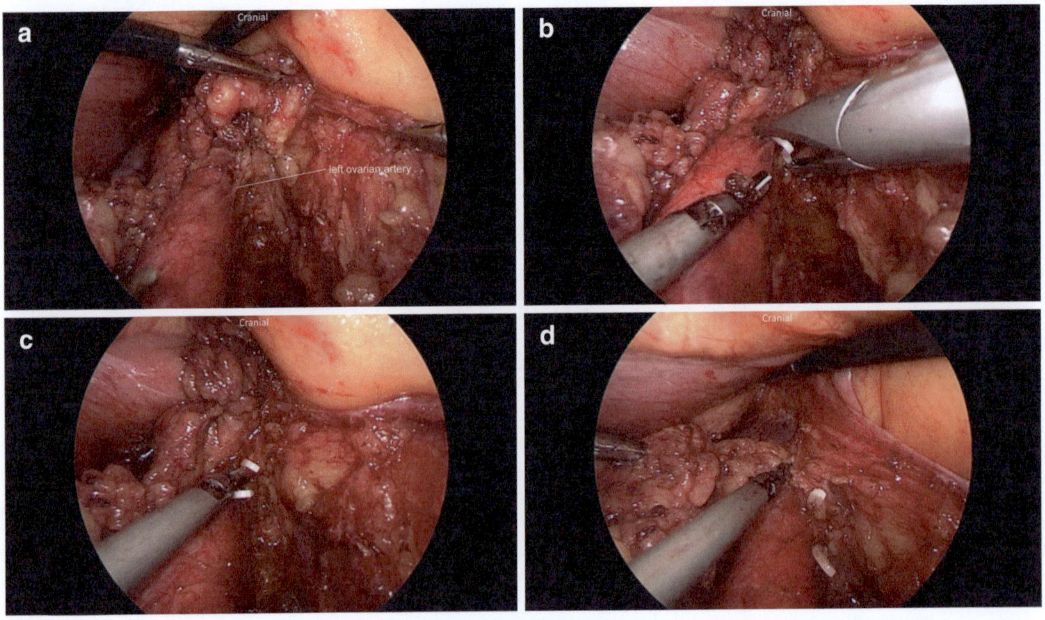

Fig. 16.26 (**a**–**d**) Clamp and transect the left ovarian artery

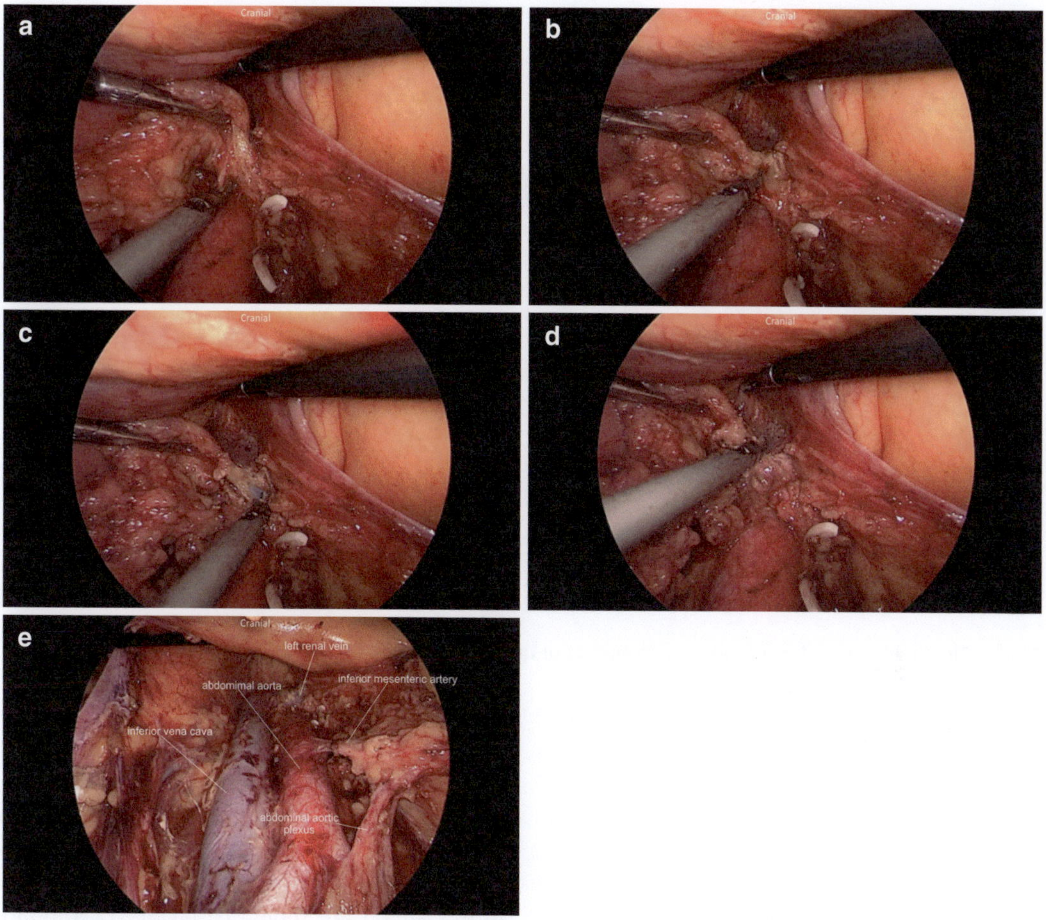

Fig. 16.27 (**a–e**) En bloc resect the lymphatic adipose tissue converging to the lower border of the left renal vein

Appendix: Surgical Staging of Cervical Cancer

According to the NCCN 2023 version 1 guidelines, patients with stage IB3, IIA2, IIB, III, and IVA cervical cancer are eligible for informed decision-making regarding staging surgery. This is particularly relevant for cases where imaging suggests pelvic lymph node involvement. Through surgical intervention, we can perform para-aortic lymph node dissection to determine the presence of metastasis. This procedure can offer valuable evidence to guide subsequent treatment decisions.

I The surgical procedure involves exposing the iliac vessels and the lower region of the abdominal aorta, with dissection extending cranially to the level of the inferior mesenteric artery and caudally to the middle segment of the common iliac vessels (Fig. 16.28a–d).

Surgical Experience and Precautions During this step, ensure the proper exposure of the cranial aspect of the duodenum and the caudal aspect of the ureter, while exercising caution to prevent any damage to both structures.

II Excise the lymphatic adipose tissue on the surface of the abdominal aorta, the surface of the inferior vena cava, and the tissue between the two vessels (Fig. 16.29a–i).

Surgical Experience and Precautions During the separation process, it is essential to focus on

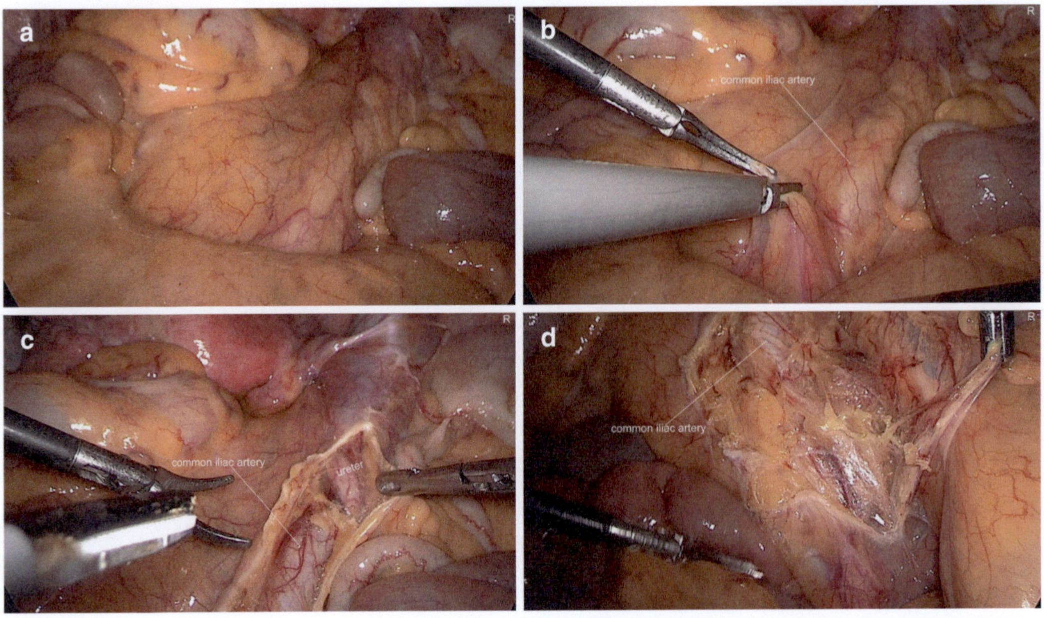

Fig. 16.28 (**a–d**) Expose lymph nodes on the surface of the iliac vessels and the lower region of the abdominal aorta

revealing the right ureter to prevent any potential damage. Additionally, during the excision of lymph nodes, it is critical to be aware that multiple venous tributaries connect the lymph nodes to both the inferior vena cava and the right common iliac vein. Managing these tributaries separately is necessary to prevent bleeding.

III Excise the lymph nodes on the surface of the left common iliac vein (Fig. 16.30a–c).

IV Excise the lymph nodes in the left region of the abdominal aorta below the level of the inferior mesenteric artery. During this procedure, it is important to first retract the lateral peritoneum laterally. Proceed to dissect along the inferior mesenteric artery from the cranial to caudal direction and from the ventral to dorsal direction, exposing the lymphatic adipose tissue in this area. Care should be taken to avoid any damage to the left ureter, lumbar arteries, and lumbar veins during the separation process (Fig. 16.31a–d).

Staging surgery procedure is demonstrated in Video 16.3.

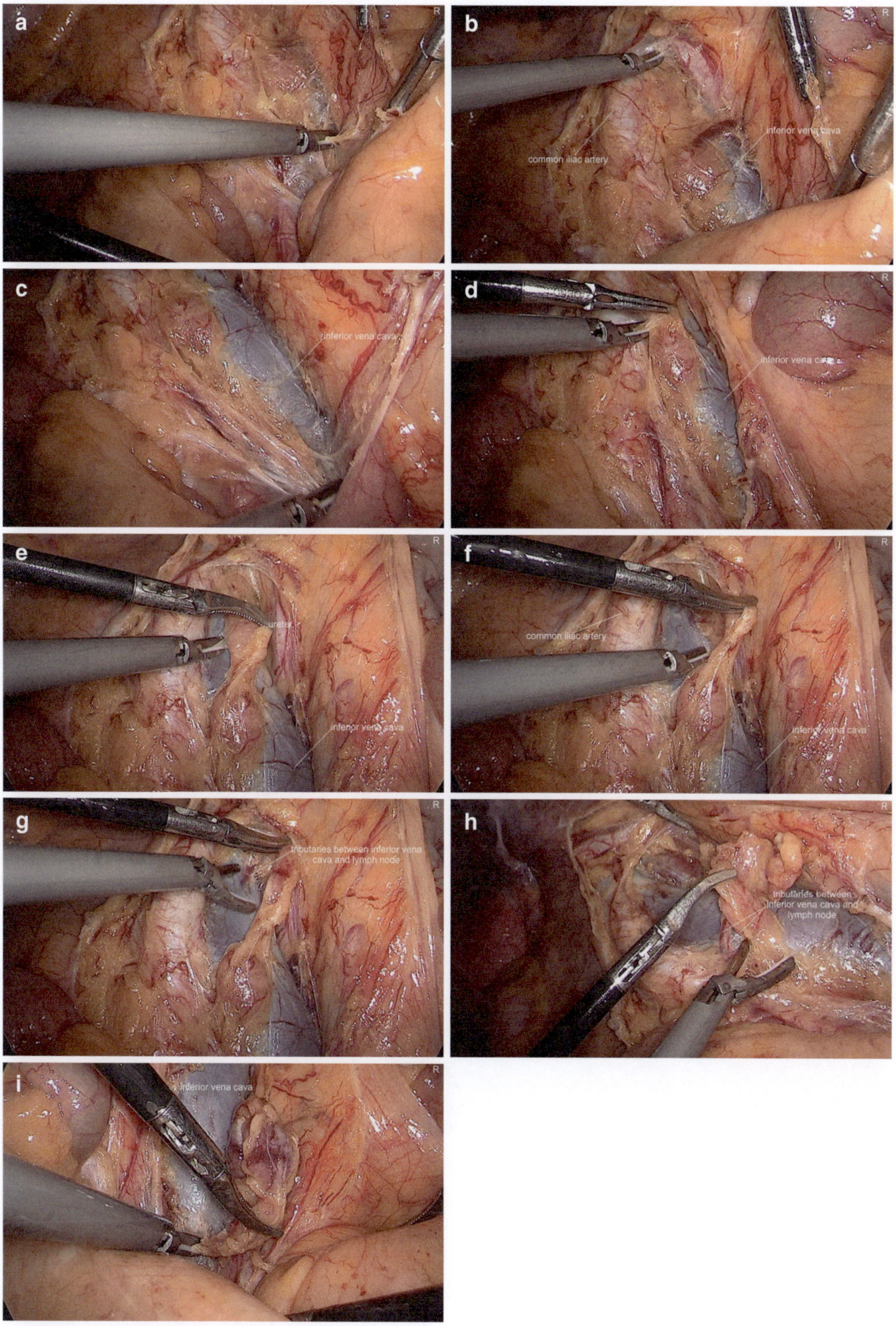

Fig. 16.29 (**a–i**) Excise the lymphatic adipose tissue on the surface of the abdominal aorta, the surface of the inferior vena cava, and the tissue between the two vessels

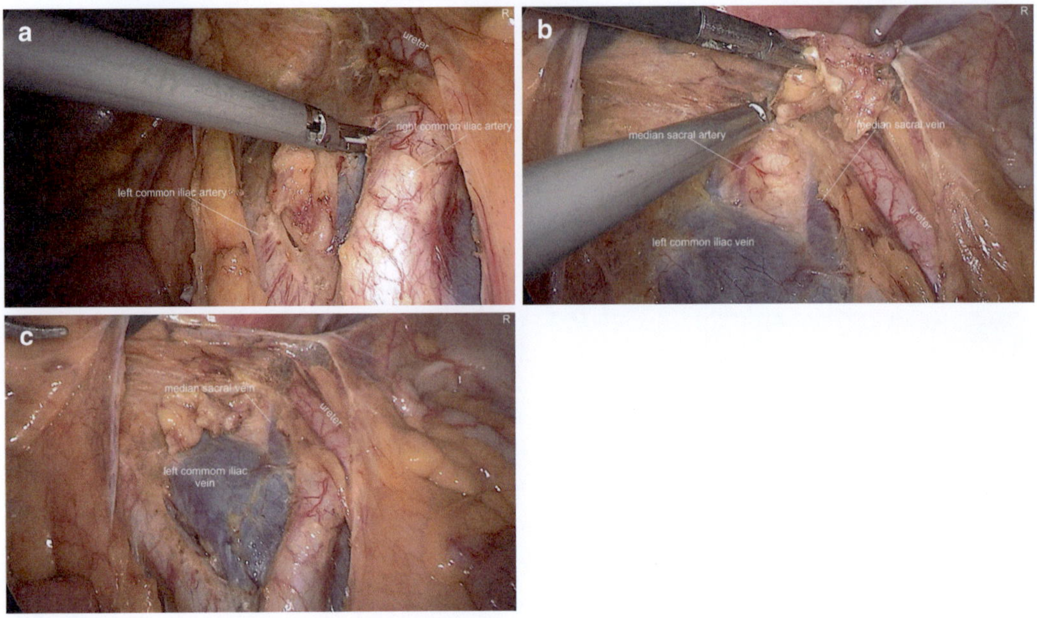

Fig. 16.30 (**a**–**c**) Resect the lymph nodes on the surface of the left common iliac vein

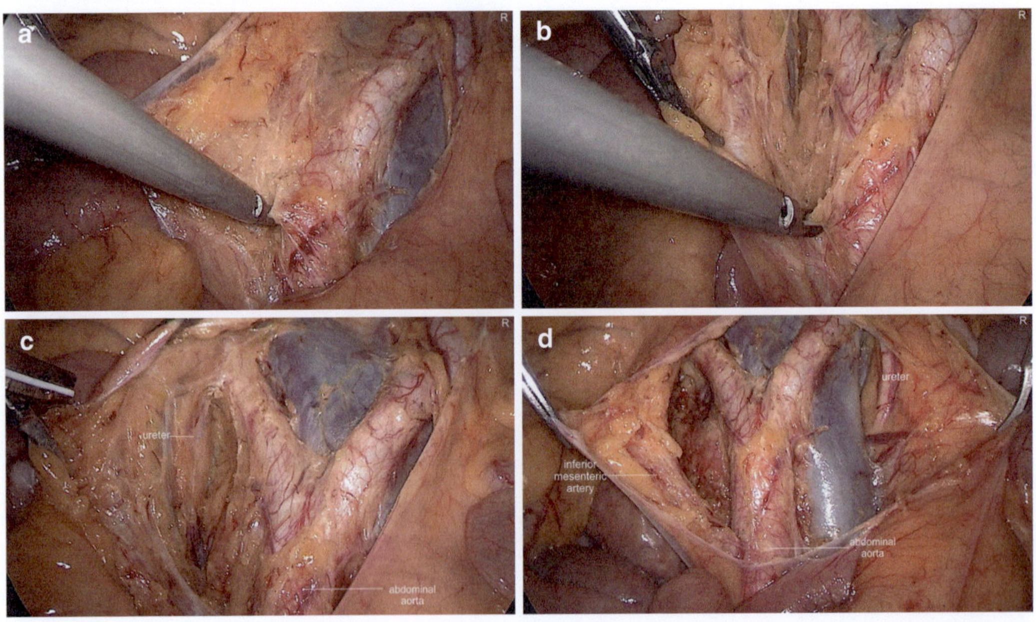

Fig. 16.31 (**a**–**d**) Excise the lymph nodes in the left region of the abdominal aorta below the level of the inferior mesenteric artery

References

1. Sakuragi N, Satoh C, Takeda N, et al. Incidence and distribution pattern of pelvic and paraaortic lymph node metastasis in patients with stages IB, IIA, and IIB cervical carcinoma treated with radical hysterectomy. Cancer. 1999;85:1547–54. Available at: http://www.ncbi.nlm.nih.gov/pubmed/10193945
2. Huang H, Liu J, Li Y, et al. Metastasis to deep obturator and paraaortic lymph nodes in 649 patients with cervical carcinoma. Eur J Surg Oncol. 2011;37:978–83. Available at: http://www.ncbi.nlm.nih.gov/pubmed/21907530

17 Sentinel Lymph Node Mapping and Dissection

Shichao Han, Jun Wang, Jing Na, Ya Li, and Xinyou Wang

Recent data indicates that Sentinel Lymph Node (SLN) biopsy could serve as a valuable strategy to reduce the necessity of performing pelvic lymphadenectomy in individuals diagnosed with early-stage cervical cancer [1, 2]. Prospective studies consistently demonstrate the viability of SLN detection in early-stage cervical cancer patients and propose that the extensive dissection of pelvic lymph nodes can be safely omitted in a substantial portion of these cases [1–10].

Sentinel lymph node dissection for cervical cancer (biopsy, mapping-based resection) is primarily employed in patients with stage IA1 accompanied by vascular tumor emboli, stage IA2, certain cases of stage IB1 with radical hysterectomy, or those undergoing radical trachelectomy. The range of tracer agents includes dyes (methylene blue, nanocarbon), radiocolloid technetium-99 (99Tc) (which possesses the potential for radiation damage but is minimally used), and fluorescent agents (indocyanine green, ICG), requiring specialized laparoscopic equipment. However, the widespread adoption of this technique in primary healthcare facilities remains challenging, prompting our team to exclusively mention the utilization of methylene blue for sentinel lymph node dissection.

17.1 Injection of the Sentinel Lymph Node

Utilize a direct cervical injection with dye into the cervix, usually at 2 or 4 points (Fig. 17.1).

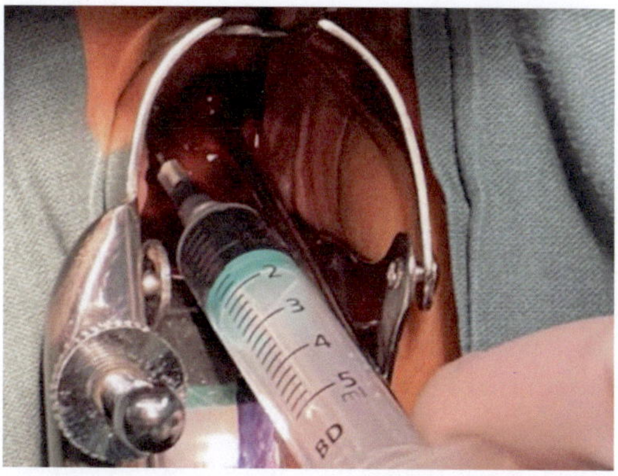

Fig. 17.1 Injection of the sentinel lymph node

Supplementary Information The online version contains supplementary material available at https://doi.org/10.1007/978-981-97-7687-0_17.

S. Han (✉) · J. Wang · J. Na · Y. Li · X. Wang
Department of Gynecology and Obstetrics, Second Affiliated Hospital of Dalian Medical University, Dalian, China

S. Han, J. Wang (eds.), *Open, Laparoscopic, and Robotic Surgery for Cervical Cancer*, https://doi.org/10.1007/978-981-97-7687-0_17

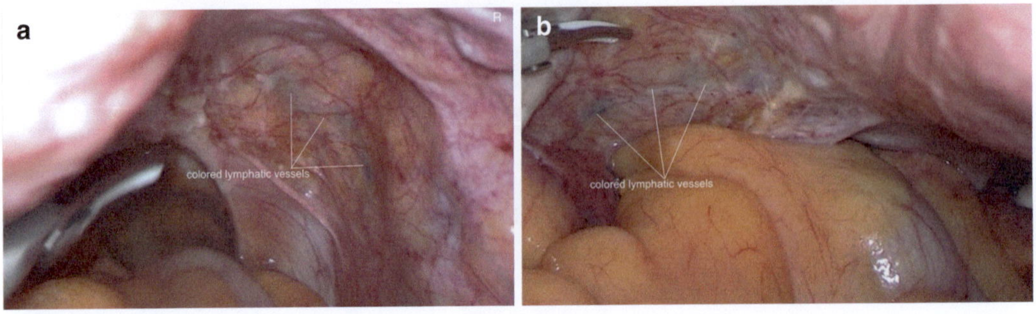

Fig. 17.2 (**a**, **b**) Exploration of the pelvic sentinel lymph node

17.2 Exploration of the Pelvic Sentinel Lymph Node

Explorate pelvic region and expose the sentinel lymph node mapping (Fig. 17.2).

17.3 Locating the Sentinel Lymph Node

Early anatomical studies identified two consistent pelvic lymphatic pathways: an upper paracervical with a course along the uterine artery with draining external iliac lymph nodes and a lower paracervical pathway running along the uterine vein to the hypogastric area and/or presacral area [11, 12].

The tracer agent is employed to visualize the upper and lower pathways of the parametrial regions separately. The lymphatic vessels of the upper parametrial region originate from the parametrial tissue adjacent to the cervix. They follow the course of the uterine artery toward the pelvic iliac vessels. After crossing the internal iliac artery, these vessels have three distribution pathways: (1) Toward the deep inguinal region. (2) Toward the obturator region, running along the interval between the external iliac artery and the psoas major muscle, and then returning toward the cranial direction along the outer edge of the iliac vessels. (3) Toward the bifurcation area of the internal and external iliac veins, and subsequently flowing cranially along the inner side of the iliac vessels.

Using an ultrasonic scalpel, make a sharp incision in the lateral peritoneum to expose the retroperitoneal space behind it. Gradually utilize this retroperitoneal space to reveal the ureter, internal iliac artery, and lymphatic vessels that have been previously enhanced with a contrast agent. Follow the contrast-enhanced lymphatic vessels to locate the enhanced sentinel lymph node (Fig. 17.3a–h). The visualization of the sentinel lymph node commonly follows the pattern of lymphatic vessels originating from the parametrial area, crossing the internal iliac artery, and flowing laterally. One pathway leads to the obturator space or the region between the internal and external iliac veins (Fig. 17.4a–l). The other pathway involves the lymphatic vessels crossing the internal iliac artery and then proceeding cranially between the surface of the external iliac vessels and the psoas major muscles.

Surgical Experience and Precautions Our team believes that it is crucial to meticulously identify every drainage pathway of the pelvic lymph nodes. The first enhanced lymph node detected along each drainage pathway can be considered as a sentinel lymph node. Therefore, the search for sentinel lymph nodes does not necessarily need to be immediate after cervical injection of the contrast agent. Waiting for a certain period before conducting the search can also be highly meaningful.

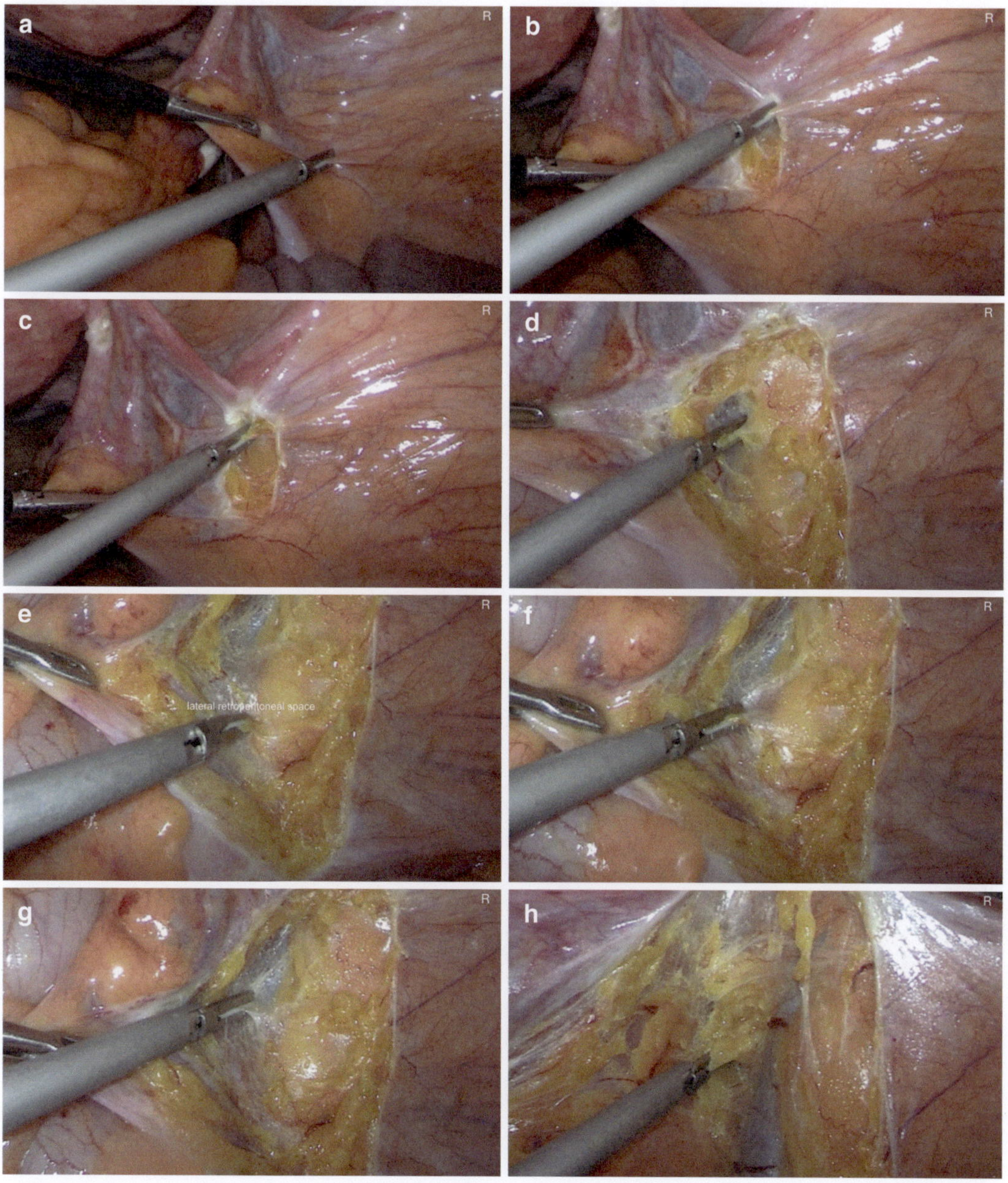

Fig. 17.3 (**a–h**) Explore the enhanced lymphatic vessels and lymph nodes

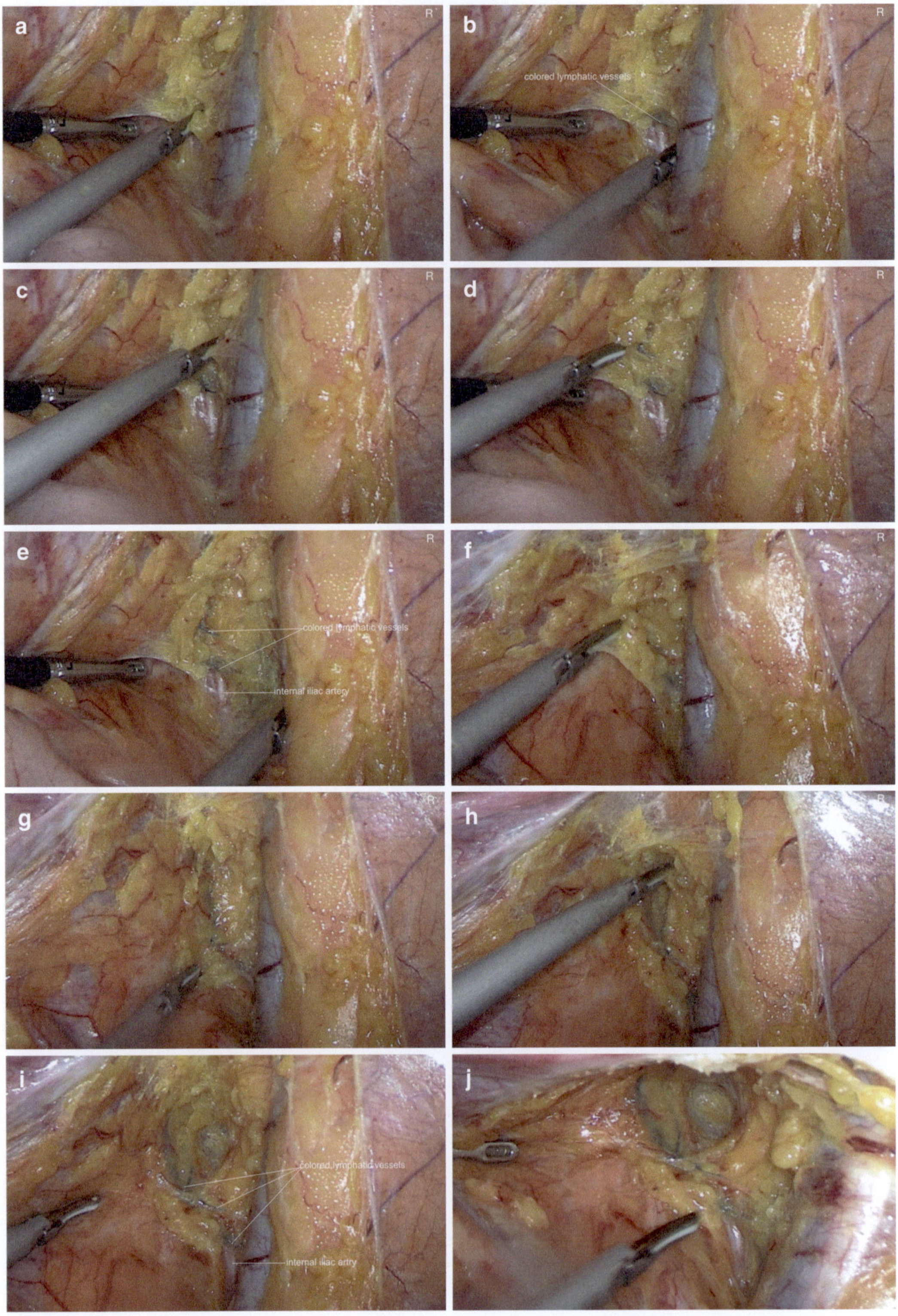

Fig. 17.4 (**a**–**l**) Paracentral lymphatic drainage: backflow laterally across the internal iliac artery to the obturator space or the region between the internal and external iliac veins

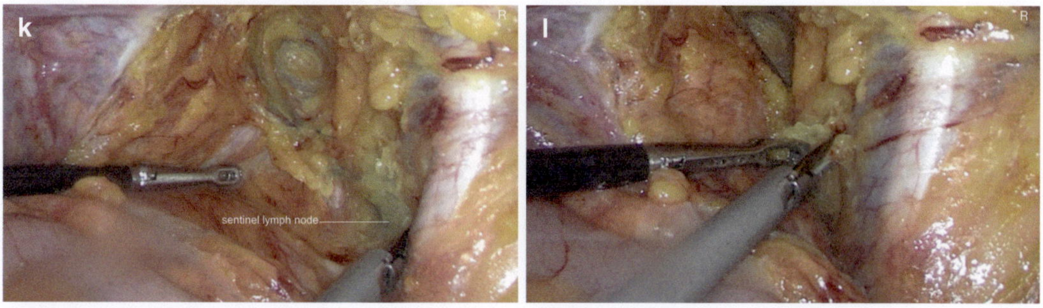

Fig. 17.4 (continued)

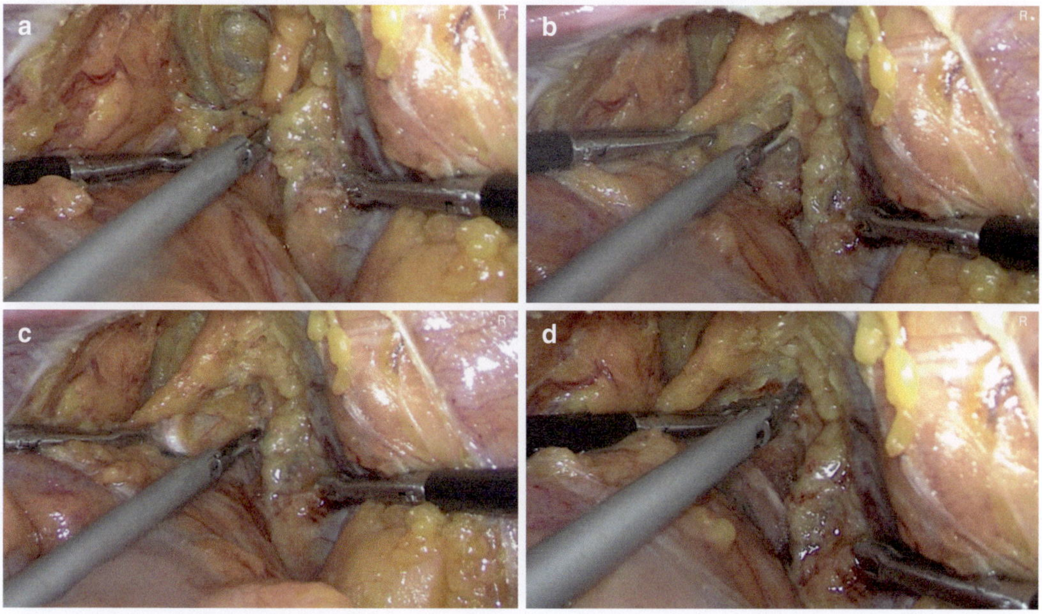

Fig. 17.5 (**a**–**d**) Dissect the sentinel lymph node and the lateral umbilical ligament

17.4 Sentinel Lymph Node Dissection Method 1

When conducting the removal of sentinel lymph nodes situated within the obturator space or the region between the internal and external iliac veins, it is crucial to ensure the intact excision of the sentinel lymph nodes while meticulously dissecting the adjacent arteries, veins, and nerves to prevent any potential damage (Figs. 17.5, 17.6, 17.7, and 17.8).

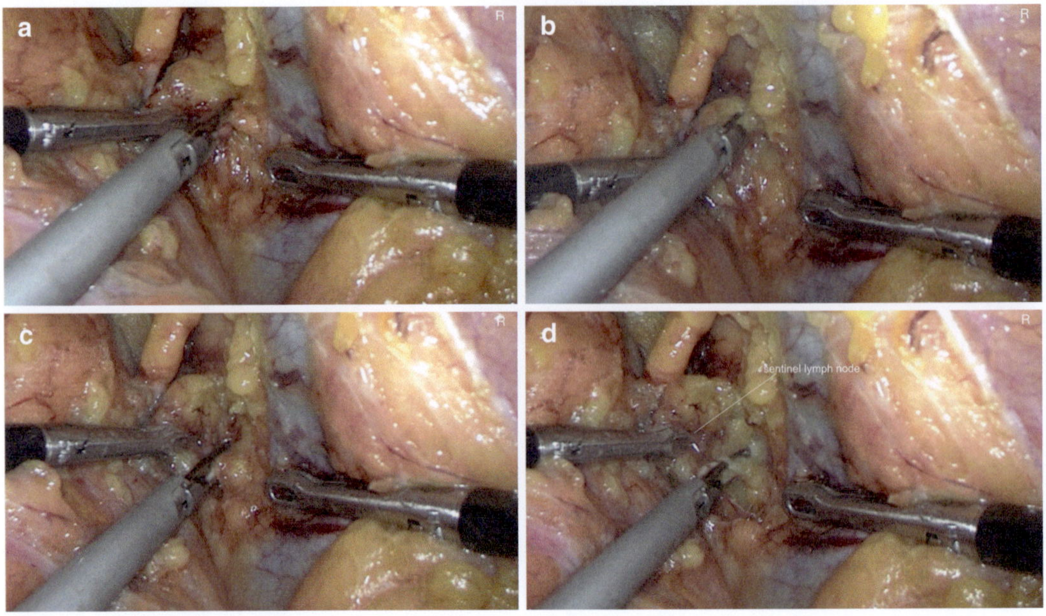

Fig. 17.6 (**a**–**d**) Dissect the sentinel lymph node and the external iliac vein

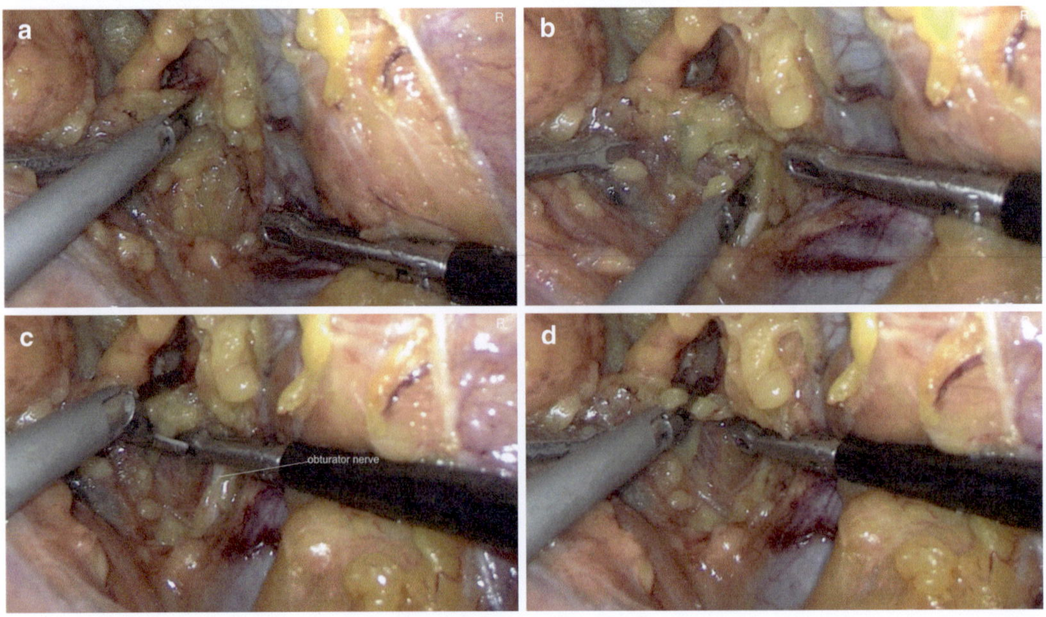

Fig. 17.7 (**a**–**d**) Dissect the sentinel lymph node and the obturator nerve

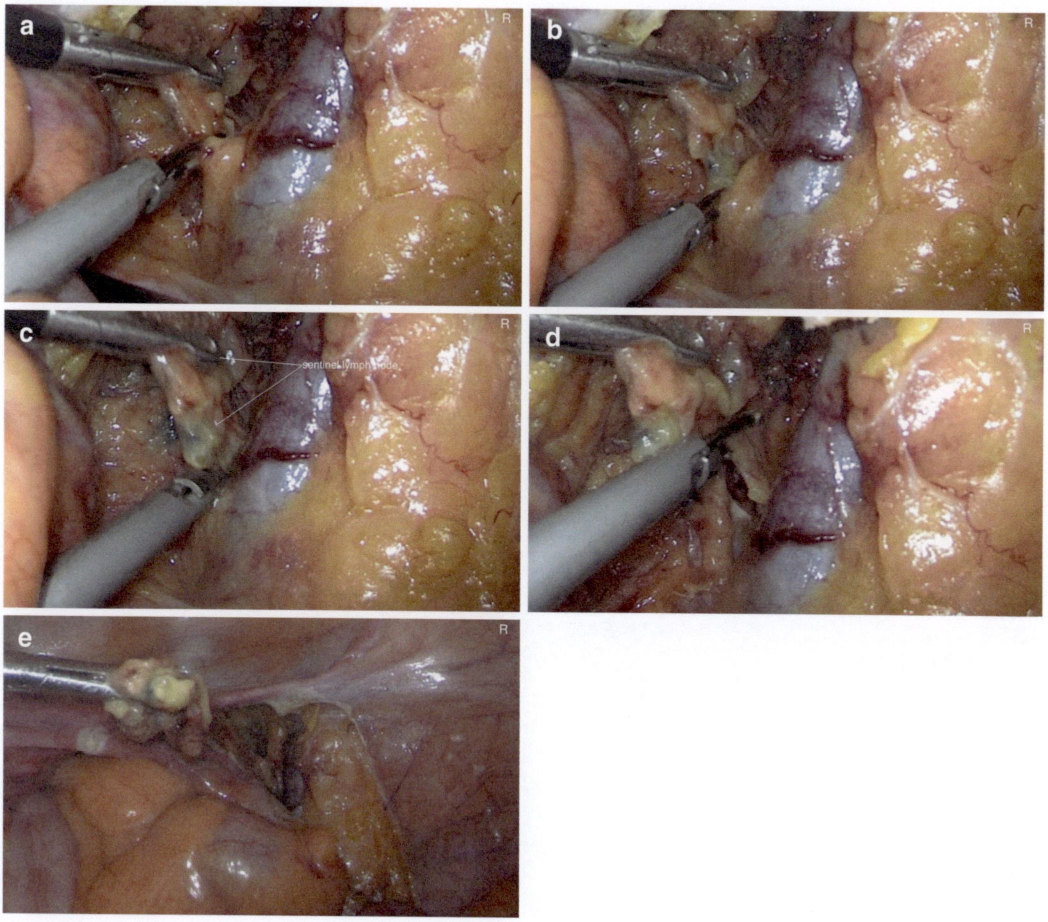

Fig. 17.8 (**a**–**e**) Complete excision of the sentinel lymph node between the obturator space and the internal and external iliac veins

17.5 Sentinel Lymph Node Dissection Method 2

Upon traversing the internal iliac artery, the sentinel lymph nodes that course cranially along the region between the surface of the external iliac vessels and the psoas major muscles are excised. During this excision process, in addition to removing the visually colored lymph nodes, meticulous attention should be directed toward inspecting the surrounding lymphatic vessels for any indications of enlarged or suspicious lymph nodes (Figs. 17.9a–d and 17.10a–j), which should also be excised.

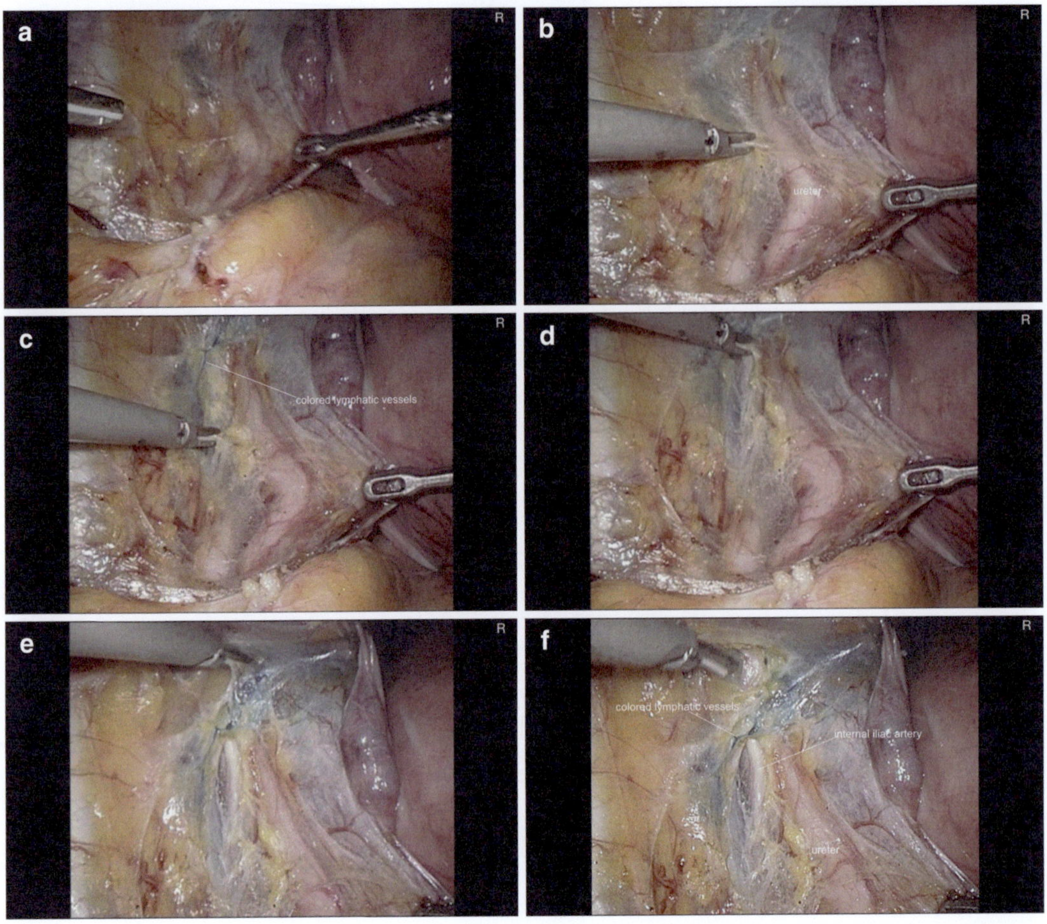

Fig. 17.9 (**a**–**f**) Paraaortic lymphatic drainage: Flowing cranially along the surface of the external iliac artery and vein after crossing the internal iliac artery

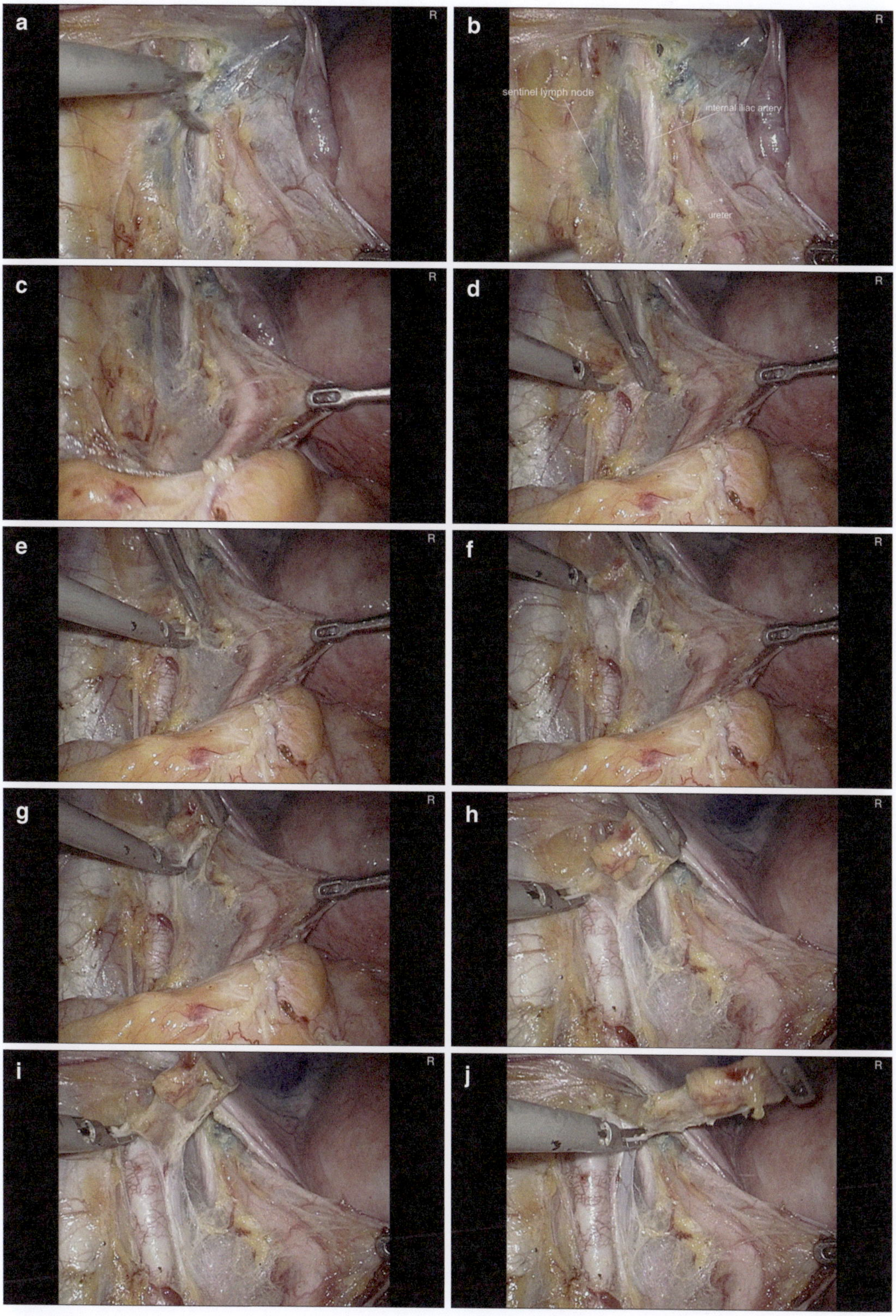

Fig. 17.10 (a–l) Complete resection of the sentinel lymph node between the external iliac artery, vein, and the psoas muscle

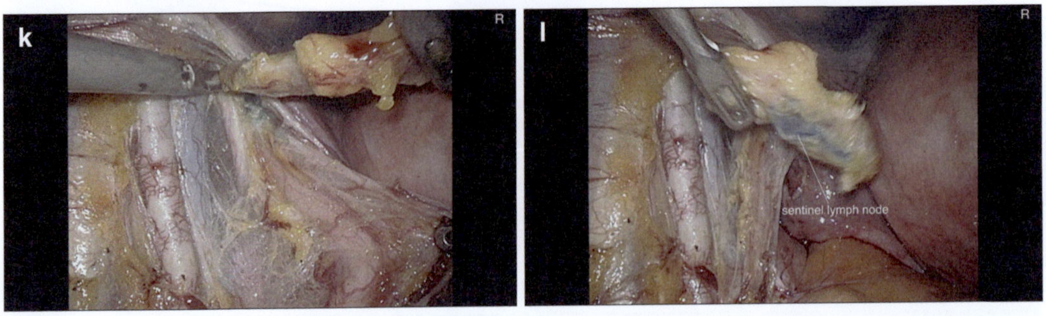

Fig. 17.10 (continued)

17.6 Sentinel Lymph Node Dissection Method 3

During the mapping-based resection of the sentinel lymph nodes, the lymph nodes that exhibit enlargement, suspicion, and enhancement along the path of the contrast-enhanced lymphatic vessels should be en bloc excised (Figs. 17.11, 17.12, 17.13, and 17.14).

Sentinel lymph node dissection procedure can be viewed in Video 17.1.

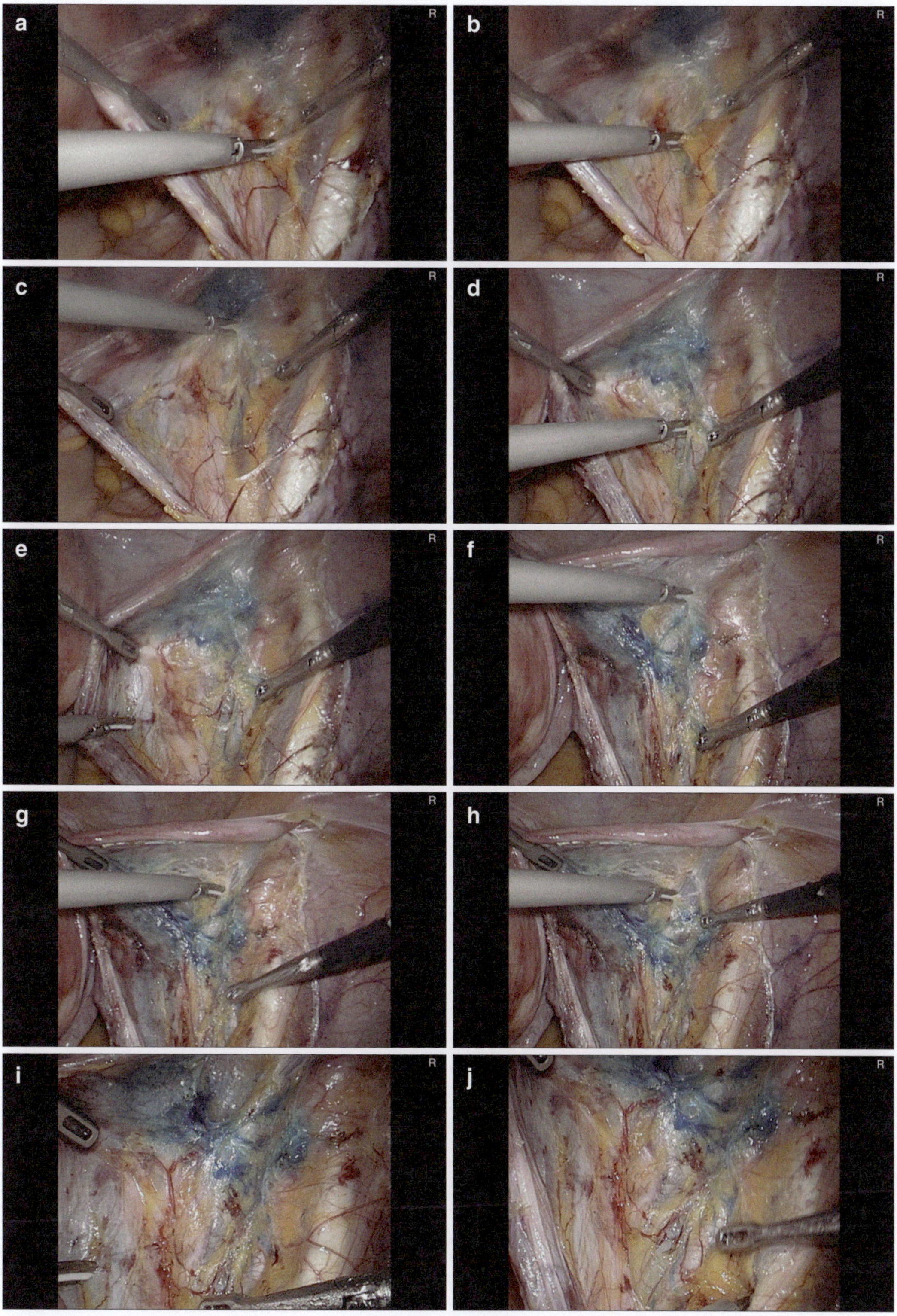

Fig. 17.11 (**a**–**j**) Adequate exposure of lymphatic drainage pathway

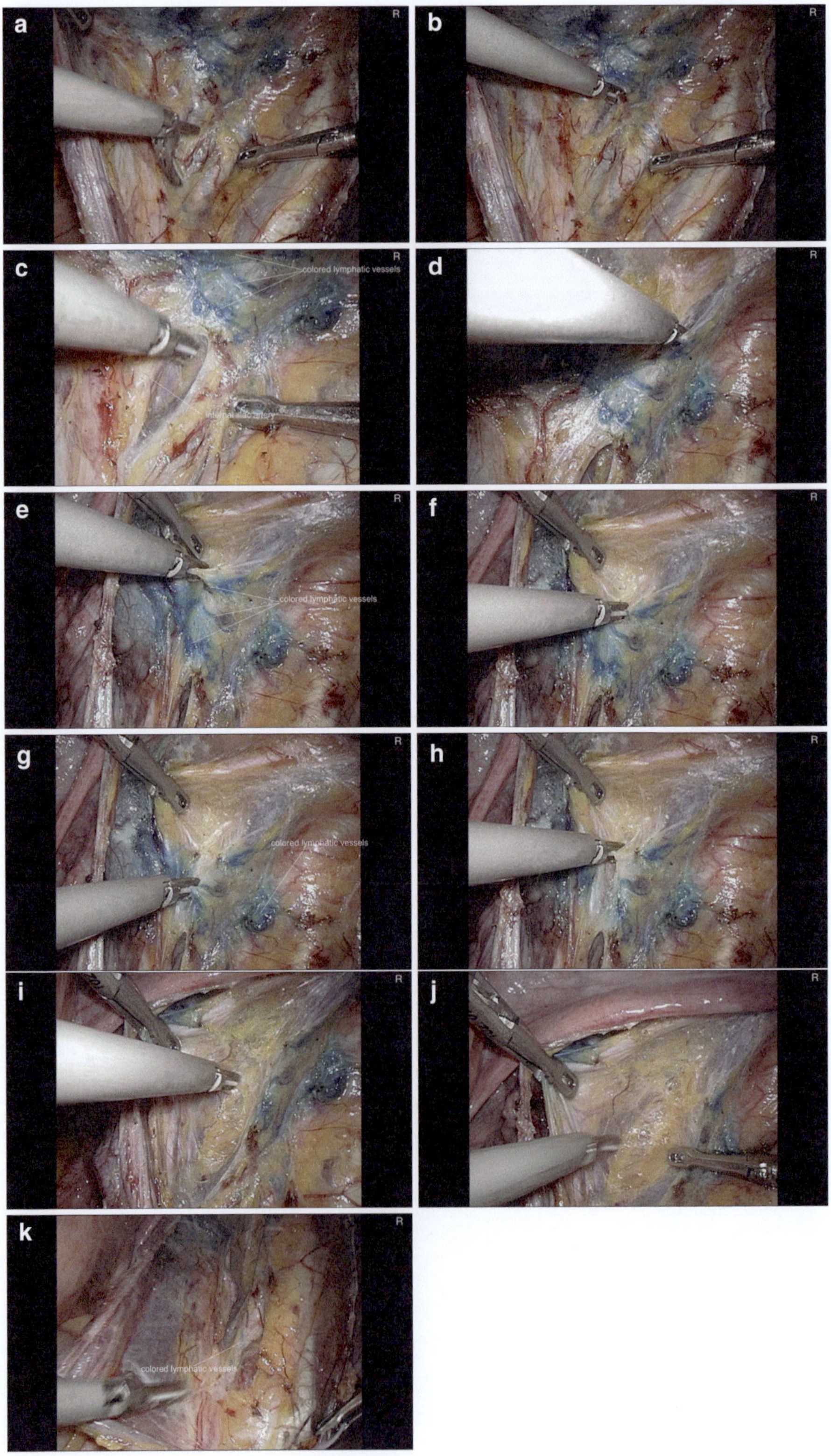

Fig. 17.12 (**a**–**k**) Adequate exposure and separation of lymph nodes along the tracer-labeled lymphatic channel

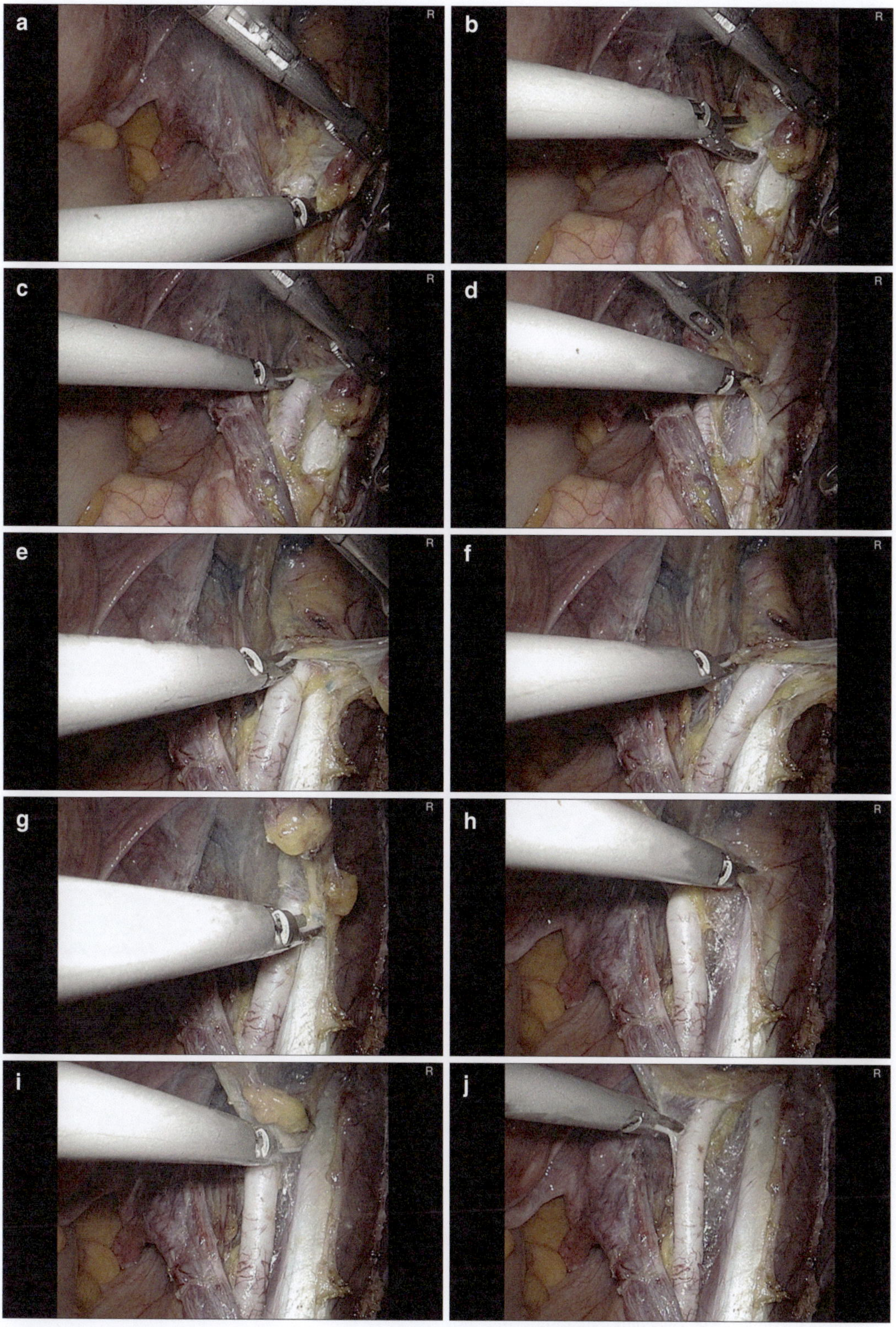

Fig. 17.13 (**a–l**) En bloc removal of sentinel lymph nodes on the surface of the external iliac artery using a mapping technique

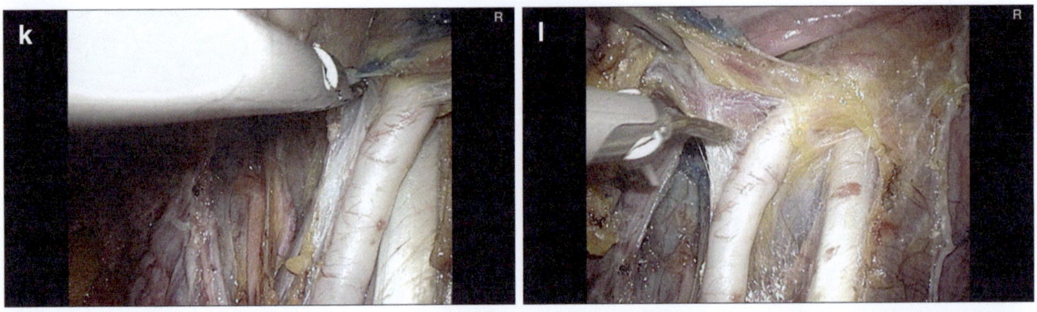

Fig. 17.13 (continued)

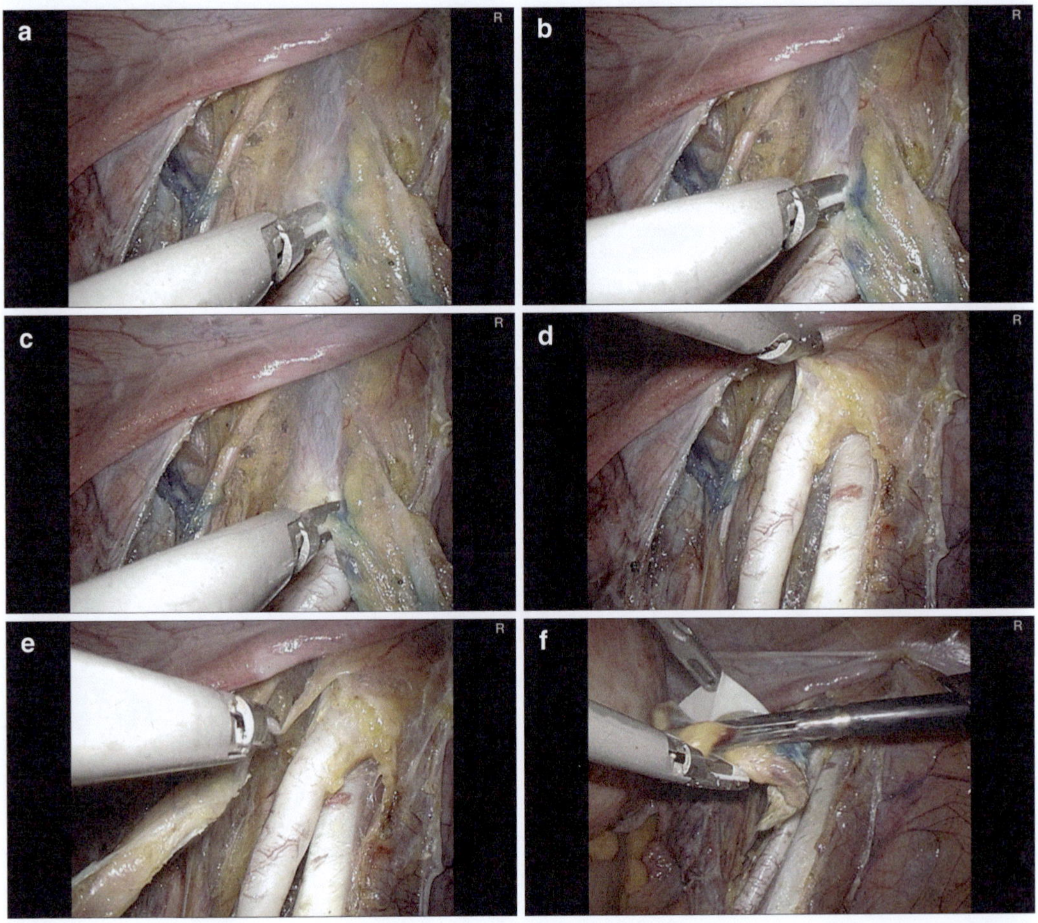

Fig. 17.14 (**a**–**f**) En bloc removal of sentinel lymph nodes using a mapping technique

References

1. Cormier B, Diaz JP, Shih K, et al. Establishing a sentinel lymph node mapping algorithm for the treatment of early cervical cancer. Gynecol Oncol. 2011;122:275–80. Available at: http://www.ncbi.nlm.nih.gov/pubmed/21570713
2. Lecuru F, Mathevet P, Querleu D, et al. Bilateral negative sentinel nodes accurately predict absence of lymph node metastasis in early cervical cancer: results of the SENTICOL study. J Clin Oncol. 2011;29:1686–91. Available at: http://www.ncbi.nlm.nih.gov/pubmed/21444878
3. Altgassen C, Hertel H, Brandstadt A, et al. Multicenter validation study of the sentinel lymph node concept

in cervical cancer: AGO Study Group. J Clin Oncol. 2008;26:2943–51. Available at: http://www.ncbi.nlm.nih.gov/pubmed/18565880

4. Bats AS, Buenerd A, Querleu D, et al. Diagnostic value of intraoperative examination of sentinel lymph node in early cervical cancer: a prospective, multicenter study. Gynecol Oncol. 2011;123:230–5. Available at: http://www.ncbi.nlm.nih.gov/pubmed/21893335
5. Bats AS, Mathevet P, Buenerd A, et al. The sentinel node technique detects unexpected drainage pathways and allows nodal ultrastaging in early cervical cancer: insights from the multicenter prospective SENTICOL study. Ann Surg Oncol. 2013;20:413–22. Available at: http://www.ncbi.nlm.nih.gov/pubmed/22911367
6. Cibula D, Abu-Rustum NR, Dusek L, et al. Bilateral ultrastaging of sentinel lymph node in cervical cancer: lowering the false-negative rate and improving the detection of micrometastasis. Gynecol Oncol. 2012;127:462–6. Available at: http://www.ncbi.nlm.nih.gov/pubmed/22943880
7. Cibula D, Abu-Rustum NR, Dusek L, et al. Prognostic significance of low volume sentinel lymph node disease in early-stage cervical cancer. Gynecol Oncol. 2012;124:496–501. Available at: http://www.ncbi.nlm.nih.gov/pubmed/22120175
8. Fader AN, Edwards RP, Cost M, et al. Sentinel lymph node biopsy in early-stage cervical cancer: utility of intraoperative versus postoperative assessment. Gynecol Oncol. 2008;111:13–7. Available at: http://www.ncbi.nlm.nih.gov/pubmed/18684499
9. Lecuru F, Bats A, Mathevet P, et al. Impact of sentinel lymph node biopsy on staging of early cervical cancer: results of a prospective, multicenter study [abstract]. J Clin Oncol. 2009;27(Suppl 18):Abstract CRA5506. Available at: http://meeting.ascopubs.org/cgi/content/abstract/27/18S/CRA5506
10. Slama J, Dundr P, Dusek L, Cibula D. High false negative rate of frozen section examination of sentinel lymph nodes in patients with cervical cancer. Gynecol Oncol. 2013;129:384–8. Available at: http://www.ncbi.nlm.nih.gov/pubmed/23395889
11. van de Lande J, Torrenga B, Raijmakers PGHM, et al. Sentinel lymph node detection in early stage uterine cervix carcinoma: a systematic review. Gynecol Oncol. 2007;106:604–13. Available at: http://www.ncbi.nlm.nih.gov/pubmed/17628644
12. Andikyan V, Khoury-Collado F, Denesopolis J, et al. Cervical conization and sentinel lymph node mapping in the treatment of stage I cervical cancer: is less enough? Int J Gynecol Cancer. 2014;24:113–7. Available at: http://www.ncbi.nlm.nih.gov/pubmed/24335661

Part IV

Complications and Postoperative Care

Complications Related to Radical Hysterectomy Surgery and Postoperative Care

18

Jun Wang, Junling Lu, and Yuemei Cui

Radical hysterectomy is the primary method for the surgical treatment of localized early-stage cervical cancer. Any surgical procedure is a double-edged sword, as it inevitably brings both benefits in treating the disease and potential risks and complications. Moreover, the characteristics of complications may vary depending on the specific surgical approach.

18.1 Vascular Injury and Hemorrhage

Intraoperative bleeding is the most common complication of surgery, with an incidence ranging from 1.8% to 4.7%. Literature reports an average blood loss of 600–800 ml during classic abdominal cervical cancer surgery (Wertheim III type) [1]. Radical hysterectomy involves many major blood vessels in the pelvic and abdominal cavities. Even a slight mishap during surgery can result in major vascular damage and uncontrollable hemorrhage, leading to surgical failure. Among these, the most common sites for significant bleeding are the uterine artery, uterine venous plexus and cardinal ligaments, the ureteric tunnel, and the vesicovaginal venous plexus. Surgeons must have a firm grasp of the anatomical knowledge, including the origins, courses, and branches of all major pelvic vessels, and maintain a clear awareness during the surgery. Careful and precise handling, along with meticulous hemostasis, is essential, and violent tearing and pulling should be avoided. Damage to pelvic vessels and bleeding often result from tearing, inadvertent cutting, or incomplete coagulation. Proper use of various dissection and coagulation instruments, along with thorough dissection and effective coagulation, is crucial in preventing damage and bleeding. When significant vascular damage and bleeding occur, it is essential to remain calm and composed. Hasty clamping should be avoided. Instead, a suction device can be used to aspirate the blood flow and expose the bleeding point. Then, attempts can be made to clamp or compress to halt the blood flow. For smaller vessels or those that need to be cut, electrocoagulation can be used for hemostasis. In the case of larger vessels that need to be preserved, laparoscopic suturing for hemostasis can be performed. In cases of massive or uncontrollable bleeding that is difficult to expose or manage, or when the surgeon is not proficient in laparoscopic vascular suturing techniques, timely conversion to open surgery for hemostasis may be necessary. When necessary, appropriate measures should be

J. Wang (✉) · J. Lu
Department of Gynecology and Obstetrics, Second Affiliated Hospital of Dalian Medical University, Dalian, China

Y. Cui
Department of Gynecology and Obstetrics, Dalian Municipal Central Hospital, Affiliated of Dalian University of Technology, Dalian, China

S. Han, J. Wang (eds.), *Open, Laparoscopic, and Robotic Surgery for Cervical Cancer*,
https://doi.org/10.1007/978-981-97-7687-0_18

taken under the guidance and assistance of vascular surgeons to avoid and minimize the occurrence of severe complications to the greatest extent possible [2].

18.2 Postoperative Infections

According to reports, the incidence of infectious complications after radical hysterectomy is 8% [3], including infections at the vaginal stump, surgical incision sites, urinary tract, and respiratory tract, among others. These infections typically manifest with fever as the primary symptom. Early postoperative symptoms may indicate ureteral, bladder, or intestinal injuries, and within a few days after surgery, the possibility of secondary infections caused by lymphatic cysts or chyle leaks should also be considered [4].

In cases where infection has already occurred, the treatment principles include:

1. *Identifying the source of infection.*
2. *Conducting microbiological examinations (cultures of sputum, urine, feces, drainage fluids, wound or vaginal secretions).*
3. *Fluid resuscitation.*
4. *Temperature control and monitoring, including regular checks of body temperature, blood tests including complete blood count, C-reactive protein, and procalcitonin levels.*
5. *Chest X-ray examination.*
6. *Pelvic and abdominal ultrasound examination.*
7. *When necessary, performing abdominal and pelvic CT and MRI scans.*
8. *Adjusting antibiotic treatment based on susceptibility testing.*

For uncomplicated pelvic infections, symptoms typically improve rapidly with intensified antibiotic therapy. If there is suspicion of pelvic or abdominal infection caused by intestinal perforation, prompt exploratory surgery is necessary.

18.3 Urinary Tract Injuries

Urinary tract injury is one of the serious complications of radical hysterectomy. Iatrogenic urinary tract injuries mainly occur in the ureter and bladder, with reported incidence rates ranging from 0.3% to 1.8%. Among these, bladder injuries are more common than ureteral injuries. Failure to detect these injuries promptly or improper management can lead to long-term damage to renal function [5]. Ureteral injuries often occur at sites where the ureters cross with the uterine artery, at the ovarious suspensory ligament, at the ureteral bladder entrance, and at the uterosacral ligament [6]. Bladder injuries are primarily located at the top, bottom, and trigone of the bladder [7]. In radical hysterectomy surgery, urinary tract injuries are often associated with factors such as radiation therapy, surgical scars, tumor involvement or invasion, reduced ureteral blood supply, thermal injury, and duplicated ureteral anomalies [8]. If there is a sudden increase in drainage volume postoperatively, the possibility of a urinary system fistula should be considered. Typically, this assessment is conducted in two steps: first, determining whether there is a urinary system fistula, and second, identifying the location of the fistula. Postoperatively, the presence of a urinary system fistula can be determined by examining the creatinine and blood urea nitrogen levels in pelvic drainage fluid. The bladder indigo carmine test can be used to differentiate between bladder-vaginal fistulas and ureteral-vaginal fistulas. Further evaluation through cystoscopy and CT urography (CTU) can clarify the side of the injury and the location of the fistula. It's important to check for complex fistulas, such as concomitant ureteral and bladder fistulas, bilateral ureteral fistulas, and multiple bladder fistulas in more than two locations.

During surgery, if there is a strong suspicion of ureteral injury, a double "J" stent can be placed via cystoscopy. It's typically removed around 1–2 months postoperatively. If it's discovered that the ureter has been inadvertently ligated or clipped, immediate correction is necessary. If the ureter appears normal in color and peristalsis, a ureteral stent can be placed for 10–12 days without the need for further intervention. However, if the ureter has been severed or if the blood supply does not restore its color and peristalsis after ligation release, resulting in ureteral dilation, then the damaged portion should be resected. Ureteral reconstruction can be performed, either end-to-end anastomosis or ureteral bladder anastomosis, with the insertion of a double "J" stent for support. The anastomosis site should be tension-free, have good blood supply, and mucosa-to-mucosa alignment to prevent postoperative ureteral stricture. When ureteral injury is discovered postoperatively, it must be managed promptly without delay.

18.4 Intestinal Injury

Intestinal injuries are relatively rare in radical hysterectomy, with a reported incidence of 0.9% [9]. These injuries typically occur during laparotomy, Veress needle insertion for laparoscopic surgery, or the placement of the first trocar when entering the abdominal cavity. The primary site of intestinal injury is the rectum, with injuries to the small intestine being extremely rare. Various factors contribute to intestinal injuries during the procedure, such as inflammation, endometriosis, difficulty in separating the rectovaginal space during extensive pelvic dissection, cervical cancer invading the vagina, and unintentional damage to the rectum during clamping or ligation of the sacrum or cardinal ligaments [10]. The management of gastrointestinal injuries depends on the location, extent, type of injury, the patient's general condition, and whether there is a history of radiation therapy. Small bowel injuries are more common in laparoscopic surgery, and if a small bowel injury is diagnosed postoperatively, immediate exploratory laparotomy is necessary. Repair is usually sufficient for the majority of small, localized small bowel injuries, but extensive injuries may require partial small bowel resection and anastomosis [11]. Treatment options for colon and rectal injuries include repair, partial segmental resection, and colostomy [12].

18.5 Venous Thromboembolism

Venous thromboembolism is a common postoperative complication in gynecological pelvic surgeries. The exact incidence of venous thromboembolism after radical hysterectomy is unclear, with a clinical diagnosis rate of around 1%. However, when more sensitive laboratory methods are used, the probability of detecting events may increase to 12% [13]. Patients with gynecological malignancies have a higher risk and should be given adequate attention. Venous thromboembolism is a multifactorial disease, and to date, the mechanism of thrombus formation remains consistent with Virchow's triad, which involves factors related to slow blood flow, vascular wall damage, and blood abnormalities [14].

Deep vein thrombosis (DVT) can occur in veins in various parts of the body, including the lower limbs, liver, pelvis, and the area around the vagina. Approximately, 90% of DVT cases occur in the lower limbs, with the majority of cases affecting the legs. The main clinical manifestations of DVT in the lower limbs include limb pain, swelling, congestion, skin erythema, local tenderness, and functional impairment. However, only about 30% of patients with DVT exhibit symptoms [15]. Diagnosis can be confirmed through B-mode ultrasound, and for patients suspected of having DVT, Doppler ultrasonography or venography can be used. Additionally, D-dimer testing can be combined for DVT screening.

Patients who are found to have deep vein thrombosis (DVT) postoperatively through vascular ultrasound and venography should receive systemic anticoagulant therapy. The goal of this treatment is to prevent further embolism, the aggregation of blood clots, and the occurrence of pulmonary embolism.

18.6 Lymphatic Reflux Disorder

Lymphatic reflux disorder is one of the common complications after regional lymph node dissection surgery, with an incidence rate of about 4.3–48% [16]. Although lymphatic cysts are not life-threatening, they often come with symptoms like fever, chronic pelvic pain, and leg swelling, significantly affecting a patient's quality of life and subsequent treatment. The treatment principles differ based on the course of the disease. In the early stages, the goal is to eliminate retained lymphatic fluid and prevent lymphatic effusion. In the later stages, the objective is to surgically remove irreparable diseased tissue or perform shunting procedures to treat localized lymphatic duct obstruction.

If pelvic lymphatic cysts are small, asymptomatic, and have the potential to resolve on their own, no specific clinical intervention may be necessary. General treatments like topical traditional Chinese medicine applications may suffice. However, if the lymphatic cyst is large, has been present for an extended period, causes compression symptoms, or leads to leg swelling that affects mobility, timely intervention is needed. Typically, this involves local puncture drainage under direct or ultrasound guidance, and a drain may be left in place after drainage. The aspirated fluid should be subjected to routine examination, biochemical analysis, chyle testing, etc., to further establish the diagnosis.

For the prevention of pelvic lymphatic cysts, several measures have been suggested in current research to potentially reduce their occurrence [17, 18].

Adequate Postoperative Pelvic Drainage This includes both abdominal wall and vaginal drainage. Drainage can help the posterior peritoneum adhere closely to the pelvic wall, reducing the formation of dead space behind the peritoneum after surgery. Additionally, when peritoneal surfaces adhere to each other, it can compress the cut ends of lymphatic vessels, preventing lymph leakage, reducing intraperitoneal fluid accumulation, and thus decreasing the formation of pelvic lymphatic cysts.

Opening the Pelvic Floor Peritoneum Opening the peritoneum at the pelvic floor during surgery can promote the participation of lymphatic fluid in intraperitoneal fluid circulation, increasing lymphatic fluid absorption and reducing lymphatic fluid accumulation.

Thorough Closure of Lymphatic Vessels During pelvic lymph node dissection, it's important to thoroughly and reliably close larger lymphatic vessels. Some studies suggest that using bipolar electrocoagulation or titanium clips (LIGACLIP) to close lymphatic vessel cut ends may reduce the risk of postoperative lymphatic cyst formation. Care should be taken to avoid excessive damage to normal lymphatic vessels and surrounding tissues, minimizing unnecessary lymphatic vessel rupture or damage to prevent postoperative lymphatic cysts.

These measures are aimed at reducing the risk of pelvic lymphatic cyst formation and should be considered during surgical planning and execution.

18.7 Tumor Dissemination and Incisional Metastasis

For cervical cancer patients who are suitable for surgical treatment, their tumors are often localized to the uterus and do not directly communicate with the abdominal cavity. Therefore, tumor dissemination and incisional metastasis are not common after radical hysterectomy. To avoid tumor detachment and contact with fresh surgical wounds, the following points should be observed during surgery:

1. Adhere to the principle of tumor-free surgery.
2. Avoid uterine perforation.
3. Avoid squeezing the tumor during manipulations.
4. Under laparoscopy, identify the vaginal incision and transition to vaginal surgery as early as possible. Use a "sleeve" method to circumcise the vagina to minimize the risk of tumor detachment into the abdominal cavity or contact with the vaginal incision.
5. Thoroughly irrigate the pelvic and abdominal cavities, as well as all surgical incisions, with a low-residue solution before concluding the surgery.
6. Postoperatively, administer adjuvant radiotherapy or chemoradiotherapy promptly to eligible patients to prevent and reduce the risk of pelvic and vaginal stump tumor dissemination, implantation, metastasis, and recurrence.

The occurrence of complications following radical hysterectomy is indeed related to the surgeon's experience. Gynecologic oncologists, who specialize in treating gynecological cancers, tend to have lower rates of surgical complications compared to general gynecologists. However, several other factors can also influence the occurrence and severity of complications, including the complexity of the surgery, the extent and approach of the procedure, and the coordination among the surgical team. Therefore, it's crucial to have an experienced surgical team, including the surgeon, assistants, and nurses, to minimize the risk of complications during a radical hysterectomy.

References

1. Yoo S, Terai Y, Tanaka T, et al. Role of the two-point pull-up technique for treating the uterine arteries during radical hysterectomy and trachelectomy. Eur J Obstet Gynecol Reprod Biol. 2013;170:544–9.
2. Asfour V, Smythe E, Attia R. Vascular injury at laparoscopy: a guide to management. J Obstet Gynaecol. 2018;38:598–606.
3. Wenzel HHB, Kruitwagen RFPM, Nijman HW, et al. Short-term surgical complications after radical hysterectomy—a nationwide cohort study. Acta Obstet Gynecol Scand. 2020;99:925–32.
4. Faro C, Faro S. Postoperative pelvic infections. Infect Dis Clin N Am. 2008;22(4):653–63.
5. Naser O, O'Connor E, Greenwell TJ. Urological complications following gynaecological surgery. Obstet Gynaecol Reprod Med. 2022;32(12):272–81.
6. Oh BR, Kwon DD, Park KS, et al. Late presentation of ureteral injury after laparoscopic surgery. Obstet Gynecol. 2000;95(3):337–9.
7. Soong YK, Yu HT, Wang CJ, et al. Urinary tract injury in laparoscopic-assisted vaginal hysterectomy. J Minim Invasive Gynecol. 2007;14(5):600–5.
8. Centini G, Labanca L, Afors K, et al. Laparoscopic dissection of the pelvic ureter: rules of engagement. J Minim Invasive Gynecol. 2019;26(4):604.
9. Rettenmaier CR, Rettenmaier NB, Abaid LN, et al. The incidence of genitourinary and gastrointestinal complications in open and endoscopic gynecologic cancer surgery. Oncology. 2014;86(5–6):303–7.
10. Boukerrou M, Lambaudie E, Collinet P, et al. A history of cesareans is a risk factor in vaginal hysterectomies. Acta Obstet Gynecol Scand. 2003;82(12):1135–9.
11. Mendez LE. Iatrogenic injuries in gynecologic cancer surgery. Surg Clin North Am. 2001;81(4):897–923.
12. Jo EJ, Lee YY, Kim TJ, et al. Management and outcome of rectal injury during gynecologic laparoscopic surgery. J Minim Invasive Gynecol. 2013;20(2):166–71.
13. Barber EL, Clarke-Pearson DL. Prevention of venous thromboembolism in gynecologic oncology surgery. Gynecol Oncol. 2017;144(2):420–7.
14. Cervantes J, Rojas G. Virchow's legacy: deep vein thrombosis and pulmonary embolism. World J Surg. 2005;29(1):S30–4.
15. Bruni-Fitzgerald KR. Venous thromboembolism: an overview. J Vasc Nurs. 2015;33(3):95–9.
16. Tsuji Y, Kawaguchi R, Haruta S, et al. Late onset of pulmonary embolism caused by lymphocyst following pelvic lymphadenectomy. J Obstet Gynaecol Res. 2007;33(5):734–8.
17. Achouri A, Huchon C, Bats AS, et al. Postoperative lymphocysts after lymphadenectomy for gynaecological malignancies: preventive techniques and prospects. Eur J Obstet Gynecol Reprod Biol. 2012;161(2):125–9.
18. Gallotta V, Fanfani F, Rossitto C, et al. A randomized study comparing the use of the Ligaclip with bipolar energy to prevent lymphocele during laparoscopic pelvic lymphadenectomy for gynecologic cancer. Am J Obstet Gynecol. 2010;203(5):483.e1–6.

MIX
Papier aus verantwortungsvollen Quellen
Paper from responsible sources
FSC® C105338

FSC
www.fsc.org

If you have any concerns about our products,
you can contact us on
ProductSafety@springernature.com

In case Publisher is established outside the EU,
the EU authorized representative is:
Springer Nature Customer Service Center GmbH
Europaplatz 3, 69115 Heidelberg, Germany

Printed by Libri Plureos GmbH
in Hamburg, Germany